EVOLUTION OF LONGEVITY IN ANIMALS

A Comparative Approach

BASIC LIFE SCIENCES

Alexander Hollaender, Founding Editor

Recent volumes in the series:

EVOLUTION OF LONGEVITY IN ANIMALS

A Comparative Approach

Edited by

Avril D. Woodhead and
Keith H. Thompson
Brookhaven National Laboratory
Upton, New York

PLENUM PRESS • NEW YORK AND LONDON

Library of Congress Cataloging in Publication Data

Brookhaven Symposium in Biology (34th: 1986: Upton, N.Y.)
  Evolution of longevity in animals.

  (Basic life sciences; v. 42)
  "Proceedings of the Thirty-fourth Brookhaven Symposium in Biology on Aging
Processes in Animals, held October 19–22, 1986, in Upton, New York"—T.p. verso.
  Bibliography: p.
  Includes index.
  1. Longevity—Congresses. 2. Aging—Congresses. 3. Evolution—Congresses. 4.
Physiology, Comparative—Congresses. I. Woodhead, Avril D. II. Thompson, Keith
H. III. Title. IV. Series.
QP85.B73   1986   591.3/74   87-29100
ISBN 0-306-42692-7

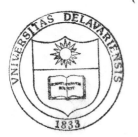

Proceedings of the Thirty-Fourth Brookhaven Symposium in Biology
on Aging Processes in Animals, held October 19–22, 1986,
in Upton, New York

© 1987 Plenum Press, New York
A Division of Plenum Publishing Corporation
233 Spring Street, New York, N.Y. 10013

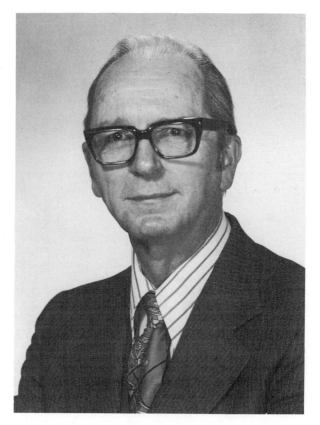

DR. GEORGE SACHER

"But I am a scholar. Why are you a scholar -
Is it not to make you happy?"

DEDICATION

In the emergence of a discipline, it is important to have someone
who organizes the inchoate mass of anecdotal bits and scattered pieces of
information available and derives from these general concepts which serve
as the springboard for the future. The efforts by Sacher provided
glimpses into the complex phenomenon that is aging, shedding light on how
different species cope with the constant onslaught of endogenous and
exogenous environmental agents. He provided an alternative framework to

look at aging, asking not "how do we die" but, "how do we live so long?" This misleadingly simple question has sparked intense interest in the protective mechanisms developed during phylogeny.

Using lifespan data, a number of different concepts of aging were tested, evaluated, discarded, or modified. The importance of metabolism and homeostatic control were emphasized. These ideas now are being detailed with the various molecular and biochemical techniques of modern science. Information from our penetrating new understandings of basic processes, such as control of growth and development, are being applied to the question of how the complex interaction, which is a mature organism, goes awry.

In applying these new techniques, George Sacher led the way, developing a new model and incorporating molecular biology. During his research life he remained a scholar, truly a person who worked because it made him happy.

Ronald W. Hart

This meeting is being dedicated to George Sacher, whom I knew for many years although we never spent a great deal of time together. Most of the times that we met in our earlier years, we were at one scientific meeting or another. George was a physicist, a radiation biologist, and an unbelievable naturalist. He had a wealth of knowledge about animals and plants. He was a comparative biologist, and most of all, a biogerontologist. Among his many awards and honors probably the one that meant most to him, was being president of the Gerontology Society of America. This is a multidisciplinary group representing not only biologists but people from clinical medicine, psychology, and sociology as well as the various proponents of social research planning and practice. George felt that this was a rather unique honor and was delighted to have been elected. George was an individual who, in contrast to many of us in science, probably had one of the most genuine qualities of humbleness that I knew. He let his work speak for itself.

George Sacher made many important contributions to comparative evolutionary biology. His refined equations gave a solid mathematical basis for a number of meaningful investigations on aging. His comparative approach to species longevity, as exemplified by his early work on brain weight/body weight relationships, to some of his later work with Ronald Hart examining the levels of DNA excision repair in a short- and long-lived strain of mouse bring unquestioning testimony to his unswerving faith in the value of the comparative evolutionary approach. He believed that in this way one can gain insight into the basic biochemical, physiological, and the molecular genetic mechanisms of aging. In short, George Sacher's perseverance, his intellectual curiosity, and his unique ability and energy to draw relevant information from diverse disciplines into functional paradigms for future research in comparative biogerentology are his legacy to us. It is one, I might add, that is far from being fully exploited. With that closing thought, I know that I can tell Dorothea, George's loving wife and friend, that she need never worry about George's last request. When George got into the ambulance that day, he called to her and asked that she not forget to say goodbye to all his friends and colleagues. I cannot really seem to say goodbye to him and I expect that the reason why we, in aging research, cannot say goodbye, is that his work is so much a part of us and will be for generations to come. Indeed, I believe it is and will remain one of the cornerstones of biogerontology.

George T. Baker, III

PREFACE AND ACKNOWLEDGEMENTS

This Symposium had its informal beginning in after-dinner talks with Dr. Alex Comfort and others at an earlier meeting on aging at Brookhaven National Laboratory. We were speaking of the remarkable growth in our understanding of the mechanisms of aging at the macromolecular and molecular level that had occurred over the last ten years. Someone pointed out that much of this information stemmed from work with a few species of rather short-lived mammals, usually laboratory rodents that are rather imperfect models for aging. Had the pendulum swung too far away from comparative approaches to aging? After all, aging is common to all metazoans.

Comparative studies have long been the poor relative in the aging field, yet as George Sacher showed, remarkable insights can be gained from such work. In this spirit of enthusiasm we decided that it was timely and would be rewarding to emphasize again the value of the evolutionary and mathematic approach to aging research. Since the field is so wide, we attempted to direct our attention to growing points; however we look forward to the day when we can include in our symposia many of the excellent areas that unfortunately we had to omit.

The Symposium was made possible through the support and generosity of our sponsors listed below. We would especially like to thank Dr. Donald Hughes of The Procter and Gamble Company for his encouragement. We shall sorely miss the late Dr. Alexander Hollaender, who did so much for this Symposium, as he did for many others held at Brookhaven National Laboratory.

Ms. Helen Z. Kondratuk coordinated the Symposium with efficiency, grace and charm and we are most grateful for her efforts in making the meeting so pleasurable for everyone. Ms. Nancy Siemon took over the thankless task of correcting the manuscripts; she worked with care and with a willingness that made life much easier for us. We thank her for her efforts. This 34th Symposium in Biology was held under the auspices of the U.S. Department of Energy.

Symposium Committee:

Avril D. Woodhead, Chairwoman
George T. Baker
Ronald W. Hart
Richard B. Setlow
Rajindar S. Sohal
Matthew Witten

Symposium Sponsored by:

The Procter and Gamble Company
Council for Research Planning, Inc.
Estee Lauder, Inc.
American Cyanamid Company
Squibb Corporation
Johnson and Johnson
Associated Universities, Inc.

CONTENTS

GENETIC AND ENVIRONMENTAL DETERMINANTS OF LONGEVITY IN DROSOPHILA

Robert Arking

Department of Biological Sciences and
Institute of Gerontology
Wayne State University
Detroit, MI 48202

INTRODUCTION

In his seminal essay, "The Duration of Life," August Weismann in 1891 posed a most perplexing question: "How is it that individuals are endowed with the power of living long in such various degrees?" As if in partial reply, he later suggested that, "In answering the question as to the means by which lengthening or shortening of life is brought about, our first appeal must be to the process of natural selection." Today, with a century's worth of hindsight available, we recognize that Weismann was correct in concept, although wrong in detail. The duration of life appears to be the resultant of both intrinsic and extrinsic, of genetic and environmental factors. That much seems certain. Our grasp of the detailed mechanisms involved, however, seems much less secure. In large part, our uncertainty stems from the lack of a commonly accepted theoretical paradigm of aging. History shows, however, that progress is possible even in the midst of uncertainty. Accordingly, the goal of this paper will be to demonstrate that a careful following of the lead provided by Weismann has allowed us to use selection procedures to create an animal model with which we can empirically define some of the specific factors involved in controlling the duration of life in Drosophila melanogaster.

In general, the identification and characterization of the mechanisms controlling the aging process has proven to be a uniquely difficult biological problem. As Francois Jacob wrote (1982), "It is truly amazing that a complex organism, formed through an extraordinarily intricate process of morphogenesis, should be unable to perform the much simpler task of merely maintaining what already exists." Many hypotheses have offered plausible explanations for senescence at a variety of different operational levels (see Hayflick, 1985). One of the more intractable problems, and one which is not always addressed by the various theories, is the conceptual difficulty of distinguishing those age-dependent changes which are causally related to the aging process from those which are not related. Many individuals believe that a genetic approach to the problem of aging might allow one to sort out the confusing correlative factors from the causal factors. Much work has been done using this approach, particularly in Drosophila, beginning with Raymond Pearl and his colleagues (1928). Yet Lints (1978) concluded that while aging was undoubtedly a genetically controlled phenomenon there were no obvious

1

tools then in existence with which to exploit this insight. Thus, despite all the fine descriptive work done with different mutants, different strains, and different species of Drosophila--each with its own characteristic pattern of longevity--it had not yet been possible to define a genetic system which unambiguously affects the aging process (Arking and Clare, 1986).

SELECTION OF AND CHARACTERIZATION OF LIFE EXTENSION MUTANTS

Following Weismann's "...appeal to the process of natural selection" (1891), my colleagues and I decided that an operational understanding of the aging process might be achieved by using artificial selection to create long lived Drosophila strains. Such strains then could be used in a genetic and molecular analysis of aging. Our choice of lifespan extension mutants, rather than lifespan reduction mutants, was based on our need to ensure that the genetic system which we would eventually isolate should be one that was affecting lifespan through a direct effect on the aging process itself. It seemed to be a reasonable postulate that there were many more ways to indirectly reduce the lifespan than there were ways in which one could indirectly increase lifespan. The probability of identifying a basic aging mechanism seemed to be higher by adopting the strategy of searching for lifespan extension mutants.

Our experiments were successful and constitute the first clear demonstration that a species specific lifespan can be significantly increased through selection (Luckinbill et al., 1984; Luckinbill and Clare, 1985; Arking, 1987), thereby vindicating Weismann's faith in "...the process of natural selection." Figure 1 summarizes the changes that occurred in the mean female lifespan of each of the independent selection strains. Our experimental design was one of indirect selection in which we selected for one trait (time of reproduction) and measured another trait (female lifespan) believed to be pleiotropically linked to the former (see Luckinbill et al., 1984.) We selected for either long life (L) or short life (E) under conditions of high larval density (NDC) or low larval density (DC). The control line (R) was bred at random times during the adult life span and individual lines raised under NDC or DC conditions. A detailed description and analysis of the survival data is given in Arking (1987). An examination of the results presented in Figure 1 show that selection for increased lifespan was effective in the high larval density environment (NDC-L) and less effective, although visibly present, in the low larval density environment (DC-L). Selection for a decreased life span was not effective in either of the two strains subjected to this regime (NDC-E and DC-E). There was some fluctuation but no net change in the lifespan characteristics of the control (R) line. There was no statistically significant difference in the mean lifetimes of the control line when raised under either NDC or DC conditions.

Conclusions based only on differences in mean values could be misleading, for there are known instances where an intervention will produce significant changes in the mean lifespan but have very little if any effect on the maximum lifespan. Success in obtaining a bona fide life extension mutant must be signaled by significant increases in both the mean and the maximum lifespan values (Balin, 1982). An analysis of the survival curve data shown in Figures 2 and 3 strongly suggests that the increased lifespan characteristic of the NDC-L females has been brought about almost entirely by a delay in the time of onset of senescence, and not by an extension of every phase of the life cycle. This interpretation is buttressed by the following facts:

1. There is no significant difference in the developmental times
    (i.e. days from egg to adult eclosion) of the L lines relative
    to the R lines (Luckinbill and Clare, 1985);

2. the 28-day difference in the reported mean lifespans of the L
    lines relative to the R lines is essentially matched by the
    26-day delay in the time when the L females enter their senes-
    cent phase (defined operationally as the time of LT10) relative
    to the controls (Figures 2 and 3; Arking, 1987);

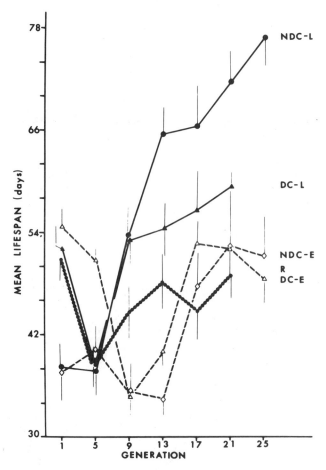

Figure 1. The alteration in the mean lifespan (± 95% confidence
          limits) of the five different strains used throughout the
          25 generations of the selection experiment. The four
          experimental strains were each subjected to two different
          selection parameters: L = strains selected for late age of
          reproduction and hence long life; E = lines selected for
          early age of reproduction and hence short life; DC = lines
          raised under controlled (low) larval density conditions;
          NDC = lines raised under uncontrolled (high) larval
          density; R = control line bred at random ages and hence not
          subject to lifespan selection. (From Arking, 1987).

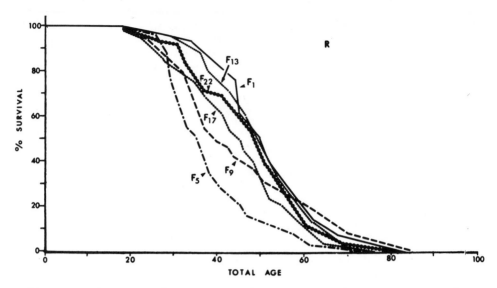

Figure 2. The survival curves for the six measured generations of the
R line. Note the lack of any temporal directionality in
the curves and their oscillation about the mean. Note also
that there are minor differences only in the LT_{10} and LT_{90}
values as well. (From Arking, 1987).

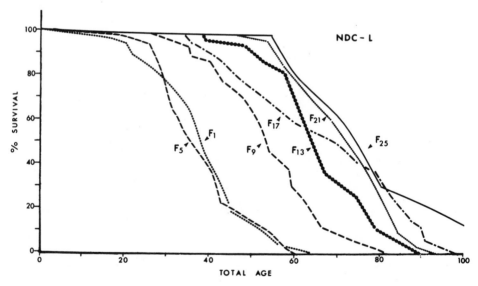

Figure 3. The survival curves for the seven measured generations of
the NDC-L lines. Note the obvious temporal directionality
in the LT_{90} values. The increased mean lifespan is clearly
accompanied by a delayed onset in the time of senescence.
(From Arking, 1987).

3. the length of the senescent period, operationally defined as the interval between LT10 and LT90, is more or less the same in both the L and the R strains (Figure 2 and 3; Arking, 1987);

4. when these survival data are analyzed with the use of Gompertz plots, the major difference between the two strains lies in the decreased value of qo (the y-intercept) and not in any significant change in the slope of the calculated line (Witten and Arking, in preparation). According to Sacher's (1977, 1978) interpretations of the Gompertz relationships, the value of qo reflects the innate vigor or genetic constitution of the organism while the slope of the line reflects the rate of aging. The logical deduction is that the affected genetic constitution of the L strain has no effect on the rate of aging, but only on the time when it begins. This tentative interpretation will be more rigorously analyzed elsewhere (Witten and Arking, in preparation).

Given these observations, it seems reasonable to conclude that the genetic system for which we have selected brings about an increase in the lifespan via an extension of one specific stage of the life cycle--and not via a non-specific "rubber band" like extension of the entire life cycle. This interpretation leads us to further deduce that the mechanism regulating the onset of senescence must be functioning as a temporally specific genetic switch. This important concept will be discussed in more detail below.

It is noteworthy that the selection experiment was done exclusively by measurement and overt selection through the female sex, yet the male lifespans also were altered in a manner identical to that of the female (Figure 4).

This selection experiment was successful but its design was not original. A similar approach was adopted by Lints and Hoste (1974, 1976) and by Rose (Rose and Charlesworth, 1981; Rose, 1984); Lints' group did not obtain any genetically based increase in life span while Rose and his colleagues had results comparable to ours. The differences in the results obtained from superficially similar experiments must be addressed and understood. In addition, one would want to understand why the high larval density regime was more successful in supporting the selection of long lived animals than was the low density regime (Figure 1), and why it was not possible to select for short lived animals under conditions in which selection for long life was successful. We have elsewhere reviewed these several different genetical approaches to experimental gerontology and given a developmental genetic explanation as to why our efforts were successful and others were not (Arking and Clare, 1986). We suggested that the use of high larval density is essential to disrupting the developmental homeostasis normally preventing the expression of the inherent genetic variability in life span. It is the phenotype, as an integrated expression of environmental and genomic interactions, which bears the effects of natural selection. If there is no phenotypic variability, then there exists no material on which selection might work. Developmental homeostasis, or "canalization" in the terminology of Waddington (1940), suppresses the expression of existing genomic variability by producing a relatively constant, or normal, phenotype. An idea of the mechanism that underlies this concept was provided by the dynamic model of gene flux developed by Kacser and Burns (1982) as discussed by Arking and Clare (1986). The work of Riska et al. (1984), for example, clearly shows that initial genetically and environmentally determined differences in growth rates of mice are progressively reduced by the convergence of their trajectories so as to yield a restricted range of "normal" phenotype. To be effective, artificial selection experiments must uncover the existing genetic variability present in each generation by destabilising those developmental processes involved in canalization and allowing the production of phenotypes which may be acted upon by selection (Luckinbill and Clare, 1985). Another observation supporting the efficacy of high larval density is the recent report of Luckinbill and Clare (1986) that there exists a density threshold for the expression of longevity in genetically identical animals such that long-lived animals reared at a low density have a decreased longevity relative to their sibs raised at high density, but one which is still longer than that of the controls. The important point is that low larval density reduced both the penetrance and the expression of the long lived phenotype, and does so by means of standard genetic mechanisms. The differences between the several experiments can now safely be attributed entirely to procedural differences, and not to any odd genetic mechanisms.

Our indirect selection for short life was ineffective in producing a strain of short-lived organisms, regardless as to whether it was implemented with high or low larval density. This observation led us to try to create short lived strains by direct selection in which we bred from the offspring of the shortest lived females (Arking, 1987). It proved relatively easy to obtain short-lived individuals but impossible to develop strains from them, as they were not healthy and often died out within a generation or two. This raised the possibility that a healthy short lived strain may be a contradiction in terms. In fact there may be a minimum species life span, in much the same way as there is a maximum species life span. If an organism is put together in a minimally effective manner such that it has no gross abnormalities and its various organ systems are coordinated with one another, then it has the intrinsic ability to survive for a certain amount of time. Decreasing this minimum time may destabilize the organism's intrinsic homeostasis and it may not be possible to do this without simultaneously creating conditions that will cause the animal to die. Kirkwood's ideas (1987) regarding the evolutionary balance in energy allocation between germ line and soma may shed further light on this suggestion. This hypothesis implies that Drosophila melanogaster is living at or near its normal minimum species life span: this deduction may be consistent with the expectations of evolutionary theory (King, 1982). Should the concept of a minimum species lifespan be valid, then one might suggest that mutants bringing about an accelerated aging may exert their effects in a very different manner and at a very different level than do mutants causing an increased life span. Their analysis may give us insight into the different types of genetic mechanisms involved in regulating the aging process in Drosophila. Both Baird and Liszczynsky (1985) as well as Grigliatti and his colleagues (Grigliatti, 1987; and Leffelaar and Grigliatti, 1984) have described sex linked temperature sensitive mutants in Drosophila which appear to reduce lifespan via an apparent acceleration of aging.

The fact that the selection experiment was successful implies that the selected phenotype is under some form of genetic control. There are certain observations that support and extend this implication.

First is the commonly agreed upon standard (Balin, 1982) that the goal of identifying a basic aging mechanism for lifespan extension requires that the longest lived survivors live to some point clearly beyond the maximum life span reported for the species under optimal conditions. The results of the experiment more than fulfill this criterion, the 77 day mean lifespan of the NDC-L F25 females clearly exceeds the LT90 lifespan of 68.5 days (F9) observed in any generation of the R

6

strain (Figures 2 and 3; also Table 1, in Arking, 1987). Therefore, the significant increased longevity is not due to a decrease in premature deaths or any other such similar cause but most likely has arisen via a genetic alteration to a basic aging mechanism.

Second, continued selection has proven to be effective in bringing about a continuous increase in the lifespan. There has been no diminution in the rate of change of the phenotype; indicating that the genetic variability of the population (implied by the success of the experiment) has not yet been exhausted by the selection process.

Third, reversed selection applied to five generations of the long lived strain (F20 to F25) resulted in a 12% decrease of the mean lifespan (Luckinbill and Clare, 1985). This ability to alter the phenotype following an alteration in the genotype further suggests that the difference between the two strains is due to allelic differences in the genes controlling this quantitative trait.

Fourth, additive inheritance for the phenotype of long life has been convincingly demonstrated by Clare and Luckinbill (1985) in a very interesting two part experiment. First, they measured the lifespan of reciprocal F_1 hybrids arising from a cross between an L line parent and an E line parent when raised under NDC conditions. The F_1's lifespan of ca. 65 days was almost exactly intermediate between the E line lifespan of ca. 53 days and the L line lifespan of ca. 77 days. The second part of this experiment involved raising the F1 hybrids at a low larval density. Surprisingly under these conditions the mean lifespan of such animals (ca. 57 days) was statistically identical with that of the short-lived parent. These data suggest that the normal or shorter lived trait is dominant under density controlled conditions but acts in an additive fashion under high larval density conditions (Clare and Luckinbill, 1985). Thus the genes controlling this delayed senescence may be modulated by specifically changing the environment in which the larvae are raised.

The most convincing evidence for genetic control would be to localize, map and characterize the gene(s) involved. We are engaged in localizing the chromosomes involved, using an approach requiring a controlled replacement of each major chromosome (Dapkus and Merril, 1977). Our preliminary data suggest that the gene(s) responsible for the expression of the long lived phenotype are mostly located on the third chromosome, but that their expression may be modulated by at least a gene(s) on the second chromosome. It does not appear as if a large number of genes are involved in the genetic regulation of lifespan in _Drosophila_: a statistical analysis of the lifespan data suggests about 5 to 8 genes (Witten and Arking, in preparation). The tentative localization of these several genes on one chromosome raises the possibility of there existing a single gene cluster, or at least a single regulatory gene site controlling a number of contiguous genes. Luckinbill, (personal communication) believes that only one genetic factor may be involved, and this suggestion is compatible with the known data. Although we have not yet succeeded in mapping the gene(s), it seems reasonable to conclude that these selection experiments have identified a gene system responsible for the control of longevity.

There are two separate approaches one may raise in analyzing this life extension mutant. One approach would be to characterize the strain from a genetic point of view; the other would involve an examination of the processes known or suspected of being able to modulate lifespan. The results of such a two pronged investigation would allow us to begin sketching in the overall genetic architecture of the system.

EXAMINATION OF PHYSIOLOGICAL DIFFERENCES BETWEEN NORMAL AND GENETICALLY
BASED LONG LIVED STRAINS

Loeb and Northrup (1917) were among the first to report that poikilothermic insects such as <u>Drosophila</u> showed an inverse relationship between
adult lifespan and ambient temperature. This observation was incorporated
by Pearl into his theory (1928) as a strong predictor of the existence of
an inverse relationship between metabolic rate and aging. Of necessity,
the experiments that tested this prediction were designed to indirectly
vary the metabolic rate (by varying ambient temperature and/or physical
activity), and then measured such effects on the lifespan (Sohal, 1986).
The predicted relationship was sustained by normal flies and by short
lived flies (Trout and Kaplan, 1970), but no tests have been done to
determine if the metabolic rate relationships would adequately predict the

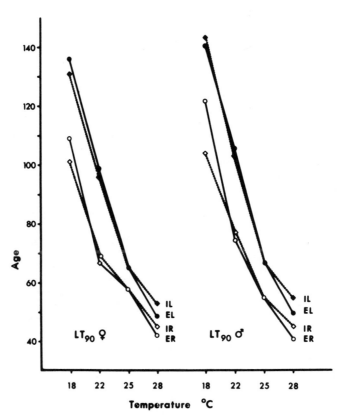

Figure 4. A graphical representation of the effects of different
         ambient temperatures on adult longevity, as indicated by
         the LT$_{90}$ survival times. All animals were raised under NDC
         conditions. L and R as in Fig. 1. I = animals raised from
         egg to adult eclosion at 25°C and then shifted to the
         indicated temperature for the remainder of their adult
         life; E = animals raised at the indicated temperature from
         oogenesis through death. Note that the temperature manipu-
         lations can affect lifespan of each strain but cannot over-
         come the genetically based higher longevities of the L
         line. (From Arking et al., 1987a).

Table 1   Lack of Effect of Developmental Time On
Adult Lifespan Parameter[1]

Strain	Developmental Period	LT10	LT50	LT90
IL18	12.5 + 2.5	63	109	131
EL18	22.0 + 7.0	75	98	136
IR18	12.5 + 2.5	54	78	101
ER18	25.0 + 7.0	52	78	109

[1]From Arking et al., 1987.

mechanism by which lifespan could be significantly extended. We were very
interested in determining how a known and effective environmental input,
such as temperature, fit into our postulated mode of an environmentally
sensitive genetic switch.

The structure of our experiment was quite simple (Arking et al.,
1987). We measured the male and female metabolic rates (expressed in
$\mu 10_2$/mg/hour) for replicate populations of both the R and the L strains at
each of four different ambient temperatures ($18°$, $22°$, $25°$ and $28°$ C). In
addition, each strain at each temperature also was tested for the effects
of developing at either $25°$C or at the same temperature at which it would
spend its adult life. Our results are based on the analysis of 16 defined
experimental groups.

Our fundamental finding from this experiment is shown in Figure 4,
where the LT90 values are seen to vary in the same manner when plotted as
a function of sex, strain, developmental treatment, and ambient temperatures. Several conclusions can be drawn from these data. First, as
expected from the past reports (see Sohal, 1986, for references), there
exists an inverse relationship between ambient temperature and lifespan.
Second, both sexes of the L lines live significantly longer than do the R
lines at each of the temperatures. Thus, the temperature treatments are
clearly incapable of overcoming the genetically based interstrain differences. We conclude that the environmental and genetic treatments exert
their effects on lifespan by affecting separate physiological compartments. We conclude further that their effects are additive. Third, there
is no consistent nor significant difference in adult lifespan between the
developmental treatments for either strain at any temperature. This
finding, that a doubling of the development time had no discernible effect
on adult lifespan (Table 1), was important and unexpected. The relationship between lifespan and developmental time long has been unclear (Lints
and Lints, 1971; Bourgois and Lints, 1982), and it simplifies matters to
realize that it is unimportant, at least in this system. Our findings
confirm the recent report of Economis and Lints (1986) who observed that
adult lifespan is roughly independent of developmental temperature.
Furthermore, this finding makes clear that temperature has no effect
during larval life, but appears to exert its effects only during
adult life.

We measured metabolic rate in these different experimental groups
(Arking et al., 1987). Figure 5 depicts the lifetime variation in the
measured metabolic rate for each sex of the two strains at $22°$C. The
pattern of the male metabolic data (not shown) is similar to, although
slightly lower than, that of their female sibs. There are no other
obvious sexually based metabolic differences. In most cases, the L strain
animals have an apparently higher metabolic rate than their corresponding
R line controls. The overlapping standard deviations suggest that this

increased rate is not statistically significant; in fact, the higher
metabolic rate of the L lines almost disappears at 18°C (Arking et al.,
1987a). However the consistency of the higher metabolic rate of the L
lines suggests that there may be some increase in a specific metabolic
compartment which our total body measurements can detect but only at a low
level of resolution. In general, the metabolic rates for both strains at
all temperatures reach a maximum during the second week or so of adult
life and then gradually decline. There does not appear to be any immediately obvious alteration in metabolic rate that might be expected if a
simple genetic switch were operating.

These impressions are confirmed when one compares the Mean Daily
Metabolic Rates (MDMR) calculated for each strain, sex, developmental
treatment and temperature (Figure 6). In general, there is a straight
line relationship between these several factors with no obvious statistical difference between any member of this family of curves. The slope
of these lines are opposite to those depicting the effect of temperature
on life span (Figure 4). Animals raised at a low temperature have a lower
MDMR and a longer lifespan that do animals raised at a higher temperature,
in agreement with the findings of many other workers. What is surprising
in our results is that there is very little, if any, difference in the
MDMR between normal lived animals and genetically selected long lived
animals. Long life involves something more than simply counting calories.

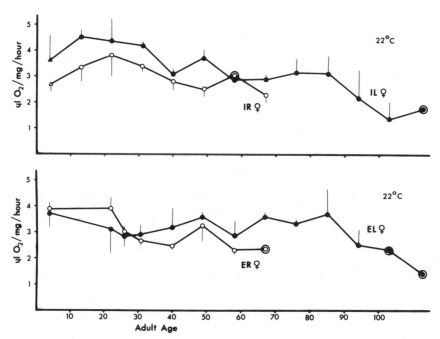

Figure 5. The top panel shows the measured metabolic rate at 22°C
          throughout the lifetimes of the L females and of the R
          females, both raised under I conditions. The bottom panel
          shows the measured metabolic rates throughout the lifetimes
          of the L females and of the R females, both raised under E
          conditions. Abbreviations as in Figures 1 and 4. The
          vertical bars are the standard deviations. (From Arking et
          al., 1987).

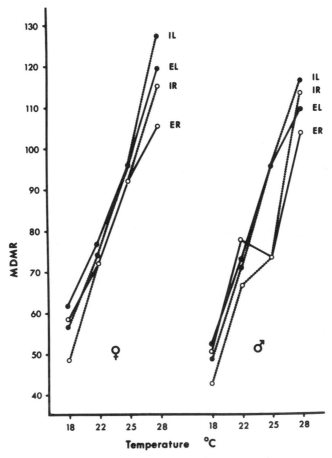

Figure 6. The variation on the mean daily metabolic rate (MDMR) as a function of strain, developmental conditions and adult ambient temperature. There appears to be no statistically significant difference in the metabolic response of the two strains to changes in these parameters. (From Arking et al., 1987).

USING BIOMARKERS OF AGING AS AN INDEPENDENT MEASURE OF PHYSIOLOGICAL CHANGES

Part of the difficulty in understanding the significance of information such as the metabolic data lies in the fact that the only biological measure of aging utilized in this experiment are those based entirely on survival data. It is very difficult to reliably sort out true age dependent processes from mere time dependent phenomenon. For example, our determination of the time of onset of senescence, a value which is essential to the logic of our biphasic gene model of lifespan regulation (see below), is based entirely on the LT_{10} survival time. We needed to develop a biological marker of the animal's physiological age, one that would allow us to critically test the predictions of the biphasic gene model without resorting to chronological survival data. As discussed elsewhere (Arking et al., 1987), we discovered that a decrease in fertility and

Table 2. Evidence that the Delayed Onset of Senescence is [1] Correlated with the Delayed Onset of Loss of Female Fertility[1]

Strain	Mean Age at Time of Fertility Drop	Fecundity Drop	Death	Length of Senescent Period
L	59.9	61.9	70.9	11.0
R	36.8	41.3	48.8	12.0
Delay (L-R)	23.1	20.6	22.1	

[1] From Arking, 1987.

fecundity is a widespread and reliable indicator of the onset of senescence and the impending death of that female. It is widespread since 83% of the R line females and 100% of the L line females display this decline several days prior to death. It is reliable since fewer than 9% of the affected females of either strain can be designated as false positives. In addition, there is an excellent correlation ($r > 0.82$) between the length of time of the period of decreased fertility and that of decreased fecundity in the individual females of either strain. We have identified a quantifiable and vital physiological process which can serve as a true biomarker of aging. Table 2 gives us some insight into the physiological processes affected by the selection regime for long life. It may be seen that in both strains there is an 11-12 day interval which elapses between

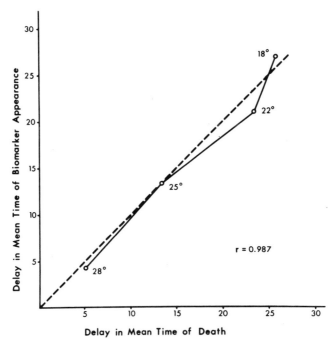

Figure 7. The correlation in days between the length of the delayed drop in fertility of the L line relative to the R line at four different ambient temperatures, and the length of the delay in the mean time of death of the L line relative to the R line at each of these temperatures. The dotted line is that expected for a perfect correlation between the two parameters. (From Arking et al., 1987b.)

12

the mean age at fertility decrease and the mean age at death. This
suggests that the physiological processes characteristic of senescence
that are set in motion by decreased fertility and which culminate in death
are similar if not identical in both strains. What is even more striking
is that the 23-day delay in the mean age of appearance of these reproductive biomarker in the L strain relative to the R strain almost exactly
corresponds to the 22-day delay in the mean age at death in the L strain
relative to the R strain. This information independently suggests that
the increased lifespan of the L strain has come about through an extension
of the pre-senescent phases of the adult life span, resulting in a con-
comittant delay in the time of onset of these biomarkers characteristic of
later life. Furthermore, the processes affected are ones which occur
prior to day 36 of adult life in the R strain. The biomarker information
is entirely compatible with the concept of a genetic switch controlling
the onset of senescence in adult life, and with the interpretation that
our selection regime has simply delayed the time of operation of this
genetic switch.

If our suggestion is correct that these biomarkers are measuring the
rate of aging, then it logically follows that their expression should be
modifiable by the environment. The simplest environmental manipulation
capable of substantially altering the life span of poikilothermic inverte-
brates is temperature. It was of great interest to determine whether, and
in what manner, the expression of these biomarkers would be altered as a

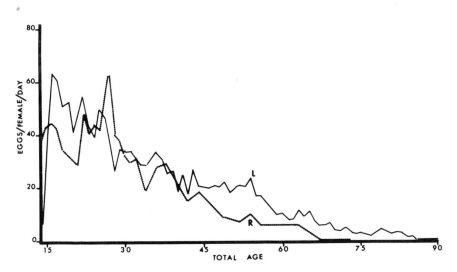

Figure 8. A comparison of the mean daily egg production as observed
in the R strain (F_{22}, N=87) and in the NDC-L strain (F_{21},
N=66). The R strain females produce 1195.4 eggs/female/
lifetime, or 24.5 eggs/female/day of mean lifetime. The
NDC-L females produce 1514.4 eggs/female/lifetime, or 21.4
eggs/female/day of mean lifetime. The 13% reduction in
daily fecundity of the L strain is more than compensated by
the 46% increase in its mean lifetime, resulting in a 26.7%
increase in lifetime fecundity of the NDC-L strain relative
to the R strain. These data imply that the L line should
out compete the R line. Since there do not appear to be
any naturally existing L strains in the wild, this then
implies that the effects of the early eggs on inclusive
fitness are probably greater than are the effects of the
later eggs. (From Arking, 1987).

function of lifetime ambient temperature. As shown in Figure 7, (Arking et al., 1987b), there exists a very tight correlation (r=0.987, P>0.001) between the temperature dependent delayed expression of the biomarker in the L strain relative to the R strain, and the delay in the mean time of death of the L strain relative to the R strain, across a wide range of physiological temperatures. Therefore we conclude that the fertility and fecundity decrease that we characterized is a true time-independent but age-dependent biomarker of physiological aging in <u>Drosophila</u>. We tested this conclusion by examining our data to see if the age at which fecundity dropped for a number of individual females could be used to reliably predict the lifespan for each of these individuals. The correlation between the actual lifespan and the predicted lifespan is very high r=0.799, P<0.001). Although it is still far from being a perfect predictor (since this value overestimates the shorter lifespans and underestimates the longer lifespans), the data strongly suggest that this particular suite of biomarkers is reflecting the rate at which an important age-dependent process is taking place (Arking et al., 1987b).

The very nature of the biomarkers involved indicates the involvement of the reproductive process in the aging process. We examined the reproductive effort of females of these two strains (Figure 8) (Arking, 1986). The data indicate that the L strain lays fewer eggs/female/day than the R strain for the first two days of adult life, an essentially equivalent amount to the R strain for the subsequent 15 days, and thereafter lays more eggs/female/day than the R strain until the end of the reproductive period. The early reproductive superiority of the control strains relative to the L strains was previously noted and reported as evidence supporting the pleiotropic gene hypothesis (Luckinbill et al., 1984; Luckinbill and Clare, 1985). The pattern of egg production in Figure 8 suggests that the R line enters reproductive decline at about day 38 while L line enters this phase at about day 54. It is of interest to note that the comparable estimates for the onset of senescence, based on survival data only, are days 31 and 57, respectively (Arking 1987). The data in Figure 8 also suggest that the L animals have evolved a plateau phase of reproduction extending from about day 25 to day 40, during which the females have a consistent output of about 20 eggs/female/day. The R line females exhibit no such plateau phase but appear to transit directly from their peak production phase to the declining senescent phase. We believe that the key to understanding the mechanism by which lifespan has been extended may involved this effective extension of the reproductive period in the L line females, and we shall return to this point in more detail.

If the suite of biomarkers that we have identified actually reflected the onset of senescence, then one might expect that physiological processes other than those associated with reproduction also would be affected. This prediction is especially forceful, since decreased reproductive activity in and of itself should not result in an increased probability of dying. In fact, quite the opposite is true (Partridge and Farquhar, 1981; Aiguki and Ohba, 1984). Given this situation, it is clear that decreased reproductive activity is a necessary but not a sufficient indicator of the onset of senescence. We therefore re-examined the metabolic data from this new perspective and calculated the MDMR of the R and the L females during the presenescent and the post-senescent intervals of their adult life, using the age of biomarker expression as the physiological indicator of the time of onset of senescence (Arking et al, 1987b). The results of this analysis are shown in Table 3. The MDMR of either strain is significantly higher in the pre-senescent phase than in the senescent phase. In other words, the pre-senescent R and L animals are much more similar to one another than they are to the post-senescent stage of the same strain. Essentially similar results are obtained when these strains are tested at other ambient temperatures (Arking et al.,

Table 3. Relationship Between Biomarker Defined Pre-Sensescent
and Senescent Lifestage Phases and Metabolic Rate

Temperature	Strain	MDMR Prior to Fecundity Drop	MDMR After Fecundity Drop	%Change
25°	R	105.4	60.9	-42.2
	L	112.1	76.9	-31.4

[1]From Arking et al., 1987.

1987b). This finding implies that there is no obvious difference in the
overall physiology of the R and L strains, save that the latter genetically delay the onset of senescence. These data strongly support the
view that longevity is an intrinsic, genetically programmed process.

None of the above findings should be misinterpreted as suggesting
that the drop in fertility is the cause of the subsequent senescence and
death, for it is more than likely that the two processes in fact are only
indirectly connected. It is certainly plausible that the extended lifespan might be due to a genetically programmed delay in the time at which
certain neuroendocrine functions would decrease below threshold values.
These decreases might result in a decreased juvenile hormone titer and a
consequent impairment of vitellogenesis (Postlewait and Handler, 1979).
This impairment would first manifest itself as an increase in the frequency of functionally abnormal eggs and only later as a decrease in the
daily numbers of eggs produced by the senescent female. This prediction
is coincident with our empirical observation of an initial drop in fertility followed by a decrease in fecundity (Arking, 1987; Arking et al.,
1987b). The actual causes of death itself, however, need not be due to
this particular neuroendocrine driven reproductive decline. This identical process cannot be the causal factor in males. At the present time, we
suggest that death may logically be attributed to some other neuroendocrine mediated process which is present in both sexes and is essential to
somatic repair and maintenance.

The metabolic data which we have presented led us to conclude that
the long lived L line animals do not bring about their increase in longevity by husbanding their calories. They expend slightly more energy than
do the controls on a daily basis (Figure 6), yet they manage to live
significantly longer (Figure 4). Clearly, the mechanisms that bring about
long life are working through some other process. This conclusion is not,
however, equivalent to stating that our data disprove the predictions of
the rate of living theory, nor do they disallow a role of metabolism in
the regulation of longevity. Sohal (1986) pointed out that a contemporary
interpretation of this theory requires us to redefine the theory's predictions to read: "The rate of aging is directly related to the rate of
unrepaired molecular damage inflicted by the by-products of oxygen metabolism, and it is inversely related to the efficiency of antioxidant and
reparative mechanisms." This redefinition stops us from examining broad
and general processes such as the overall metabolic rate and instead
focuses our attention on specific mechanisms, such as the various antioxidant repair mechanisms suspected of playing a vital role in the aging
process. We believe it to be more than coincidental that a null mutant
recently isolated at the cSOD locus in Drosophila melanogaster has been
reported as being a short lived semi-lethal mutant (Hilliker et al.,
1986).

The problem facing us is to be able to integrate these environmental, physiological and genetical results into a coherent, logical and reasonable model. Creation of such a model runs the not inconsiderable risk of generalizing beyond the data. The risk may be amply repaid, however, if the model serves to organize and to guide the experiments designed to disprove the theory. This is in keeping with Whitehead's advice (1919) to "Seek simplicity and distrust it." What follows, then, is our current view of the genetic and physiological interactions which together might regulate the longevity of <u>Drosophila</u> (Figure 9). It should be viewed as a plausible hypothesis waiting to be disproved; not as a fact which has been verified.

During larval life, there takes place a gene-environment interaction which programs the organism with respect to the eventual time of onset of the senescent period (Clare and Luckinbill, 1985). This appears to require the specific environmental input of high/low larval density, thus it is possible that it might involve some specific metabolic product(s). The genes involved in this interaction are termed the larval stage genes. A logical analysis of their F1 hybrid longevity data leads to the conclusion that these genes must be composed of both cis- and trans- acting regulatory genes. These larval stage regulatory genes are postulated to regulate the time of repression of the adult stage structural genes. The genes which bring about the onset of senescence are believed to act during adult life, at a time prior to the onset of senescence (Arking, 1987). These adult stage genes may be structural genes, and may or may not be contiguous to the larval stage genes. The timing of the onset of senescence (i.e., gene repression) appears to be controlled by the larval stage regulatory genes. The structural genes presumably affect processes which are suspected on the basis of other evidence to be causally involved in controlling the aging process. The intimate involvement of the reproductive process in the onset of senescence, strongly argues for the involvement of the neuroendocrine system since it is this system which appears to regulate the female reproductive activities (Jowett and Postlethwait, 1980). It is possible therefore that the adult stage genes may be exerting their effects through the neuroendocrine system, thereby leading to a strain specific onset of senescence. Our data (Figure 4) strongly suggest that the effect of temperature on lifespan is mediated in an additive manner through some mechanism or compartment other than the genetic one: hence, our suggestion that the ambient temperature is working at the neuroendocrine level or later. The neuroendocrine changes, however they are brought about, lead to a reproductive senescence and physiological senescence. These are envisioned as being two separate processes that may well share some common early step which functionally links them together. The reproductive senescence in the female, is postulated to be mediated via juvenile hormone regulation of oogenesis. The physiological senescence, which presumably operates through the same mechanisms in both sexes, may be mediated through the neuroendocrinological regulation of anti-oxidant enzyme concentrations and/or activities. The failure of such presumably important repair and maintenance activities may play the most important role in bringing about the decrement of physiological functions known as senescence. For example, the ca. 30% drop in MDMR observed in post-senescent animals of either strain (Table 3) might result from oxygen byproduct damage to the mitochondria. In this view, senescence itself does not appear to be under direct genetic control, but may be determined in a stochastic manner. Once the processes that constitute senescence have been set in motion by the gene system described here, then the length of the senescent period may be the resultant of the organism's past physiological history. This speculation is consistent with our information on the temperature dependency of the senescent period (Figure 7) and its approximately equivalent length, in both the R and the L strain (Figures 2 and 3). The non-identity of the mechanisms controlling the pre-senescent and the senescent periods suggests that very different interventions will be required for the modification of each phase of the life cycle.

There is strong evidence in a variety of organisms that suggests the widespread existence of gene systems formally similar to that described above. For example, Paigen and his collaborators showed that a trans-acting regulatory locus (Gus-t) within the b-glucoronidase gene complex of the mouse controls the temporal sequence of gene activity at this locus and also displays additive inheritance (Luis et al., 1983). There is a formal similarity between this system and our own model. The Gus locus is a single gene locus. The similarity in the patterns of additive inheritance seen at that locus and in our own data should caution us from simply assuming that multiple genes must inevitably be involved in the genetic

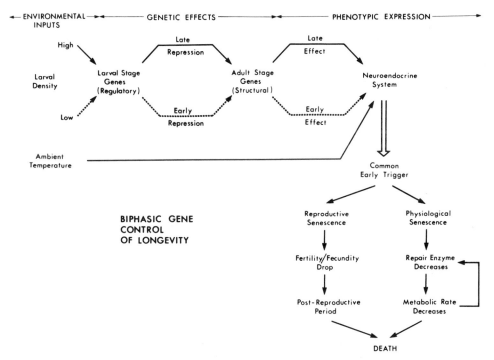

Figure 9. A model for the genetic regulation of senescence and longevity as deduced from the several experiments presented in
this paper. It is based on the premise that longevity is
inherited and is controlled via the timing of the onset of
senescence. There are two phases of gene action, larval
and adult. Environmental factors are believed to act on
the larval stage regulatory genes and this interaction
results in a temporal programming of the adult stage structural genes, which may or may not be contiguous to the
larval stage genes. Repression of previously active genes,
particularly those affecting the neuroendocrine system,
might bring about reproductive and physiological senescence. Senescence itself is not postulated to be under
genetic control and may well be a stochastic process dependent on the organism's past history (After Arking, 1987).

control of delayed senescence. The data are compatible both with single
gene models, as evidenced by the mouse work, or with models involving only
a small number of genes (Thompson, 1975). In addition, similar trans-
acting temporal gene systems have been described for mouse b-galactosidase
(Luis and Paigen, 1978); mouse a-galactosidase (Berger et al., 1979);
Drosophila amylase (Abraham and Doane, 1978); maize catalase (Lai and
Scandalios, 1980); and maize alcohol dehydrogenase (Scandalios et al.,
1980). These systems are able to produce age-dependent tissue specific
changes in the transcriptional activity of structural genes and thus may
be viewed as primed examples of the type of system involved in the genetic
control of senescence. In addition, Cutler's work on the evolution of
longevity has led him to conclude that the observed increase in mammalian
lifespan is almost certainly the result of regulatory gene evolution
(Cutler, 1982).

Thus our model flows logically from the data and is consistent with
the experimental and theoretical conclusions obtained by other researchers
with other systems. The similarity in the genetic architecture between
these different biological systems give us hope that the study of aging in
Drosophila may lead us to insights regarding the genetic control of aging
and senescent in other organisms. Can we interpret this as portending
that there actually exists one universal mechanism of aging? We can, but
we should not. There is no one single mechanism by which a fertilized egg
transforms itself into an adult. We are acquainted with the different
methods of cleavage and germ layer formation, that together lend diversity
to the study of embryos. There is no a priori reason to believe that
there will not similarly be a multiplicity of aging mechanisms. On the
other hand, it is incumbent to point out that there is not an overwhelming
number of different paths that eggs traverse in their journey towards
adulthood. The tens of thousands of animal species do very nicely with a
very finite--even small--number of basic developmental mechanisms.
Furthermore, the existence of "homeoboxes" and their role in gene processes controlling embryonic segmentation in both dipteran and mammalian
embryos suggests that even the few diverse developmental processes may
retain genetic traces of their common evolutionary heritage. Thus, our
reasoning by analogy (a risky business in any event) suggests that there
may exist a small number of different aging mechanisms. The model proposed in Figure 9 might illustrate the outlines of only one such mechanism. One intriguing aspect of this model is that its overall genetic
architecture is similar to the overall architecture of the mechanisms
independently suggested as being operative in mammals, in the sense that
it integrates the regulatory genes (Cutler, 1982) with the neuroendocrine
system (Finch, 1985) while still allowing for environmental modulation.

As stated elsewhere in this volume (Templeton, 1987), it is not clear
as to whether the genes involved in aging will prove to be "aging genes"
or simply "genes with aging effect." Our model and the data on which it
is based can be made compatible with either point of view. Perhaps our
future researches will permit us to rephrase the questions and move away
from dichotomous dilemmas.

The other more important aspect of interest is that the model sets up
specific and testable predictions. Our model (Figure 9) undoubtedly
contains both major and minor errors, both of omission and commission.
For example, it does not spell out the details of gene regulation nor is
it clear how this gene system would be integrated with the already identified gene system believed to bring about accelerated aging in the adult
Drosophila (Baird and Liszczynsky, 1985; Leffelaar and Grigliatti, 1984).
But it does suggest, for example, that there should exist a discrete
larval period during which the larval stage genes may be programmed by
specific environmental cues, and that after this period, one might expect

the environment to be without effect on lifespan. It further predicts that the central nervous system is involved, a finding consistent with the observations of Grigliatti (1987), that antioxidant enzyme values should show significant alterations only after the time of fertility drop, and so forth. Therefore it is the specificity of the predictions made by the model which are important, for by focusing our research efforts on these predictions, it may be possible to refine the errors out of our concepts and thereby perhaps gain a more accurate perception of reality.

It is appropriate to end this review in the same manner as I started it, with a quotation from Weismann (1891): "And so, in discussing this question of life and death, we come at last--as in all provinces of human research--upon problems which appear to us to be, at least for the present, insoluble. In fact it is the quest after perfected truth, not its possession, that falls to our lot, that gladdens us, fills up the measure of our life, nay! hallows it."

Acknowledgements

The selection experiment was done in collaboration with Prof. Leo S. Luckinbill and was supported by NIH grant AG01812 and by a WSU-NIH Grant in Aid to L.S.L. and R.A. The other experiments referred to in the paper were supported by a WSU-NIH Grant in Aid to R.A. and by the generous long term support of the WSU Institute of Gerontology to R.A. I thank Steven Buck, Stephen Dudas, Robert Pretzlaff and Robert A. Wells for their spirited technical support and involvement in the work, and Drs. R.S. Sohal and G. Baker for their stimulating discussions and probing questions.

REFERENCES

Abraham, I. and Doane, W.W., 1978, Genetic regulation of tissue- specific expression of Amylase structural genes in Drosophila melanogaster,Proc. Natl. Acad. Sci. USA 75: 4446-4450.

Aigaki, T. and Ohba, S., 1984, Effect of mating status on Drosophila virilis lifespan, Exp. Gerontol., 19:267.

Arking, R., 1987, Successful selection for increased longevity in Drosophila: analysis of the survival data and presentation of a hypothesis on the genetic regulation of longevity, Exp. Gerontol., In press.

Arking, R. and M. Clare 1986, "Genetics of Aging: Effective selec tion for increased longevity in Drosophila." In Comparative Biology of Insect Ageing: Strategies and Mechanisms, K. Collatz and R. Sohal (eds.) Springer-Verlag, Berlin.

Arking, R., Buck, S., Wells, R.A. and Pretzlaff, R., 1987, Metabolic rates in genetically based long lived strains of Drosophila, Submitted.

Arking, R., Wells, R.A., Buck, S. and Pretzlaff, R., 1987b, A biomarker of senescence and impending death in Drosophila melanogaster, Submitted.

Baird, M.B. and J. Liszczynskyj 1985, Genetic control of lifespan in Drosophila melanogaster, Exp. Gerontol. 20:171-177.

Balin, A. K. 1982, "Testing the free radical theory of aging" in
    Testing the Theories of Aging, R.C. Adelman and G.S. Roth (eds),
    CRC Press, Boca Raton, Florida.

Berger, F.G., G.A.M. Breen and K. Paigen 1979, Genetic determination of
    developmental program for mouse liver B-galactosidase: involvement
    of sites proximate to and distant from the structural gene, Genetics
    92:1187-1203.

Bourgois, M. and Lints, F.A. 1982, Evolutionary divergence of growth
    components and lifespan in subpopulations of Drosophila melanogaster
    raised in different environments, in "Advances in Genetics, Devel-
    opment and Evolution of Drosophila," S. Lakovaara, ed., Plenum Press,
    New York.

Campbell, S.D., Hilliker, A.J. and Phillips, J.P., 1986, Cytogenetic
    analysis of the cSOD microregion in Drosophila melanogaster,
    Genetics, 112:205.

Clare, M.J. and L.S. Luckinbill 1985, The effects of gene-environment
    interaction on the expression of longevity, Heredity: 55:19-29.

Cutler, R.G. 1982, "Longevity is determined by specific genes: Testing
    the hypothesis" in Testing the Theories of Aging, R.C. Adelman and
    G.S. Roth (eds). CRC Press, Boca Raton, Florida.

Dapkus, D. and Merrel, D.J., 1977, Chromosomal analysis of DDT- resistance
    in a long term selected population of Drosophila melanogaster,
    Genetics 87:685.

Economos, A. C. and Lints, F.A., 1986, Developmental temperature and life
    span in Drosophila melanogaster I. Constant developmental
    temperature: evidence for physiological adaptation in a wide
    temperature range, Gerontology 32:18.

Finch, C.E. and Landfield, P.W., 1985, Neuroendocrine and autonomic
    functions in aging mammals, in "Handbook of the Biology of Aging"
    (second edition), C.E. Finch and E.L. Schneider, eds., Van Nostrand
    Reinhold, New York.

Grigliatti, T.A., 1987, Genes that act late in adulthood and mutations
    that appear to accelerate aging, in "Aging Processes in Animals,"
    Brookhaven Symposia in biology number 34, Plenum Press, New York.

Hayflick, L., 1985, Theories of Biological Aging, Exp. Gerontol., 20:145.

Jacob, F., 1982, "The Possible and the Actual," Pantheon Books,
    New York.

Jowett, T. and Postlethwait, J.H., 1980, The regulation of yolk
    polypeptide synthesis in Drosophila ovaries and fat body by
    20-hydroxyecdysone and a juvenile hormone analog, Develop. Bio.,
    80:225.

Kacser, H. and Burns, J. A., 1981, The molecular basis of dominance,
    Genetics 97:639.

King, C. E. 1982, The evolution of life span, in "Evolution and Genetics
    of Life Histories," H. Dingle and J. P. Hegmann, eds.,
    Springer-Verlag, New York.

Kirkwood, T.B.L., 1987, Immortality of the germ line versus disposability of the soma, in "Aging Processes in Animals," Brookhaven Symposia in Biology Number 34, Plenum Press, New York.

Lai, U.K. and J.G. Scandalios 1980. Genetic determination of the developmental program for maize scutellum alcohol dehydrogenase: Involvement of a recessive trans-acting temporal regulatory gene, Developmental Genetics 1:311-324.

Leffelaar, D. and Grigliatti, T.A., 1984, A mutation in Drosophila that appears to accelerate aging., Develop. Genetics, 4:199.

Loeb, J. and Northrup, J.H., 1917, On the influence of food and temperatures on the duration of life, J. Bio. Chem., 32:103.

Lints, F.A. 1978, Genetics, Experientia 37:1046-1050.

Lints, F.A. and Hoste, C. 1974, The Lansing effect revisited. I. Life-span, Experimental Gerontology 9:51-69.

Lints, F.A. and Hoste, C. 1976, The Lansing effect revisited. II. Cumulative and spontaneously reversible parental age effects on fecundity in Drosophila melanogaster, Evolution 31:387-404.

Lints, F.A. and Lints, C.V. 1971, Influence of preimaginal environ ment on fecundity and aging in Drosophila melanogaster hybirds. III. Developmental speed and life span., Exp. Geront. 6:427-445.

Luckinbill, L.S., Arking, R., Clare, M.J., Cirocco, W.C., and Buck, S.A. 1984, Selection for delayed senescence in Drosophila melanogaster, Evolution 38:996-1003.

Luckinbill, L.S. and Clare, M.H. 1985, Selection for lifespan in Drosophila melanogaster, Heredity 55: 9-18.

Lusis, A.J. and K. Paigen 1978, Genetic determination of the B-galactosidase developmental program in mice, Cell 6:3710-378.

Lusis, A.J.; V.M. Chapman, R.W. Wangenstein and K. Paigen 1983, Transacting temporal locus within the B-glucoxidase gene complex, Proceedings National Academy Science (USA) 80:4398-4402.

Partridge, L. and Farquhar, M., 1981, Sexual activity reduces lifespan of male fruitflies, Nature, 294:580.

Pearl, R., 1928, "The Rate of Living," University of London Press, London.

Postlethwait, J.H. A.M. Handler 1979, The roles of juvenile hormone and 20-hydroxyecdysone during vitellogenesis in isolated abdomens of Drosophila melanogaster, J. Insect Physiol. 25:455-460

Riska, B., W.R. Archley and J.J. Rutledge 1984, A genetic analysis of targeted growth in mice, Genetics 107:79-101.

Rose, M.R. 1984, Laboratory evolution of postponed senescence in Drosophila melanogaster, Evolution 38: 1004-1010.

Rose, M.R. and B. Charlesworth 1981, Genetics of life history in Drosophila melanogaster. II., Exploratory selection experiments, Genetics 97: 187-196.

Scandalios, J.G., D.Y. Chang, D.E. McMillen, A. Tsuftaris and R.H. Moll 1980, Genetic regulation of the catalase developmental program in maize sculellum: identification of a temporal regulatory gene, Proceedings National Academy Science (USA) 77:5360-5364.

Sohal, R. S., 1986, The rate of living theory: A contemporary interpretation, in "Insect Aging: Strategies and Mechanisms," K.G. Colatz and R.S. Sohal, eds., Spring-Verlag, New York.

Templeton, A.R., 1987, The proximate and ultimate control of aging in Drosophila mercatorum, in "Aging Processes in Animals," Brookhaven Symposia in Biology Number 34, Plenum Press, New York.

Thompson, J.N., Jr. 1975, Quantitative variation and gene number, Nature 258:665-668.

Trout, W.E. and Kaplan, W.D., 1970, A relationship between longevity, metabolic rate and activity in shaker mutants of Drosophila melanogaster, Exp. Gerontol. 5:89.

Waddington, C.H. 1980, The genetic control of wing development in Drosophil, Journal of Genetics 41:75.

Weismann, A., 1891, "Essays upon Heredity and Kindred Biological Problems," 2nd ed., Vol. 1., Clarendon Press, Oxford.

Whitehead, A.N., 1919, "The Concept of Nature," University of Michigan Press, Ann Arbor (1957).

INFORMATIONAL STRUCTURE OF THE DEVELOPMENTAL TREE OF

MULTI-CELLULAR ORGANISMS

Simon Y. Berkovich

The George Washington University
Washington D.C. 20052

INTRODUCTION

From an abstract mathematical point of view, an evolving organism at
the cellular level can be described in terms of developmental trees where
cells can be conceived of as terminal nodes of a binary tree initiated
with a zygote as a root. Information associated with the process of cell
differentiation can be expressed by means of labeling the branches of the
developmental tree. Specificity of a given cell is determined by the
history of its divisions which is represented by a path leading to this
cell from the root. In this paper a formal scheme for the construction
of a developmental tree is considered and its several biological
implications are discussed.

A specific feature of a cell system is that it is a dynamic
population of elements with a distributed control. This type of control
in a developing organism implies that each cell must be equipped with its
own "memory" mechanism to keep track of the history of divisions. The
idea of the presence of such a mechanism, the internal cellular clock,
was promoted by Hayflick's[1] discovery on the limited division resources
of normal cells. The biological significance of the internal cellular
clock is two-fold. On one hand, it is involved in the control of cell
differentiation and organism development. On the other hand, it
determines a limit on cell division and thus establishes the upper bound
on the longevity of multi-cellular organisms, supposingly this mechanism
is required for regulating the constancy of cell populations.

This paper considers a hypothetical cell-labeling mechanism for the
developmental tree of multi-cellular organisms previously analyzed.[2] It
is assumed that the process of copying DNA is associated with changes
which represent not random errors but predetermined information-carrying
messages. The cell-labeling information is supposed to originate because
the DNA strands are complementary rather than identical. Thus, in the
course of semiconservative replication, a pair of copied DNA strands can
carry different information content to newly created pairs of
chromosomes.

Daughter cells receive random combinations of copies of each
individual chromosome from their mother cells. The control information
accumulated in the internal cellular clock is created by independent
combinations of these choices. Some possible patterns of chromosomal

interactions performing clock functions were analyzed by means of mathematical theory of reliability and were compared with the Hayflick limit on cell division (50 ± 10). This allows us to estimate the replicative potential of individual chromosomes.

The developmental tree is considered in two extreme situations combining the two apparently different phenomena of cancerogenesis and monozygotic twinning. Failure of the internal cellular clock removes the limitation on replication resources of dividing cells, a factor stabilizing constancy of cell populations and supposedly preventing cancerogenesis. The model yields estimates for the cumulative and threshold effects in this process. In particular, it was found that in this model the threshold value for a carcinogenic factor is approximately inversely proportional to Hayflick's limit for different species. The suggested cell-labeling procedure provides similar labeling for some classes of cells, contributing to their biochemical equivalence. Under certain circumstances the equivalent labeling can be provided to the zygote's offsprings. This is considered as a necessary condition for monozygotic twinning. The model predicts that the probability of the appearance of monozygotic twins equals an integer power of 1/2. Analysis of the available data gives some support to this result.

A MODEL OF CELL-LABELING PROCEDURE

To explain the origin of non-symmetry of cells at the microlevel, we accept the hypothesis that the process of cell division is associated with some registration of DNA replication. A logical scheme is developed here for the cell-labeling procedure based on this hypothesis. The question about the physical nature of the hypothetic DNA changes during replication is open. For example, one may rely on the hypothesis of a so-called marginotomy, according to which the copied DNA undergoes shortening,[3] or developmental clocks may depend on the enzymic modification of specific bases in repeated DNA sequences as suggested by Holliday and Pugh.[4] The cell-labeling ability of this process which determines the non-symmetry in the information content of daughter cells arises because the nucleotides in DNA molecules are arranged in complementary strands. Hence, the hypothetical replicative changes appear in different components. Such a type of hypothesis has been supported by recent experimental findings by Klar.[5]

Let a chromosome in the original cell with two complementary strands of DNA be denoted as AB (Fig. 1). After the first division there will be cells containing AB' and A'B ('denotes a newly formed strand). After the second division there will be cells containing AB', A"B', A'B", and A'B. If one strand accumulates i changes, then its complement may have only (i-1) or (i+1) changes. This scheme of DNA labeling is similar to that considered by Wassermann[6] for his process algorithm in semiconservative replications.

The described process of DNA replications only partially traces the history of their states because various paths may lead to the same collection of changes. This mechanism of the internal cellular clock creates certain equivalent classes of cells. It provides an approximate count to the number of cell divisions.

The termination of function of a chromosome in the clock mechanism is assumed after a finite number of replications. However, the exhaustion of the replication resource of a certain chromosome need not be followed by a cell's death because the state of this chromosome may be non-essential for the functioning of the cell. One may assume different

24

structures of interaction of chromosome changes from the point of view of their influence on the cell's functioning. The performance of such kinds of structures using the ideas and techniques of the mathematical theory of reliability was investigated by Berkovich.[2] A summary of these results is presented here.

PROBABILITY CHARACTERISTICS OF THE CELLULAR CLOCK FUNCTIONING

First, one has to determine the probability of faultless performance of a chromosome in the course of its reproduction. Let us denote this probability after m replications by $p(m)$. The total number of a cell's descendants after m divisions will be 2^m. The portion of them containing a given chromosome, say AB, with i and i±1 changes; i.e., A^iB^{i+1} and $A^{i+1}B^i$, is denoted by $Q_m(i,i+1)$. As a result of the first division, two new cells appear, each having in a given chromosome the original DNA and a copy with one change; i.e., $Q_1(0,1)=2$, $Q_2(0,1)=2$, and $Q_2(1,2)=2$ (see Fig. 1). The subsequent values of $Q_m(i,i+1)$ will arise according to the rule of construction of Pascal's triangle, so that

$$Q_m(i,i+1) = 2\binom{m-1}{i}.\tag{1}$$

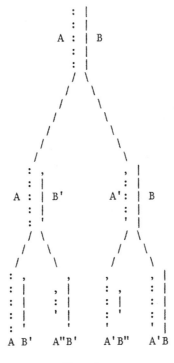

Fig. 1

Chromosomes labeling mechanism
of the cellular clock model

Let the replication resource of a chromosome be r; i.e., its performance will not fail until the number of changes in DNA exceeds r. Then p(m) under the assumption r>>1 may be written as

$$p(m) = 1/\sqrt{2\pi} \int_{-\infty}^{\frac{(2r-m)}{\sqrt{m}}} \exp(-x^2/2)dx. \tag{2}$$

The mean time to first failure (MTTF) for an element with a known probability of faultless performance, p(m), is represented by the integral:

$$MTTF = \int_{0}^{\infty} p(m)dm. \tag{3}$$

Changing the order of integration of (3), we obtain a relationship between r and a mean number of possible replications of a chromosome ($\bar{m}$) as:

$$\bar{m} = 2r + \frac{1}{2}. \tag{4}$$

If P designates the reliability of an element (a chromosome), then the reliability of the system as a whole (the cellular clock) will be represented by the so-called reliability function, h(p). To obtain an estimate for a replicative resource of a chromosome, we will consider different possible variants of the cellular clock mechanism with some structures of chromosome interaction typical for the theory of reliability:

1. All 2N chromosomes "are connected in series."

2. One definite pair of homologous chromosomes determines the cell's vitality, both of these chromosomes "being connected in parallel."

3. Certain k pairs of homologous chromosomes are "connected in series" while the chromosomes in each pair are "connected in parallel."

The first and second variants present extreme situations. In the first case the efficacy of all chromosomes is required for the vitality of the cell, while in the second case it is sufficient that at least one of the homologous chromosomes in a definite pair should be efficacious. The third case is to a certain extent more realistic. The vitality of the cell depends on the simultaneous efficacy of some subset of pairs of its homologous chromosomes. The reliability functions for these variants are as follows:

$$
\begin{aligned}
&1. \quad h_0 = p^{2N} \\
&2. \quad h_1 = 1-(1-p)^2 = 2p - p^2 \\
&3. \quad h_k = [h_2(p)]^k \quad (k=1,2,\ldots,N)
\end{aligned}
\tag{5}
$$

As soon as p is a function of m, the reliability functions (5) will present survival probability functions in the process of cell reproduction. These functions for all three variants as well as p(m) (denoted 0) are depicted in Fig. 2. We have chosen N=23, the number of chromosome pairs in human cells, and K=8 as a specific example for the third variant (see section on MZT). The unknown parameter r, the replication resource of a chromosome, is adjusted for each function to fit MTTF=50, the Hayflick limit for human cells. The values of r: 25, 23, 34 and 27 satisfy this condition for the above structures as presented in Fig. 2. Although the structure of interaction of chromosome changes in the internal cellular clock is unknown, we have an estimate of r with a reasonable accuracy.

The dispersion of the possible number of cell divisions, M, can be estimated through MTTF using a general formula from the theory of reliability for the standard deviation, σ, which is valuable for any system composed of aging elements

$$\sqrt{M} < \sigma < \sqrt{2M}. \tag{6}$$

The confidence interval for the possible number of cell divisions M±ΔM may be estimated by

$$\Delta M \sim \alpha\sqrt{M} \tag{7}$$

where α is some coefficient with an order of magnitude of about 2. Uncertainty of (7) is the consequence both of the general nature of the relation (6) and the arbitrary choice of confidence coefficients. Hayflick's experiments revealed that the number of cell divisions up to destruction is within the limits of 50 ± 10, which is apparently in agreement with this result.

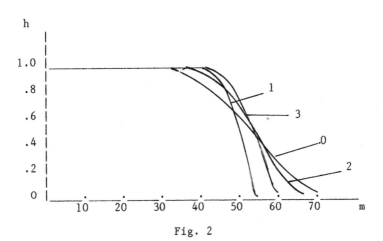

Fig. 2

The survival probability for different
clock structures (MTTF = 50)

PROBABILITY CHARACTERISTICS OF THE CELLULAR CLOCK FAILURE

Each element of a population with distributed control makes its own "decision" of replication or death. This decision can be based only on the local information, and in the absence of centralized control a desired level of systems elements cannot be easily maintained.

The constancy of the number of cells can be regulated by two different mechanisms: at the system level through a stabilization feedback (a chemical activity which increases chances for cell disappearance via lysis when their number goes up and increases the rate of mitosis when their number goes down) and at the elements level through an internal restriction for cell reproduction. For a long period of time a stabilized condition of nearly constant population may not be achieved using only the control mechanism at the system's level and must be supported by an internal mechanism limiting cell reproduction.

Cancerogenesis implies that regulation of the constancy of the number of cells in a certain part of the organism breaks down. This occurs as a result of failure of both regulating mechanisms: at the system level (physiological mechanism) and at the elements level (genetical mechanism). Failure of only one of these mechanisms may not be sufficient.

In this paper we obtain estimates of the probability of the breaking of the internal cellular clock. A more profound analysis of the regulation of the constancy of cell populations should take into consideration the self-stabilization properties of the system.

If some combination of chromosomes contributes to the normal clock functioning, then the failure of this combination will contribute to cancerogenesis. Normal chromosome functioning inside the clock mechanism and the ability of this clock mechanism to withstand chromosome failures due to outside factors are presented by so-called dual structures. If the reliability function of the former is $h(p)$, then that of the latter will be $1-h(1-p)$. For example, elements connected in series in one structure are connected in parallel in the dual structure and vice versa. Let q denote the probability that a chromosome preserve its clock's facilities under a certain external deterioration. This probability depends on the intensity of external factors such as concentration of cancerogenes, level of radiation and so on. The probability for a cellular clock to withstand the external deterioration for a period of time (0-t) will be: $1-h[1-q(t)]$.

The transformation of a normal cell into a cancer cell occurs when the cellular clock has not reached its replication limit, but the clock mechanism is somehow destroyed so it will not be able to provide signals to stop future cell reproductions. The probability of this situation at a given moment of time is $h[p(m)]h_t'[1-q(t)]dt$, so the probability, $R(t)$, of the cancer transformation for the period (0-t) will be

$$R(t) = \int_0^t h[p(m)]h_t'[1-q(t)]dt. \tag{8}$$

The value of (8) depends on the relation of speeds of two processes: normal termination of cell reproduction which is determined by the reliability function of the clock, $h[p(m)]$, and the possiblility of the clock's failure in a destructive environment as described through the dual structure $h_t'[1-q(t)]$. When the former process is faster, then $R \approx 0$ since cells die before their clocks could be destroyed. When the latter process is faster, then $h[p(m)] \approx 1$ and $R \approx h[1-q(t)]$. In this latter case the probability of clock failure depends on the integral probability of chromosomes to withstand destruction during the whole interval (0-t) and thus exhibits cumulative effect.

28

The probability of cancerogenesis, R, for the whole period of cell life (t=∞) will be:

$$R = \int_o^\infty h[p(m)]h_t'[1-q(t)]dt = -\int_o^\infty h_t'[p(m)]h[1-q(t)]dt. \qquad (9)$$

When the chances of chromosome destruction due to external factors are relatively small, then $q(t)$ can be presented as

$$q(t) = \exp(-\lambda t) \qquad (10)$$

where λ is some measure of the intensity of the destructive external factors. To present this uncertain parameter in a tractable manner, we introduce the probability, Z, of the chromosome destruction during the time between consecutive cell divisions, t_o:

$$Z = 1 - \exp(-\lambda t_o). \qquad (11)$$

As can be seen from (9), the probability, R, will remain approximately equal to 0 if $h[p(m)]$ surpasses the number of possible cell replications, $M+\alpha\sqrt{M}$, while $h[1-\exp(-\lambda t)]$ does not yet reach the point of the rapid increase of the reliability function. This situation is due to the fact that the region where $h_t'(p(m))$ is essentially different from 0 will correspond to the approximate 0 value of the term $h(1-q(t))$. The condition when this situation is changed allows us to estimate the threshold value, Z_T, when the cellular clock mechanism is breaking:

$$Z_T \approx \frac{\ln(3-2/k)}{M + \alpha\sqrt{M}} \sim \frac{1}{M}. \qquad (12)$$

The threshold value Z_T is rather insensitive to the structure of the reliability function and is roughly proportional to the inverse of Hayflick's limit, M.

Formula (12) implies that if the probability to destroy chromosome clock functions by some factor between two consecutive cell divisions in humans is less than a value of about 1/50, then there will be practically no cancerization even under the permanent influence of destructive factors. In the opposite situation the probability of the cancerization will rapidly increase. This consideration can be used to extrapolate the results on cancerogenic activity of different factors obtained on other species to humans.

EQUIVALENCE IN CELL LABELING AND MONOZYGOTIC TWINNING

Determination of monozygotic twins (MZT) presumably occurs just at the beginning of cell differentiation when few processes involved in the organism's development have been activated. Therefore, investigation of the probability of MZT may provide insight into the structure of the cellular counting mechanism.

The initial step in MZT formation, separation of the embryo into two parts, occurs at a very early stage of development.[7] The mechanical

partition of the embryo is thought to occur during the late blastula
stage. However, the control information which preceeds this mechanical
partition is obtained at an earlier time. When an organism starts its
development the internal cellular clock starts counting immediately from
the zygote stage. The cells of the embryo acquire different states of
their clock mechanisms which determine the initializations towards the
organism construction. If an embryo as a multi-cellular system is
destined to produce two organisms, the initializations of its cells have
to be changed accordingly. To obtain such harmonious changes when the
control is distributed over all the elements of the system is less likely
than when all the control development information is concentrated within
the zygote. The most simple situation in which MZT may occur is when the
initial zygote division is not associated with the advancement of the
cellular clock.

The situation is radically different when MZT are produced
artificially in vitro. There are many studies reporting formation of MZT
by mechanical splitting of embryos. Such experiments indicate that the
embryonic cells in question retain the genetic information necessary for
formation of an entire organism. This has no relevance, however, to the
mechanism of embryonic splitting that is reponsible for MZT formation in
vivo. In the in vitro experiments the external intrusion superimposes a
form of centralized control which in the native embryo could probably
have been endogenously exercised only close to the zygote stage.

The zygote is destined to produce MZT when its division is not
associated with "advancement" of the cellular counting mechanism. The
described model suggests a way in which this may happen. A pair of
homologous chromosomes of the zygote {AB, ab} can be reproduced in the
daughter cells in one of two modes: as likewise ({A'B, a'b} and {AB',
ab'}) combinations or crosswise ({A'B, ab'} and {AB', a'b}) combinations
(Fig. 3). Assuming homologous chromosomes to be equivalent in their
genetic control, the latter combination may not contribute to the change
of the informational content of the cell control mechanism; i.e., to the
advancement of the cellular clock mechanism. Therefore, if the cellular
clock consists of K pairs of homologous chromosomes, then the probability
of its "non-advancement" due to simultaneous occurrence of all K
crosswise combinations will be $(1/2)^K$.

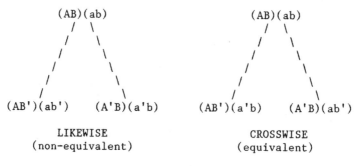

Fig. 3

Possible cell-labeling combinations of the homologous
chromosomes at the initial zygote division

Review of data on MZT frequency has been presented by Berkovich and Bloom.[8] Available data, though scant, supports the hypothesis that the MZT probability is $(1/2)^K$, where K is a species-specific integer parameter. For humans[9] MZT occurs in about four of 1000 births which is close to one occurrence in 2^8 births; i.e., K=8.

In a rigorous study of MZT in mice,[10] it was found that the 95% confidence limits for frequency of MZT were 0.2% and 2.6%, giving a calculated mid-range of 1.4%. The breadth of this range reflects the rarity of MZT. The mid-range value is close to one occurrence in 2^6 births, which is 1.56%.

This concept apparently contradicts the theory of retarded development as the etiological factor in MZT which seems to operate under some extreme experimental conditions.[9] This contradiction can be obviated if we consider that environmental factors can play a selective role for genetically controlled processes in ontogenesis as they do in phylogenesis. For example, environmental factors, directly or through retardation in embryo development, could promote survival of monozygotic embryos which might otherwise have died. In this case, incidence of MZT would be induced from practically zero to some finite value. Assuming our hypothesis, this value must be in the form $(1/2)^K$. The above scheme conforms with experimental findings[11] which have shown that MZT in rabbits can be induced by delayed ovulation. Being exceptional under natural conditions, the induced MZT in rabbits was observed in 6 out of 387 embryos; i.e., in about 1.5%, an induced frequency close to one occurrence in 2^6 births which is 1.56%.

CONCLUDING REMARKS

This paper presents an abstract model of the internal cellular clock based on the assumption that the labeling procedure of cell divisions is associated with some registration of DNA replication. The suggested model provides a workable hypothetical mechanism which can be applied to the investigation of the informational structures related to the processes of cell reproduction.

To ascertain the biological significance of the considered hypothetical mechanism of registration of DNA replications, it is necessary to analyze what happens with such a mechanism in other cases when biological objects, presumably, do not exhibit changes in DNA molecules during subsequent replications. There may be different explanations in various cases. For example, Olovnikov[3] hypothesized that DNA in bacteria do not undergo changes like shortening because they are in a circular form. The replicative changes in DNA must be to a certain extent of reversible nature because a number of phenomena and experiments presumably exhibit restorative properties of some differentiated cells. The existence of restorative mechanisms is especially important for meosis; as a matter of fact, in some cases of meiosis[12] retardation in the replication of a small part of DNA was observed.

The restorative mechanisms can be incorporated in the model by assuming that replicative changes in DNA are asymmetric being associated only with one of the pair of complimentary strands. This point was elicited by the ideas of the work.[5] Consider a chromosome where one DNA strand, A, can reproduce its complement, B, without changes; but on the

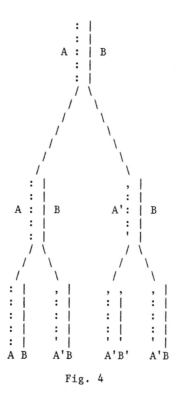

Fig. 4

Asymmetric labeling which can conserve the whole
information contents in certain chromosomes

other hand, B will reproduce A with changes. The scheme illustrating
such replications is presented in Fig. 4. We see that in the course of
cell reproduction certain chromosomes can maintain the wholeness of their
initial information.

The occurrence of MZT may not be completely determined by
the above simple scheme of equivalent labeling of zygote's offsprings.
With further considerations of possible replicative changes in DNA, in
particular considering asymmetric changes, one may reveal a finer
structure of the internal cellular clock. It is interesting to note that
in the majority of observed cases the probability of MZT is an even power
of 1/2, so it is actually a power of 1/4. In the asymmetric scheme of
DNA changes a pair of homologous chromosomes can provide equivalent
labeling at the level of zygote's grandchildren after second divison in
one fourth of possible outcomes. Thus, a cellular clock containing four
pairs of such chromosome may yield equivalent labeling at the initial
stage of zygote development with the probability of 1/256 corresponding
to the MZT probability of humans.

The unlimited replication potential of cancer cells does not have to
be associated with determinate restorative processes.

REFERENCES

1. L. Hayflick, The limited in-vitro lifetime of human diploid cell strains, Exp. Cell Res., 37:614 (1965).

2. S. Berkovich, A cybernetical model of the internal cellular clock, Medical Hypotheses, 7:1347 (1981).

3. A. M. Olovnikov, Principle of marginotomy in the synthesis of polynucleotides at a template, Dokl. Biochem., 201:226 (1971).

4. R. Holliday and J. E. Pugh, DNA modification mechanisms and gene activity during development, Science, 187:226 (1975).

5. A. J. S. Klar, Differentiated parental DNA strands confer developmental asymmetry on daughter cells in fission yeast, Nature, 326:466 (1987).

6. G. D. Wassermann, "Molecular Control of Cell Differentiation and Morphogenesis," Marcel Dekker, Inc., New York (1972).

7. C. E. Boklage, On the timing of monozygotic twinning events, in: "Twin Research 3, Twin Biology and Multiple Pregnancy," Alan R. Liss, Inc., (1981).

8. S. Berkovich and S. Bloom, Probability of monozygotic twimming as a reflection of the genetic control of cell development, Mechanisms of Aging and Development, 31:147 (1985).

9. M. G. Bulmer, "The Biology of Twinning in Man," Claredon Press, Oxford (1970).

10. M. E. Wallace and D. A. Williams, Monozygotic twinning in mice, J. Med. Genet., 2:26 (1965).

11. O. Bomsel-Helmreich and E. Papiernik-Berkhauer, Delayed ovulation and monozygotic twinning, Acta Genet. Med. Gemellol, 25:83 (1976).

12. L. Market H. Upsprung, "Developmental Genetics," Prentice-Hall, New York, (1967).

GENETIC AND ENVIRONMENTAL MANIPULATION OF AGING IN *Caenorhabditis elegans*

Richard L. Russell and Renée I. Seppa

Department of Biological Sciences
University of Pittsburgh
Pittsburgh, PA 15260

INTRODUCTION

For aging studies, the small soil nematode *Caenorhabditis elegans* offers the potential advantages of a short life span and ease of culture in large numbers, coupled with a reproductive mode (self-fertilizing hermaphroditism) which facilitates mutant isolation and thus might make possible a genetic dissection of the aging process[1,2]. To use these advantages productively and in a generalizable way, we decided some time ago, in collaboration with our colleague Lewis A Jacobson, that three additional conditions would have to be met. First, it would have to be established how general *C. elegans* aging is, i.e. to what extent it exhibits properties observed during aging in other organisms, especially mammals. Second, aging in *C. elegans* would have to be operationally defined, in a way which would permit it to be measured during manipulations aimed at altering the aging process; our view, in contrast to that of others working on many different systems, was that mere measurement of mortality (survival) statistics was **not** an adequate operational definition for this purpose. Third, it would have to be established whether useful genetic aging variants could be obtained in *C. elegans*; useful variants in this sense meant to us variants with only single-gene alterations (so that the basis of the aging effect would have some reasonable prospect of becoming understood) and in which related effects were demonstrable on more than just one of the processes which change with age (so that the genetically affected step would have a reasonable prospect of being central, rather than peripheral, to aging).

Satisfaction of these additional conditions has been a goal toward which we and others have worked over the past several years[3-7], and we now believe that the conditions have been met. The work has entailed measurement of a number of potentially age-dependent variables, separation of those which are age-dependent from those which are not, identification among the age-dependent variables of a subset which are reliable and convenient aging markers, use of these markers to characterize some environmental perturbations of aging, and finally the isolation and characterization of single-gene aging variants which do affect multiple aging processes. Below we describe these results in more detail and discuss their future applications.

RESULTS

Standard Conditions

Our work began with a choice of standard conditions under which to study aging in *C. elegans*. After trying many variations of both liquid and solid phase culture, we settled on culture on an agar surface, using a lawn of *E. coli* as food source; this resembles the natural soil habitat more closely and facilitates observation, but it is somewhat less convenient than liquid culture as regards nutritional manipulation. As our standard strain we chose, following Klass[5], the temperature-sensitive spermato-genesis-defective strain DH26, carrying the allele *b26* of the gene *fer-15*; this strain can be propagated conveniently at 20°C, but at 25.5°C is sterile for lack of sperm. In *C. elegans* aging studies with other strains, progeny production by the usual self-fertilizing hermaphroditism consti-tutes a problem; until reproduction ceases, even isolated individuals must be frequently separated from their progeny, requiring extra effort and increasing opportunities for contamination. However, with DH26 at our standard temperature of 25.5°C, no progeny production occurs and these steps are eliminated.

In our experience, the wise choice of, and strict adherence to, a set of standard conditions is essential. There appears to be intrinsic vari-ation among individuals in the aging process, against which the limited effects due to intentional manipulation are already hard enough to monitor without additional variations due to lax standardization. By the same token, standardized methods for measuring age-dependent variables are equally important, and we have established such methods for each of the variables discussed below.

Age-Dependent Variables

Our initial choice of variables amongst which to look for good aging markers was influenced by several factors. Some variables were chosen because of prior reports that they changed with age, either in *C. elegans* or in the closely related *C. briggsae*. Other were chosen because they appeared to change with age in several other species. Still others were chosen because of the relative ease, reproducibility, and sensitivity with which they could be measured in *C. elegans*. Initially, and in our final choice of markers as well, we tried to include variables at different organizational levels, from the level of the whole organism down to the biochemical level. Table 1 summarizes the results of our search, with the variables grouped roughly into three different organizational levels, "behavioral", "physiological", and "biochemical". At each level,

Table 1. Variables Examined for Possible Age-Dependence

Level	Age-Dependent	Age-Independent
Behavioral	Movement Wave Frequency Defecation Frequency	
Physiological	"Lipofuscin" Level	$^3[H]_2O$ Efflux Rate
Biochemical	Acid Phosphatase Level β-D-Glucosidase Level β-N-acetyl-D-Glucosaminidase β-D-Glucuronidase Level β-D-Galactosidase Level β-D-Mannosidase Level	Acetylcholinesterase Level Choline Acetyltransferase Level α-D-Glucosidase Level

age-dependent variables have been identified[3,4], although others (including some initially reported to be age-dependent[8]) have been shown to have little or no age-dependence on close examination.

The age-dependent variables provide some evidence that aging in *C. elegans* resembles aging in other organisms. For instance, at the behavioral level, both movement wave frequency (a general measure of mobility) and defecation frequency decline significantly with age, in keeping with the general finding of declining motor performance in aging individuals in many species (9,10). Likewise, in keeping with reported "lipofuscin" increases in many species (11), a pigment with broadly similar fluorescence properties shows a significant increase with age in *C. elegans*.

Among the age-dependent variables, we sought as markers those which could meet all or most of the following criteria.

1) Measurement of the marker's value on a given individual or cohort (as appropriate) should yield a quantitative result of adequate resolution.
2) Where possible, short-term repeat measurements on a given individual or cohort (as appropriate) should yield reproducible results.
3) Measurement, at a given age, of different individuals or cohorts (as appropriate) should yield results of only limited dispersion.
4) The measured value of the marker should change gradually throughout the lifespan.
5) Overall, the measured value of the marker should change by a factor which is large, particularly with respect to any measurement errors.

All of these properties were needed, we believed, to maximize a marker's ability to distinguish on the basis of age. In addition we hoped, for practical reasons, that the marker could meet the following supplementary criteria.

6) Measurement of the marker's value should be straightforward and fast, to facilitate data collection.
7) Measurement should be possible on a single individual, to allow assessment of inter-individual variability.
8) Measurement should be non-destructive, to allow repeat measurements longitudinally on identified individuals or cohorts (as appropriate).

(The last two criteria might seem automatic to those accustomed to other organisms, but an adult *C. elegans* is 1.4 mm long, weighs about 4 μg, and has no vascular system from which fluid samples can be taken.)

Currently we have chosen as markers five variables, drawn from all three levels of organization; these markers meet the above criteria to varying degrees. Each of these is described in more detail below.

Movement Wave Frequency. On an agar surface *C. elegans* normally lies on its side, held down by the surface tension of surface film of water. In this position it moves in a sinusoidal wiggling fashion by propagating down its body antiphasic contractile waves within the dorsal and ventral groups of longitudinal body muscle cells. For reproducible measurement of the frequency of these waves we have established standard conditions[3], including preparation of agar plates of controlled hydration, tail stimulation to elicit maximum frequency, and triplicate measurements of defined duration separated by rest periods also of defined duration. Under these conditions, the frequency of these waves is highly reproducible in successive repeat measurements of a given individual, and the variation between individuals of a given age is quite small. As shown in Figure 1,

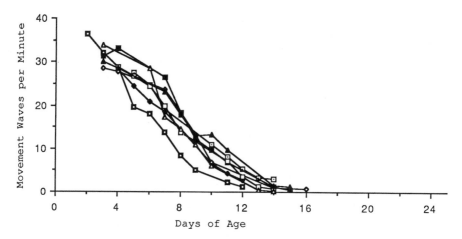

Fig. 1. Movement Wave Frequency of Strain DH26 Grown @ 25.5°C. Frequency measured after tail stimulation, on bacteria-free
movement agar, at 20°C, as described by Bolanowski et al.[3],
except that "movement waves" signifies complete waves (two
changes of head sweep direction) rather than half waves (one
change). 20 animals per age point, 3 replicate trials of 30
sec each, per animal, separated by 60 sec recovery periods.
Each symbol is for one of 8 experiments done over 17 months.

this frequency declines progressively with age from early adulthood to, and
even beyond, the mean time of death. The change is gradual, the overall
factor of change is large (at least 10-fold), and the measurements are
quite reproducible across experiments. The measurements are also non-
destructive and are inherently made on individuals, and therefore movement
wave frequency meets all of our criteria. Indeed, it is probably the best
overall marker so far identified.

β-D-Glucosidase Level. Several different enzyme activities, demonstrated to be lysosomal in other species, can be measured sensitively and
relatively easily by a common fluorescence method in which non-fluorescent
4-methylumbelliferyl substrates are enzymatically cleaved to yield fluorescent 4-methylumbelliferone as a product. In C. elegans, activity levels
for these enzymes are such that reliable values can be obtained if 5
animals are assayed for 1 to 4 hr, using standardized conditions which we
have established[4]. Maximal sensitivity is achieved by transferring animals
directly into a very small assay volume, within which they are then
homogenized, without volume losses, by repetitive freezing and thawing.
Figure 2 shows the age-dependent change (increase) in one such activity,
β-D-glucosidase; for this enzyme the variability is relatively small,
although perhaps a bit greater than for movement wave frequency, the change
is fairly gradual, and the factor of change is large, about 10-fold. Thus
this enzyme's activity level exhibits our essential features (accurate
measurement and large, gradual change) but not our additional desirable
ones; its measurement is intrinsically destructive and current assay
sensitivity requires about 5 individuals rather than 1.

β-N-acetyl-D-Glucosaminidase Activity Level. Another enzyme exhib-
iting a large factorial change with age is β-N-acetyl-D-glucosaminidase; as
with β-D-glucosidase, this enzyme has an acid pH optimum, and appears in a
lysosomal fraction upon subcellular fractionation[4]. Variation in

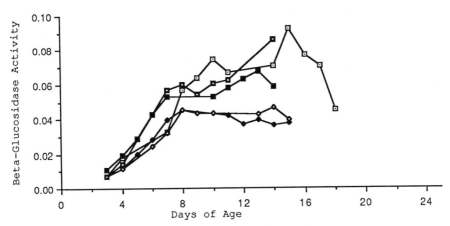

Fig. 2. β-D-Glucosidase Activity of Strain DH26 Grown at 25.5°C.
Quadruplicate 4 hr assays for each age point; 5 animals in
25 μl of 100 mM acetate buffer, pH 5.0, 0.2% NP40, 0.2% BSA,
10% glycerol, freeze-thawed 5 times to homogenize, started
with 75 μl of 0.33 mM 4-methylumbelliferyl-β-D-glucopyrano-
side, stopped with 1.0 ml 0.5 M glycine buffer, pH 10.3,
1.0 mM EDTA, fluorescence read at 455 nm, excitation at 365
nm. 1 activity unit = 0.55 pkatals. 5 expts over 8 months.

assayed activity levels is quite low; in practice standard assays have used
5 animals, but the activity level is high enough that single animals could
almost certainly be assayed accurately. Figure 3 shows the age-dependent
increase of this enzyme; the factor of increase is about 10-fold. In
general, the level of this enzyme meets all of our essential criteria, and
although its assay is intrinsically destructive, it could probably meet our
criterion of assayability on individuals.

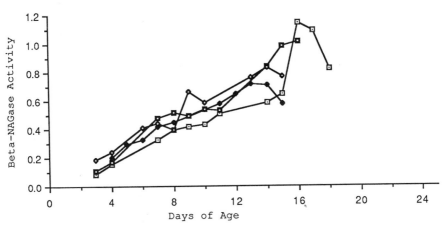

Fig. 3. β-N-acetyl-D-Glucosaminidase Activity of Strain DH26 Grown
at 25.5°C. Assays performed as in Figure 2, but starting the
reaction with 75 μl of 0.83 mM 4-methyl-umbelliferyl-β-N-
acetyl-D-glucosaminopyranoside and using a 1 hr assay time.
4 experiments conducted over 8 months.

"Lipofuscin" Level.   Many organisms exhibit an age-dependent increase
in a pigment or pigments known loosely as lipofuscin[11]. The properties of
these pigments seem to vary somewhat from source to source, making it
unclear how heterogeneous they may be, both across and within species.
Although the pigments do fluoresce with broadly similar excitation and
emission spectra, and a case has been made for a Schiff base as the primary
fluorophore in all cases[12], they have never been isolated in sufficient
purity to establish, even broadly, their chemical identity(ies).

    In *C. elegans*, initial work on this sort of pigment was reported by
Klass[5], who used a standard extraction method followed by fluorescence
quantitation to show a marked age-dependent increase. Subsequently our
laboratories (C. Link, L. A. Jacobson, and R. L. R., unpublished) carried
out a systematic fluorescence survey, both of *C. elegans* extracts and of
intact animals (using a microspectrofluorometer). Both methods revealed
three major classes of fluorescence, one having the properties expected for
tryptophan incorporated into protein, a second having the properties
expected for flavins, and the third having properties broadly similar to
those of "lipofuscin" in other systems. More or less simultaneously,
Davis, Anderson, and Dusenbery carried out a similar survey using total
luminescence spectroscopy[13], and identified the same three fluorescence
classes.

    When *C. elegans* is examined microscopically, using excitation and
emission filters to maximize selective detection of the third fluorescence class, the fluorescence is concentrated in the 34 intestinal cells,
within granular inclusions which we have shown to increase in both size and
number during aging (data not shown). These inclusions are apparently
lysosomes, capable of incorporating external substances by phagocytosis;
Clokey and Jacobson[14] have shown that when *C. elegans* is fed macromolecules (e.g. BSA) which are fluorescently tagged with distinguishable
fluorophores (e.g. RITC), each such inclusion exhibits both its endogenous
"lipofuscin" fluorescence and that appropriate for the new macromolecule.

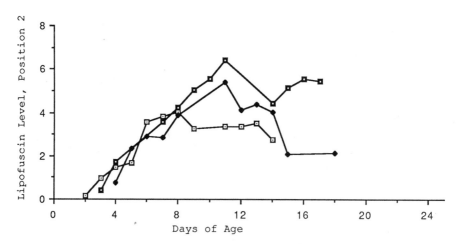

Fig. 4. Posterior Intestine Lipofuscin Level of DH26 Grown at 25.5°C.
         For each age point, 20 animals mounted on slides, heat
         killed (6 min, 60°C), and measured 3 times by epifluor-
         escence with a Leitz MPVII microspectrofluorometer over the
         posterior intestine, just anterior to the anus. Excitation,
         340-380 nm; emission, 470 nm. Results in volts read from
         the instrument, after standardization against a fixed
         thickness of quinine sulfate (@ 0.2 mg/ml) in 0.1 N H_2SO_4.

"Lipofuscin" content throughout the *C. elegans* life cycle has been quantitated in two ways, both of which show large (and comparable) age-dependent increases. The first is by chemical extraction and subsequent fluorescence quantitation (data not shown), and the second is by micro-spectrofluorometry of individuals, as shown in Figure 4. The latter method has been chosen as standard because it is simpler and can be performed on individuals. Much has been done to maximize reproducibility in this method, including the use of epifluorescence to minimize sample thickness differences, the choice of a standard location for recording (over the posterior intestine), the use of heat killing to increase the detected fluorescence level and make it more reproducible, and the use of a standard fluorescence slide to normalize the detecting photomultiplier sensitivity for each measurement series. Nonetheless, there are still day-to-day variations which are larger than desirable and appear to arise from differences in the exciting arc lamp from one ignition to the next. These variations do not compromise measurements made on a given day, as for instance when differently treated populations of the same age, run in parallel, are compared. However, they do hamper the longitudinal following of a given population over the lifespan, enough to make it unclear how well lipofuscin as a marker might meet some of our criteria. We hope to reduce these variations in the future; if we are successful, it seems likely that lipofuscin will meet all criteria except non-destructive measurement, and even that could probably be met if heat-killing could be abandoned (although the effort involved in recovering an individual and maintaining sterility after measurement would be considerable).

Survival. The variable most commonly used in other studies, survival, is also useful in *C. elegans*. While survival can obviously be determined for individuals, it clearly changes abruptly for an individual at the time of death, and is really of value only as a populational variable. Within a population, the percentage of individuals surviving can be determined quite accurately, using our defined standard criteria of death[3]. In order to ensure adequate resolution in survival data, we have adopted as standard the procedure of monitoring 96-animal cohorts, divided equally among the 24 wells of a micro-culture dish; the limit of 4 animals per well ensures adequate food supply and simplifies bookkeeping. Within a population, the change in percentage survival is fairly gradual, and survival curves are fairly reproducible, as shown in Figure 5.

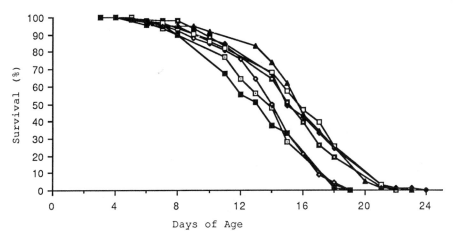

Fig. 5. Survival of Strain DH26 Grown at 25.5°C. Each curve based on a 96-animal cohort, maintained as described in text. Each symbol is for one of 7 experiments done over 14 months.

Strong effects of both temperature and nutrition on **lifespan** have been reported in *C. elegans*[5]. Given the gradual, regular nature of change in the above biomarkers over the lifespan under our standard conditions, we decided to ask whether temperature and nutrition would exhibit parallel effects on all or some of the markers. In this way we sought to test whether the markers could vary independently, and we also sought to discover how extensively the kinetics of marker change could be altered, as a prelude to analysis of genetic variants.

Effects of Temperature. In addition to our standard temperature of 25.5°C, we have followed the 5 biomarkers described above at 20°C and 16°C. At the lower temperatures, the temperature-sensitive spermatogenesis of strain DH26 cannot be used to prevent progeny production, and thus physical removal from progeny was employed. In addition, in the same experiments we compared DH26 with N2, the commonly used wild type strain from which DH26 was derived, as a check against possible unintended variations with DH26. Figure 6 shows, for clarity, only the results for 25.5°C and 16°C, the two extremes. In all cases, the measured biomarker changes considerably more slowly with age at 16°C, as generally anticipated. In addition, any differences between DH26 and N2 are small, and most likely within the range of variation observed in repeat experiments with DH26. In general, as well, the shape of the age-dependence curve appears not to be altered between the two temperatures, with the exception that lipofuscin apparently accumulates to somewhat higher levels at 16°C (Figure 6D). Given these facts, it is possible to estimate by what factor the progress of each biomarker is slowed at 16°C, by rescaling the time axis of the 16°C curve until maximal correspondance with the 25.5°C curve is obtained; an example of this scaling is presented in Figure 6F, for survival. In this case, the best scaling factor is 0.68, indicating that at 16°C, survival drops at a rate only 68% of that at 25.5°C. Similar correspondances can be achieved for the other biomarkers, but the required scaling factors are lower than for survival; the range is from 0.44 for β-N-acetyl-D-glucosaminidase to 0.50 for lipofuscin.

Effects of Nutrition. Using different (liquid suspension) culture conditions, Klass[5] reported extension of *C. elegans* **lifespan** by nutritional restriction, accomplished by reduced concentration of a bacterial food supply. Under our standard conditions, i.e. on an agar surface, bacterial concentration is much less effective in controlling nutritional level because the animals move around and can detect local concentrations and respond to them effectively. As one response to this problem, we have established inactivating treatments (heat-killing and UV irradiation) which, when applied to food bacteria, reduce nutritional value sufficiently to extend *C. elegans'* lifespan, even when the bacteria are used on agar as a lawn without dilution (G. Grossman, L. A. Jacobson, and R. L. R., unpublished). However, use of these treatments is cumbersome, and for the current experiments we instead exposed animals to alternating 24 hr periods of full feeding and complete starvation. Figure 7 shows how each of the five biomarkers was affected, compared to fully fed controls followed in parallel. The effects are less marked than for temperature (Figure 6), but each marker is affected in the same direction; its rate of change is slowed by the nutritional restriction regimen. In addition, the general shape of each curve is not significantly altered, permitting the same sort of time scaling as in Figure 6. Figure 7F shows an example of scaling for survival, in which case the best factor is 0.86. As in the case of temperature, the changes in the other markers can also be scaled, with generally quite close correspondances. However, the best scaling factors vary from marker to marker, from a low of 0.45 for β-N-acetyl-D-glucosaminidase to a high of 0.79 for movement.

42

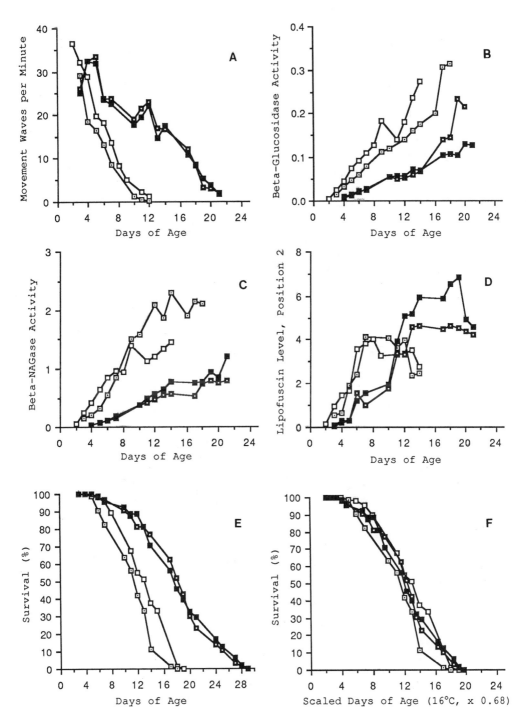

Fig. 6. Effects of Temperature on Marker Changes with Age in DH26 and N2. All markers measured as in Figures 1-5, on animals maintained either at 25.5°C (open symbols) or at 16°C (filled symbols). Dotted symbols, N2; undotted symbols, DH26. Time is scaled in F.

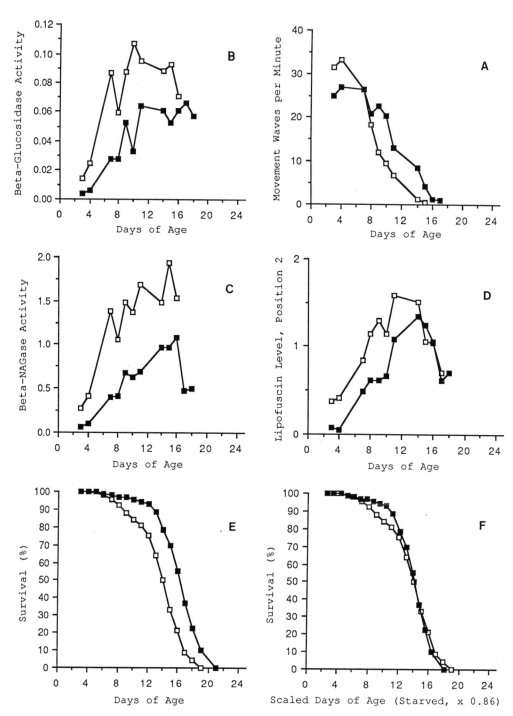

Fig. 7. Effects of Nutrition on Marker Changes with Age in DH26. Markers measured as in Figures 1-5, on animals maintained in parallel either fully fed, (open symbols), or nutritionally restricted, by alternating 24hr of normal feeding and 24 hr starvation (filled symbols). Two staggered populations of restricted animals used so that markers could be measured daily, but always after feeding.

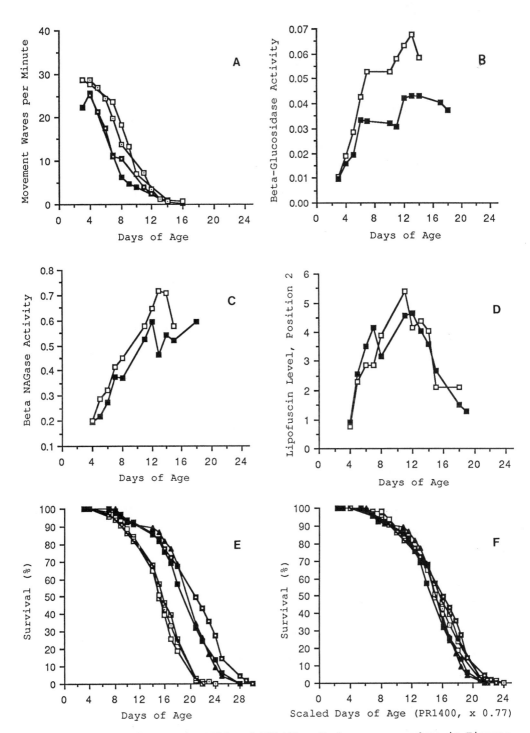

Fig. 8.   Marker Changes in DH26 and PR1400.   Markers measured as in Figures
1-5, on populations maintained in parallel at 25.5°C.   Open
symbols, DH26; closed symbols, PR1400.   Panel A, 2 experiments
done over 4 months.   Panel E, 3 experiments done over 5 months.
In panel F, time is scaled as shown for PR1400.

Genetic Manipulation of Aging

Following the methods of Klass[6], we have used a "replica-plating" method to screen amongst F2 progeny of EMS-mutagenized DH26 for new variants with extended lifespans. Details of this search will be published elsewhere, but we have characterized one of the resulting lifespan variants, strain PR1400, as an initial test of the usefulness of the above markers for analyzing the nature of genetic changes. Figure 8 shows how the markers change in PR1400, compared to their changes in DH26 populations maintained in parallel. The lifespan extension of PR1400 is reproducible and fairly sizable, about 30% as judged from Figure 8F. However, in contrast to the situation with both temperature and starvation, the effect on the other markers is much less striking. Indeed, for movement, PR1400 actually exhibits a decline which is slightly but reproducibly **more** rapid than that of DH26. This result indicates that the genetic change in this case is different from that exerted by either temperature or starvation. It also suggests that lifespan effects can be produced by genetic changes which may be rather peripheral, in the sense that they do not broadly affect the whole aging process. These points are discussed further below.

DISCUSSION

With respect to the initial goals described above, the five markers we have described help, first, to establish that aging in *C. elegans* has features in common with aging in other organisms. In particular, the steady decline in movement wave frequency (and the similar decline in defecation frequency[3], not used as a marker) demonstrate that *C. elegans*, like other organisms, exhibits declining motor performance with age. Also, the steady and large increase in fluorescent "lipofuscin" in *C. elegans* is another aging property shared in common with many other species, even though the chemical nature of this pigment remains uncertain. Lastly, survival curves in *C. elegans* appear rather typical of those already compiled for species of many different phyla.

The markers also help to provide an operational definition of aging that can be used in studies aimed at manipulating the aging process. The five markers chosen represent a spectrum of organizational levels, yet all are similarly slowed, if not to exactly the same extent, by two broad manipulations, temperature reduction and nutritional restriction. In view of these observations, we believe that the best operational definition of aging for future studies should be one based on these markers, rather than on survival alone. In essence, we argue that aging should be defined as the process which leads to joint change in **all** of these markers. A corollary of this definition is that any attempted manipulation of aging should be judged by the extent to which it affects the markers jointly. One which affects just a single marker, such as survival, seems much less likely to affect a process which is central and fundamental to aging than one which affects all or most of the markers jointly.

The initial genetic variant which we have characterized with respect to our chosen markers shows an effect different from those of temperature and nutrition. While its lifespan is significantly extended, the other markers do not follow suit. By the criteria described above, then, this variant seems unlikely to affect a central and fundamental process of aging, and we interpret it thus. While this variant is therefore not of prime interest for understanding such processes, if indeed they exist, it does serve the very important function of showing that the chosen biomarkers **can** vary independently of survival.

Future efforts, we believe, should now be directed toward identifying any genetic variants and/or pharmacological treatments which affect the chosen markers jointly. Among genetic variants, some attention should be paid, no doubt, to the recombinant inbred lines of *C. elegans* described by Johnson and Wood[7]. These lines are reported to exhibit a 3-fold range of lifespans, but no data regarding the markers is yet available; at the very least it seems likely that these lines would be useful for further establishing the degree to which the markers can vary independently. Probably of greater promise, however, are the apparently single-gene lifespan variants initially isolated by Klass[6] and recently charac- terized genetically by Friedman and Johnson[15]. Preliminary experiments with one of these variants (data not shown) indicates that it does show joint effects on several markers, not just on lifespan, and thus may come closer to affecting a putative central process of aging.

ACKNOWLEDGEMENTS

We gratefully acknowledge support of our work by grant No. AG 01154 from the National Institutes of Health in the U. S. Dept. of Health and Human Resources. We thank Lewis A. Jacobson for discussions and sugges- tions throughout, Gregory Grossman for early work establishing standard conditions of culture and standard methods of assay for some of the markers described, and Thomas E. Johnson for communication of results before publication.

REFERENCES

1. S. Brenner, The genetics of *Caenorhabditis elegans*, Genetics 77:71 (1974).
2. B. M. Zuckerman, ed., "Nematodes as Biological Models," Academic Press, New York (1980).
3. M. A. Bolanowski, R. L. Russell, and L. A. Jacobson, Quantitative measures of aging in the nematode *Caenorhabditis elegans*: I. Populational and longitudinal studies of two behavioral parameters, Mech. Ageing Dev. 15:279 (1981).
4. M. A. Bolanowski, L. A. Jacobson, and R. L. Russell, Quantitative measures of aging in the nematode *Caenorhabditis elegans*: II. Lysosomal hydrolases as markers of senescence, Mech. Ageing Dev. 21:295 (1983).
5. M. R. Klass, Aging in the nematode *Caenorhabditis elegans*: Major biological and environmental factors influencing life span, Mech. Ageing Dev. 6:413 (1977).
6. M. R. Klass, A method for the isolation of longevity mutants in the nematode *Caenorhabditis elegans* and initial results, Mech. Ageing Dev. 22:279 (1983).
7. T. E. Johnson and W. B. Wood, Genetic analysis of lifespan in *Caenorhabditis elegans*, Proc. Natl. Acad. Sci. USA 79:6603 (1982).
8. D. G. Searcy, M. J. Kisiel, and B. M. Zuckerman, Age-related increase of cuticle permeability in the nematode *Caenorhabditis elegans*, Exp. Aging Res. 2:293 (1976).
9. C. E. Finch and E. L. Schneider, eds., "Handbook of the Biology of Aging," 2nd ed., Van Nostrand Reinhold, New York (1986).
10. A. T. Welford, Motor Performance, in: "Handbook of the Psychology of Aging," J. E. Birren and K. W. Schaie, eds., Van Nostrand Reinhold, New York (1977).
11. M. Rothstein, "Biochemical Approaches to Aging," Academic Press, New York (1982).
12. A. L. Tappel, Lipid peroxidation damage to cell components, Fed. Proc. 32:1870 (1973).

13. B. O. Davis, Jr., G. L. Anderson, and D. B. Dusenbery, Total luminescence spectroscopy of fluorescence changes during aging in *Caenorhabditis elegans*, Biochemistry 21:4089 (1982).

14. G. V. Clokey and L. A. Jacobson, The autofluorescent "lipofuscin granules" in the intestinal cells of *Caenorhabditis elegans* are secondary lysosomes, Mech. Ageing Dev. 35:79 (1986).

15. D. B. Friedman and T. E. Johnson, Characterization of four mutants that extend both mean and maximum life span of *Caenorhabditis elegans*, submitted for publication.

SCALING OF MAXIMAL LIFESPAN IN MAMMALS:

A REVIEW

John Prothero[1] and Klaus D. Jürgens[2]

[1]Biological Structure, University of Washington, Seattle,
Washington, USA and [2]Zentrum Physiologie, Medizinische
Hochschule, Hannover, West Germany

INTRODUCTION

The study of maximal lifespan in mammals is a topic of considerable
interest. Recent comparative studies have demonstrated a correlation
between efficiency of DNA repair and maximal lifespan [1], an inverse
correlation between cytochrome P-448 content and maximal lifespan[2], a
correlation between the ratio of superoxide dismutase to specific energy
metablism and maximal lifespan[3], and a correlation between in vitro
cellular proliferative potential and maximal lifespan[4]. Another well
known example is the maximal lifespan-brain weight correlation discussed
by Sacher[5]. Such correlations may serve to stimulate the formulation of
hypotheses as to the nature of the factors influencing maximal lifespan.

The most extensive analysis of maximal lifespan in mammals reported
thus far is that of Sacher[5]. More recent but less extensive analyses
have been reported by Economos[6,7], Western[8], Blueweiss et al.[9], and
Boddington[10]. None of these authors draw on all of the several existing
large compilations of maximal lifespan. With the exception of
Economos[6,7], these authors do not critically examine the data or the
analytical methods employed in lifespan studies.

There were several motives for undertaking this study of maximal
lifespan in mammals. The subject is of intrinsic interest from the
standpoint of achieving a unified understanding of the mechanisms of
aging. No review of maximal lifespan in mammals with any claim to com-
pleteness had been undertaken. In a more practical vein, we were concerned with the possibility of a systematic bias in the lifespan data.
For example, the issue of whether maximal lifespan is greater in females
than males, as has sometimes been suggested (e.g., Rockstein et al.[11].
has not been carefully examined. A significant difference in lifespan
as a function of gender could confound a regression analysis in which
this factor was ignored. Again, Sacher[5,12] is not explicit about the
criteria he adopted in selecting data from different sources. A bias
could be introduced due to improvements in animal husbandry (see Snyder
and Moore [13]). Much of the data of Flower[14], which Sacher[12] draws upon
to an unspecified degree, are based on nineteenth century zoo records,
whereas the rest of his data are derived mainly from twentieth century
zoo records.

We also felt it timely to review several other matters. The relationships between mean and maximal lifespan, or between maximal lifespan in the wild and in captivity have as yet received little attention. Sacher's[12] finding that maximal lifespan is better correlated with brain weight than body weight has been the subject of much discussion (Hofman[15,16], Cutler[17], Western and Ssemakula[18], Economos[6,7], Sacher[19], Mallouk[29], Zepelin and Rechtschaffen[21]). It was felt important to re-examine this contention.

In a separate study[22] we compared the relationship between maximal lifespan in bats (order Chiroptera) with that in mammals generally. In this paper we survey maximal lifespan in mammals generally; we look at maximal lifespan in several orders, and compare these results with maximal lifespan in bats and birds.

Data Base

We made detailed regression analyses of lifespan (maximal, mean) in mammals (captive, wild) as a function of body or organ (brain, kidney) weight. We drew on five substantial (N > 150) data bases[14,23-26] (see also[27]) as well as a smaller one[8]. At least two of these data bases[14,23], are independent, but the others may overlap to some degree. Where the data permit, separate analyses have been made for male and female mammals. Regression lines also were computed for aquatic mammals[28-30], artiodactyls, carnivores, marsupials, primates and rodents. Each data base was analyzed independently of the others, to reduce the chances of introducing a systematic bias, prior to aggregating the data. The extent of the mammalian data base which has been analyzed and the parameters of the analysis are set forth in Table 1. In addition, we computed a regression line for maximal lifespan in wild birds using the graphical data of Lindstedt and Calder[31] as recovered by digitization[32].

All the lifespan data were taken from secondary sources (see Table 1). With the exception of the data of Western[8], none of these sources supply paired values of maximal lifespan and body weight. We employed representative values of body weight for each species, principally taken from Walker[33], Boitani and Bartoli[34], Dorst and Dandelot[35], Whitaker[36]. Where a range (minimum and maximum) of body weights is given, as is commonly the case, we have used the arithmetic mean. Occasionally, only a maximum weight is given, and here we multiplied this value by the ad hoc factor of 0.55 to reduce the possibility of introducing a systematic bias (since maximum weights are normally given only for larger mammals). For example, one source gave the mean weight of the Asian elephant as 2730 Kg and another a maximum weight of 5000 Kg, giving a ratio of 0.55. Failure to use such a correction factor would lead to least squares regression lines with slopes slightly below the values reported here. Where weights for males and females only are given for a species we have computed the arithmetic mean. Brain weights were taken from Crile and Quiring[37] and Martin[38]. Kidney weights were taken from Crile and Quiring[37].

We rejected those values of maximal lifespan where the species name given by an author could not be found in Corbet and Hill (39). (In a few cases ambiguities as to species name were resolved by referring to Honacki et al.[40].) For the values of maximal lifespan we employed the highest values reported, tabulating the data for males and females separately where available (see Table 1). (As improved statistics are collected, it is inevitable that many values for maximal lifespan will increase, in some cases dramatically.) Coordinate values for body weight were not available always, so that our data sets are smaller than the original lifespan data sets. Brain and kidney weights were available to us only for a much smaller sample. We omitted cases where the

Table 1. Summary of database[a]

	Maximal									Mean	
	Captivity							The Wild		Captivity	
Lifespan in as a function of in	Body Weight					Brain Weight	Kidney Weight	Body Weight		Body Weight	Source of Lifespan Data
	Males & Females	Artiodactyls	Carnivores	Primates	Rodents	Mammals	Mammals	Mammals	Aquatic Mammals	Mammals	
	Mammals										
	+	+	+	+	+	+	−	−	−	+	[14]
	−	+	+	+	+	−	−	−	−	+	[23]
	+	+	+	+	+	+	+	−	−	−	[24]
	−	+	+	+	+	+	+	−	−	+	[25,27]
	−	+	+	+	+	+	+	−	−	+	[26]
	−	+	+	+	+	−	−	−	−	+	[8]
	−	−	−	−	−	−	−	+	+	−	[28–30]

[a]Maximal or mean lifespan in captive or wild mammals, as a function of organ or body weight is analyzed in seven data sets identified in the right column. The various subgroups analyzed are identified in the fourth row.

51

maximal lifespan was given as less than one year in species with adult
weights of more than several hundred grams, on the presumption that
these data reflect infant mortality.

It should be noted that the lifespans reported for captive mammals
are often not the true lifespans, since zoos frequently acquire young
animals of unknown age. Furthermore the lifespan data are probably
biased against males, which zoos keep in smaller numbers than females[14].

From each separate data source we used the largest value of lifespan
given for each species that could be taxonically identified in Corbet
and Hill[39] and for which a documented value of body weight was available.
Apart from the few cases noted above, no values of maximal lifespan were
omitted in drawing up the data base. We have not drawn on the significant but very scattered literature which provides maximal lifespan
values for individual species.

METHODS

For each separate data base (see Table 1) the taxonomic, lifespan,
body and organ weight data were assembled and carefully checked before
any regression analyses were undertaken. In each case we report the
number of orders and species in the sample, as a measure of taxonomic
diversity (there are about 20 orders and more than 4000 species of mammals altogether). Where lifespan for males and females are both represented in the data, the number of points entering into a regression
calculation will exceed the number of species. Where gender is not
distinguished the number of points and species are the same.

As is customary in scaling studies, we assumed that a power function
is the best two-parameter representation of the data. Thus the model we
employ is:

$$y' = ax**b \qquad (1)$$

where x and y' are the variate and covariate respectively, 'a' is the
weight coefficient (or intercept) and 'b' is the exponent (or slope).
In this study 'x' is either a body or organ weight, measured in kg, and
y' is a mean or maximal lifespan, measured in years. We use '**' to
denote exponentiation.

As a rule, the accuracy with which the coefficients "a" and "b" in
equation (1) can be estimated is determined by the weight range spanned
by the data. The weight range also indicates how representative a data
set is with respect to the weight range covered by mammals generally.
We have used the notation pWR to denote the logarithm of the ratio of
the maximum to the minimum weight found in any given data set:

$$\overline{pWR} = logarithm \text{ (maximum weight/minimum weight)} \qquad (2)$$

For mammals generally (shrews to blue whales), pWR is about 8.

In addition, as a way of further characterizing each regression
line, we report the (geometric) mean weight, Wp, calculated from the
relation:

$$\overline{Wp} = sqrt(Wmin* Wmax) \qquad Kg \qquad (3)$$

where '*' denotes multiplication. To the extent that a power law actually governs empirical scaling relations, a geometric mean is a better

measure of centrality than an arithmetic mean.

In each case the data were expressed in logarithmic form and submitted to linear least squares regression analysis[41]. A mean percent
deviation (% Dev) between the data points and each regression line was
calculated from the relations:

$$y_i' = a*(x_i**b) \tag{4}$$

$$\% \ Dev = 100/n \ \sum_{i=1}^{n} \left| y_i' - y_i \right| /y_i \tag{5}$$

where x_i is the ith value for body or organ weight, y_i is the ith value
for observed maximal lifespan, y_i' is the value of y_i predicted from
equation (4), 'a' and 'b' are as given above (see equation (1)), and 'n'
is the number of data points.

The mean percent deviation, provides a simple – and readily
interpretable – measure of goodness-of-fit, whereas the correlation
coefficient (squared) measures simply the extent to which variation in y
is due to variation in x. Note that a high correlation coefficient may
be associated with an unreasonably high mean percent deviation. Hence,
these two statistics reflect different aspects of the degree to which a
regression line adequately represents a (logarithmically transformed)
set of data.

For each regression line we report the correlation coefficient,
the mean percent deviation and the number of points lying above and
below the regression line (for normally distributed data the points will
be disposed symmetrically about the regression line). The above
measures of taxonomic diversity, weight range, goodness-of-fit, etc.,
associated with a single regression line are referred to as the
'regression characteristic'.

Two unusual findings were made in the course of computing these
regression lines. First, a significant number of points deviate from
the calculated regression line by more than one hundred percent. (In
prior studies with reasonably 'clean' data sets [i.e., data uniformly
distributed approximately]) we have found that the mean deviation is
typically 20 to 30%[42-44]. The large deviations found here raise
questions as to whether the data are, in fact, "clean." Second, without
exception, all of these highly deviant points fell below the computed
regression line.

For a uniformly distributed data set the dispersion (here measured
by mean percent deviation) will be nearly the same on both sides of the
regression line. Points deviating by one hundred percent or more from a
regression line appear to exceed 'typical' biological variation by a
factor of at least three to five (see above). This asymmetric distribution and large dispersion does not appear to be attributable to normal
biological variation. Because of this markedly skewed distribution of
the data, we adopted the practice of first computing a 'primary'
regression line with the full data set (FDS), and then deleting all the
points deviating by more than 100%, thereby generating a reduced data
set (RDS). A 'secondary' regression line was then computed using the
RDS for all cases where one or more points deviated by at least 100%.

It is reasonable to suppose that the asymmetric distribution and the
large dispersion are due to sampling errors which bias the data on the
side of younger animals. Although an RDS may still contain points

deviating (negatively) from the regression line by 100% or more, we believe that the RDS is a better approximation to a 'clean' data set and is likely to be more representative of 'true' maximal lifepans than is an FDS.

RESULTS

The regression characteristics for lifespan (maximal or mean) as a function of body weight in mammals generally are reported in Table 2 for six different data sets. In two cases we show the regression characteristics for both the full (FDS) and reduced data sets (RDS) (see rows 1,2,3,4 of Table 2). Note that the regression characteristic for mean lifespan as a function of body weight is given in row 10 of Table 2. (Due to an error in our software, discovered after the calculations for this paper were completed, the values for the standard error in the intercept in this (and previous papers from our laboratory) are too low by an estimated 10% to 15%).

Table 3 gives the regression characteristics for maximal lifespan as a function of body weight in male and female mammals, as well as for artiodactyls, carnivores, primates and rodents, drawing on subsets of the data summarized in Table 2. Even when we employ the RDS to compute a 'secondary' regression line, points may still deviate from the regression line by more than 100% (see Table 3, rows 1 and 5, column 12). The reason is that the 'secondary' regression line always lies above the 'primary' regression line (see Fig. 1). A few points which deviate by a little less than 100% from the 'primary' regression line may thus come to deviate by a little more than 100% from the 'secondary' regression line. This fact emphasizes the arbitrary nature of using 100% (or any other percentage) as a threshold for data exclusion.

Table 4 gives maximal lifespan as a function of body or organ (brain, kidney) weight in captive or wild mammals. Table 5 gives the regression characteristics for mean lifespan as a function of body weight in artiodactyls, carnivores, primates and rodents. The number of points deleted prior to the computation of 'secondary' regression lines is reported in column 12 of Tables 2,3,4 and column 11 of Table 5.

In Table 6 we report the results of an analysis in which, for each species, we abstracted the single largest value for maximal lifespan, drawing from each of the five major data sets (14,23-26) (see Table 2). This gave a full data set (FDS) of 578 and a RDS of 494 species. A breakdown of Table 6, by source, is given in Table 7.

In analyzing the results obtained with this aggregated data set it was noted that 12 of the 13 points for the bat species lie above the regression line, with a mean deviation of 58% and that all of the five points for the edentates lie above the regression line, with a mean deviation of 40%. We therefore deleted the bats and edentates from the sample and computed a new regression line. The results are given in Table 6 (row 3).

In the various data sets used in this study the points are often distributed unevenly along the regression line. In order to produce a more even distribution, using the aggregated data set, we divided the data into 16 groups, each extending over an approximate two-fold weight range. We computed a (logarithmic) mean for each individual weight range and an (arithmetic) mean of the maximal lifespans in each weight range, using the FDS. We then fitted a regression line to this data set. The results are given in Table 6 (row 4).

Table 2. Regression characteristics for lifespan (maximal or mean) as a function of body weight in captive mammals by source[a]

	Orders	Species	Points	pWR	W̄p	a	Log(a) ± se	b ± se	r	% Dev	+/-	Points Deleted	Comments	Ref.
	1	2	3	4	5	6	7	8	9	10	11	12	13	14
1	14	166	202	5.9	5.4	8.14	0.911 ±0.012	0.156 ±0.010	0.729	33	107/95	0	Maximal lifespan Full data set (FDS)	[14]
2	13	158	192	5.9	5.4	8.76	0.943 ±0.010	0.149 ±0.009	0.774	26	93/99	10	Maximal Lifespan Reduced Data Set (RDS)	[14]
3	16	355	355	5.6	4.6	5.30	0.724 ±0.014	0.174 ±0.012	0.605	57	190/165	0	Maximal Lifespan FDS	[23]
4	14	311	311	3.9	4.6	6.24	0.795 ±0.011	0.168 ±0.010	0.706	39	153/158	44	Maximal Lifespan RDS	[23]
5	13	232	285	3.45	10.2	9.94	0.997 ±0.010	0.147 ±0.009	0.699	30	141/144	26	Maximal Lifespan RDS	[24]
6	20	236	236	5.5	8.5	14.15	1.151 ±0.011	0.116 ±0.009	0.641	30	111/125	22	Maximal Lifespan RDS	[25]
7	14	151	151	5.8	3.8	9.97	0.998 ±0.014	0.153 ±0.011	0.746	34	75/76	13	Maximal Lifespan RDS	[26]
8	6	48	48	2.1	20.2	10.10	1.006 ±0.021	0.155 ±0.022	0.718	26	20/28	0	Maximal Lifespan FDS	[8]
9	10	188	233	3.45	10.2	9.15	0.961 ±0.010	0.156 ±0.009	0.743	28	109/124	26	Maximal Lifespan Bats, primates, aquatic mammals omitted, RDS	[24]
10	16	312	312	5.6	4.6	3.43	0.535 ±0.010	0.127 ±0.009	0.636	34	140/172	21	Mean Lifespan RDS	[23]

[a]The model is y' = a*(x**b), where x is body weight in kg, and y' is the predicted lifespan, measured in years. Columns 1, 2 and 3 specify the number of orders, species and points, respectively. Columns 4, 5, 6 and 7 give the logarithm of the weight range and the geometric mean weight, the intercept and the logarithm of the intercept plus or minus the standard error, respectively. Columns 10,11,12 and 13 report the exponent, the correlation coefficient, the mean percent deviation and the distribution of points above (+) and below (-), the regression line for the reduced data set (RDS), the parameter computed (maximal or mean lifespan) and the data set used (FDS or RDS). Column 14 gives the data sources. See text for details.

55

Table 3. Regression characteristics for maximal lifespan as a function of body weight in selected groups of captive mammals[a]

	Orders	Species	Points	pWR	W̄p	a	Log (a) ± se	b ± se	r	% Dev	+/-	Points > -100%	Comments	References
	1	2	3	4	5	6	7	8	9	10	11	12	13	14
1	9	65	65	4.5	20.1	8.85	0.947 ±0.017	0.142 ±0.017	0.715	25	30/35	1	Males Reduced data set (RDS)	[14]
2	11	78	78	5.0	14.8	9.29	0.968 ±0.015	0.149 ±0.015	0.742	25	39/39	0	Females RDS	[14]
3	1	61	61	2.9	127.7	9.79	0.991 ±0.013	0.163 ±0.022	0.690	19	33/28	0	Artiodactyls RDS	[25]
4	1	53	63	3.5	8.0	8.95	0.952 ±0.015	0.170 ±0.021	0.721	23	33/30	0	Carnivores RDS	[14]
5	1	47	47	3.1	4.4	17.70	1.248 ±0.021	0.195 ±0.029	0.706	26	23/24	2	Primates RDS	[25]
6	1	28	28	3.5	0.89	11.0	1.042 ±0.030	0.127 ±0.030	0.64	29	13/15	0	Rodents RDS	[25]
7	18	76	76	5.3	8.1	13.9	1.142 ±0.022	0.155 ±0.017	0.727	38	41/35	6	Maximal Values in each of 76 families (RDS)	[25,27]

[a]See legend for Table 2. Column 12 identifies the number of points lying below the "secondary" regression lines which deviated by more than 100% (see text).

Table 4. Regression characteristics for maximal lifespan in wild or captive mammals as a function of body or organ weight[a]

	Orders	Species	Points	pWR	$\overline{W}p$	a	Log(a) ± se	b ± se	r	% Dev	+/-	Points > -100%	Variate	Comments	Ref.
	1	2	3	4	5	6	7	8	9	10	11	12	13	14	15
1	9	90	108	4.0	0.059	31.7	1.501 ±0.014	0.255 ±0.021	0.770	28	54/54	1	Brain Weight	Captive mammals Reduced data set (RDS)	[24]
2	7	32	36	4.7	0.084	26.3	1.420 ±0.024	0.240 ±0.024	0.866	28	17/19	0	Kidney Weight	Captive mammals RDS	[24]
3	6	20	20	6.1	23.9	9.10	0.959 ±0.028	0.201 ±0.020	0.924	24	9/11	0	Body Weight	Mammals in the wild RDS	[28]
4	3	15	15	3.2	745.5	11.0	1.072 ±0.028	0.173 ±0.028	0.866	20	7/8	0	Body Weight	Aquatic mammals in the wild (FDS)	[28,29,30]

[a]See legends, Tables 2 and 3.

Table 5. Regression characteristics for mean lifespan as a function
of body weight is selected groups of captive animals[a]

	Species	Points	pWR	$\overline{Wp}$	a	Log (a) ± se	b ± se	r	% Dev	+/-	Points > -100%	Comments	References
	1	2	3	4	5	6	7	8	9	10	11	12	13
1	64	64	2.15	101	2.46	0.390 ±0.018	0.185 ±0.038	0.528	27	30/34	0	Artiodactyls RDS	[23]
2	80	80	3.54	7.92	3.30	0.518 ±0.022	0.162 ±0.031	0.511	38	42/38	3	Carnivores RDS	[23]
3	50	50	3.38	3.17	3.27	0.515 ±0.023	0.188 ±0.033	0.635	31	25/25	1	Primates RDS	[23]
4	75	75	3.88	0.61	3.34	0.524 ±0.021	0.103 ±0.025	0.435	35	31/44	2	Rodents RDS	[23]

[a]See legends, Tables 2 and 3.

Table 6. Regression analysis of aggregated data base[a]

	Orders	Species	Points	pWR	$\overline{W}p$	a	Log(a) ± se	b ± se	r	% Dev	+/-	Points > -100%	Comments
	1	2	3	4	5	6	7	8	9	10	11	12	13
1	20	578	578	6.2	5.8	8.15	0.911 ±0.012	0.187 ±0.009	0.637	63	324/255	83	Mammals generally Full data set (FDS)
2	204	494	494	6.0	4.8	10.1	1.006 ±0.009	0.170 ±0.007	0.726	38	245/249	33	Mammals generally Reduced data set (RDS)
3	18	476	476	5.9	5.4	9.7	0.988 ±0.009	0.181 ±0.007	0.752	36	240/236	25	Bats and Edentates Deleted (RDS)
4	-	-	16	5.3	8.8	9.9	0.997 ±0.016	0.168 ±0.011	0.973	12	8/8	0	Mammals generally Grouped data (see text)(FDS)
5	1	115	115	3.0	115.0	4.9	0.690 ±0.018	0.264 ±0.031	0.623	38	65/50	8	Arteriodactyls (FDS)
6	1	99	99	3.0	114.6	7.16	0.855 ±0.012	0.209 ±0.021	0.713	22	51/48	0	Arteriodactyls (RDS)
7	1	113	113	3.5	8.0	8.0	0.905 ±0.022	0.244 ±0.034	0.564	51	66/47	11	Carnivores (FDS)
8	1	103	103	3.5	8.0	10.2	1.007 ±0.015	0.188 ±0.023	0.632	29	56/47	2	Carnivores (RDS)
9	1	43	43	3.6	0.88	5.9	0.768 ±0.048	0.250 ±0.050	0.615	76	28/15	7	Marsupials (FDS)
10	1	33	33	3.6	0.88	8.3	0.917 ±0.029	0.198 ±0.029	0.770	31	15/18	0	Marsupials (RDS)
11	1	87	87	3.4	3.2	12.2	1.086 ±0.028	0.237 ±0.040	0.538	60	57/30	12	Primates (FDS)
12	1	83	83	3.1	4.4	13.6	1.133 ±0.023	0.214 ±0.034	0.577	43	49/34	9	Primates (RDS)
13	1	132	132	4.0	0.61	7.3	0.864 ±0.021	0.200 ±0.025	0.575	51	67/65	17	Rodents (FDS)
14	1	107	107	4.0	0.60	8.9	0.950 ±0.018	0.208 ±0.020	0.712	35	56/51	5	Rodents (RDS)

[a]Regression characteristics for maximal lifespan as a function of body weight computed from an aggregated data set. (14,23-26). Column 12 gives the number of points deviating from the regression line by more than -100%.

59

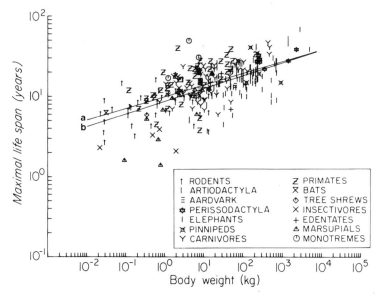

Fig. 1. Maximal lifespan as a function of body weight in mammals
generally. The lines (a) and (b) are the regression lines for
the reduced and full data sets respectively (see text). The orders
represented in the full data set are indicated. See Table 2, row 5.

For this aggregated data set we further analyzed maximal lifespan
for arteriodactyls, carnivores, marsupials, primates and rodents using
both the reduced and full data sets(see Table 6, rows 5-14).[*]

Table 8 summarizes the regression characteristics reported in prior
studies for lifespan (mean or maximal) as a function of body or organ
weight in both mammals and birds. We have recomputed the regression
characteristics for two cases, shown in Table 8, namely that of Western
(8) for mammals and that of Lindstedt and Calder (31) for birds.

A plot of the data of Crandall (24), for maximal lifespan in captive
mammals as a function of body weight, showing the FDS, and giving the
best-fit least squares regression lines for both the FDS and RDS, is
shown in Fig 1 (see Table 2, row 5). In Figure 2 we have plotted the
best-fit regression lines obtained for the five major RDS (see Table 2,
rows 2,4,5,6 and 7). Figure 3 shows the data and best fit regression
lines for maximal lifespan in artiodactyls, carnivores, primates and
rodents. Figure 4 displays the regression lines for maximal lifespan in

[*]The RDS derived from the aggregated data has been deposited with the
National Auxiliary Publications Service (American Society for Informa-
tion Science, c/o Microfiche Publications, P.O. Box, 3513, Grand
Central Station, NY 10163, USA) as Document No. 04467.

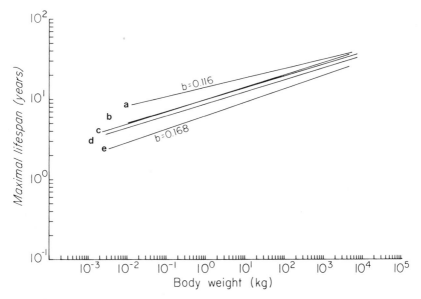

Figure 2. Regression lines for maximal lifespan as a function of body weight in mammals generally calculated from reduced data sets (see text). The lines (a), (b), (c), (d) and (e) correspond to Table 2, rows 6,5,7,2 and 4, respectively. The values for the smallest and highest slopes are indicated.

(captive) artiodactyls, carnivores, rodents, and aquatic (wild) mammals along with a best-fit regression line for maximal lifespan in (captive) mammals generally, (see Table 3, rows 3,4,6; Table 4, row 4 and below). Figure 5 (a,b) shows the FDS and the RDS derived from the aggregated data set (see Table 6, rows 1,2). The best-fit regression lines for the FDS and the RDS are shown in each plot.

Figure 6 allows one to compare the best-fit regression line for mean lifespan with that for maximal lifespan in captive mammals (see Table 2, row 10). Also shown in Figure 6 are the regression lines for maximal lifespan in wild bats and birds and captive primates (see Table 8, rows 11,15 and Table 3, row 3).

It is neither practicable nor useful to report all of the results obtained in this study . For each of the cases where we have multiple data sets (see Table 1) we have sought to report the regression characteristics for the line that is taxonomically the most representative, covers the greatest weight range, has the highest correlation coefficient, the lowest mean percent deviation and the most even distribution of points about the regression line. As a rule, no single regression line was superior by all these criteria, so that a certain degree of arbitrariness was inevitable in the selection of the 'best' regression lines.

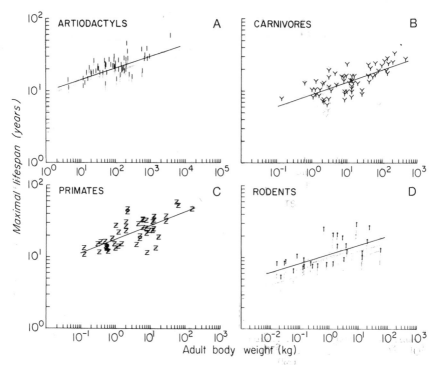

Fig. 3. Regression lines for maximal lifespan as a function of body weight calculated from reduced data sets (see text). Lines (a), (b), (c) and (d) correspond to maximal lifespan in artiodactyls, carnivores, primates and rodents, respectively. (See Table 3, rows 3,4,5,6.)

Discussion of Regression Analyses

Maximal and mean lifespan in mammals generally. The correlation coefficient (r) for maximal lifespan as a function of body weight, calculated for each of the five major RDS, varies from 0.641 to 0.774, meaning that body weight accounts for only 41 to 60% of the variance (r**2) in maximal lifespan in captive mammals (see Table 2, column 9, rows 2,4,5,6,7). This finding is consistent with the results obtained by Sacher (5) (see Table 8, row 2).

The slopes of the regression lines for maximal lifespan as a function of body weight vary from 0.116 to 0.174 (see Table 2, column 8, rows 1-9). The fact that the slope (0.127) for the regression of mean lifespan on body weight is in the same range (see Table 2, column 8, row 10) suggests that maximal and mean lifespan reflect rather similar aspects of the same underlying life-history behaviour (see also Fig. 4).

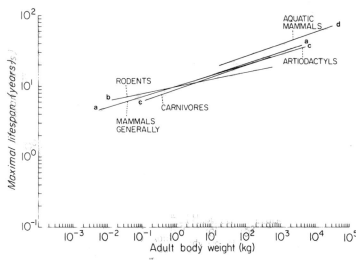

Fig. 4. Regression lines for maximal lifespan as a function of body weight calculated from reduced data sets. Lines (a), (b), (c), (d) and (e) correspond to maximal lifespan in mammals generally, and in rodents, carnivores, aquatic mammals and artiodactyls, respectively. (See text equation (6); Table 3, rows 6,4; Table 4, row 4, Table 3, row 3.)

Table 7. The number of species in the FDS and RDS and the weight range, arranged by source. The parenthetical value for the upper weight limit is for the RDS. (breakdown of Table 6 by source)

NUMBER OF SPECIES		WEIGHT RANGE	REFERENCE
FDS	RDS	Kg	
47	45	0.006 - 1000	14
128	79	0.02 - 250 (97.5)	23
132	119	0.0225 - 900	24
205	192	0.015 - 4850	25
66	59	0.0047 - 3000	26

63

Table 8. Regression characteristics for lifespan as determined in prior studies[a]

	Orders	Species	Points	pWR	W̄p	a	b ±se	r	+/-	Variate	Covariate	Comments	Ref.
	1	2	3	4	5	6	7	8	9	10	11	12	13
1	7	63	63	5.1	7.1	11.6	0.198 ±0.021	0.77	-	Body Weight	Maximal Lifespan	Mammals	[12]
2	12	239	239	-	-	10.4	0.172 ±0.010	0.739	-	Body Weight	Maximal Lifespan	Mammals	[5]
3	-	-	62	6.7	-	5.58	0.17	0.75	-	Body Weight	Mean Lifespan	Mammals	[9]
4	-	-	40	6.1	2.5	9.7	0.23 ±0.03	0.79	-	Body Weight	Maximal Lifespan	Mammals	[10]
5	6	48	48	4.2	20.2	10.1	0.155 ±0.022	0.718	20/28	Body Weight	Maximal Lifespan	Mammals (Recomputed)	[8]
6	11	170	170	5.6	7.9	10.4	0.172	0.792	-	Body Weight	Maximal Lifespan	Mammals	[7]
7	12	239	239	-	-	35.5	0.282 ±0.012	0.843	-	Brain Weight	Maximal Lifespan	Mammals	[5]
8	1	43	43	-	-	59.8	0.379 ±0.039	0.83	-	Brain Weight	Maximal Lifespan	Anthropoidea	[5]

	Orders	Species	Points	pWR	W̄p	a	b ± se	r	+/-	Variate	Covariate	Comments	Ref.
	1	2	3	4	5	6	7	8	9	10	11	12	13
9	–	40	40	4.3	0.7	23.3	0.24	0.780	17/23	Liver Weight	Maximal Lifespan	Mammals	[7]
10	–	40	40	4.4	0.004	91.7	0.27	0.81	21/19	Adrenal Weight	Maximal Lifespan	Mammals	[7]
11	1	28	28	2.2	0.048	19.4	0.077 ±0.063	0.234		Body Weight	Maximal Lifespan	Bats	[22]
12	1	34	34	2.5	23.7	10.0	0.193	0.598	14/20	Body Weight	Maximal Lifespan	Carnivores	[7]
13	1	39	39	3.5	3.3	15.7	0.236	0.836	19/21	Body Weight	Maximal Lifespan	Primates	[7]
14	1	27	27	3.2	0.5	8.8	0.252	0.846	12/15	Body Weight	Maximal Lifespan	Rodents	[7]
15	–	–	150	3.5	0.2	16.9	0.189 ±0.013	0.778	73/77	Body Weight	Maximal Lifespan	Wild birds* 1 point deleted	[31]

aSee legend, Table 2. Some of the data have been recovered from graphs and therefore the regression characteristics are not exact.

*Data recovered by digitization.

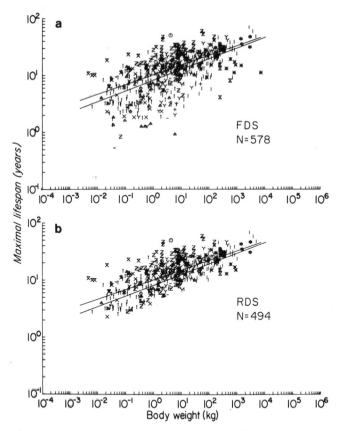

Fig. 5. Regression lines for maximal lifespan as a function of body
weight in mammals generally, using the full data set (FDS) and reduced
data set (RDS) derived from the five major aggregated data bases (see
Table 6, rows 1,2). The top panel is for the FDS and the lower panel
is for the RDS. The lower and upper solid lines are the best-fit
regression lines for the FDS and the RDS, respectively.

It is true that mean lifespan is generally considered to be an unreli-
able statistic. However in this large sample (n = 312), derived from
one source (23), the regression characteristic is not notably different
from those for maximal lifespan (e.g., compare row 10 with rows 3 and 6
of Table 2). This internal evidence suggests that the effects of
disease and variations in animal husbandry do not bias mean lifespan in
a way fundamentally different from maximum lifespan. At the same time
we recognize that data from an independent large sample would be of
value.

It is clear from Fig. 2 that of the five major maximal lifespan data
sets analyzed in Table 2, three have best-fit regression lines which lie
quite close to one another (see Table 2, rows 2,5,7). One data set (25)
has a smaller slope and lies everywhere above the other four regression
lines (see Table 2, row 6). Another data set (23) has a steeper slope
and lies entirely below the other four regression lines (see Table 2,
row 4). It seems reasonable to use the three regression lines which lie
close together as a basis for computing a global best-fit line for maximal lifespan as a function of body weight.

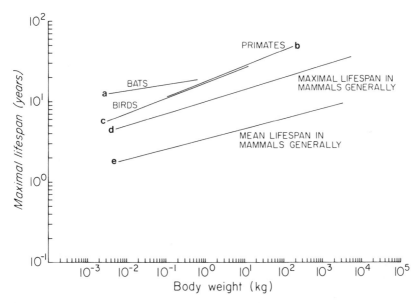

Fig. 6. Regression lines for mean and maximal lifespan as a function of body weight calculated from reduced data sets. Lines (a), (b), (c), (d) and (e) correspond respectively to maximal lifespan in bats, primates and birds, and maximal and mean lifespan in mammals generally. (See [Table 6, row 11]; Table 3, row 5; Table 6, row 15; text equation (6); and Table 2, row 10).

Our job is to compute mean values of the slope and intercept from the values obtained for the three (3) most congruent data sets. In order to allow for differences in the reliability of the values for slope and intercept, we computed six weighting factors, each equal to the inverse of the relevant standard error. A 'best' slope and intercept were then calculated from the weighted values for the three slopes and the logarithm of the three intercepts (e.g., see (55)). The result of this computation of the best-fit function for maximal lifespan (MLS) is:

$$MLS = 9.97*(x**0.15) \qquad (years) \qquad (6)$$

where 'x' is body weight in Kg.

By way of comparison, Sacher (5) obtained the values 10.4 and 0.172 for the intercept and exponent respectively (see Table 8, row 2). We have used equation (6) to compute the best fit regression line for maximal lifespan as shown in Figs. 4 and 5.

For comparative purposes we have also computed a 'best-fit' regression line by a different method. It might be supposed that the skewness in the data could be reduced by choosing an appropriate subset of the data. One reasonably objective way to accomplish this is to select out one single value of maximal lifespan for each family represented in a data set (there are about 130 families of mammals altogether (39)). Accordingly, we picked out the largest value of maximal lifespan for each family represented in the data of Jones (25,27) and computed the best-fit regression line (see Table 3, row 7).   It is curious that the mean percent deviation and the asymmetry in the distribution of data points are both still very high (see Table 3, row 7, columns 10,11). However, the slope (0.155) of the best-fit regression line calculated in this way is very close to the value (0.15) obtained above (see equation (6)), whereas the intercept (13.9) is significantly higher. For the aggregated data set (see Table 6, row 2) we find a slope of 0.170, very close to the value of 0.172 reported by Sacher (5) and somewhat above the values of 0.15 and 0.155 just obtained above by two different methods. At the same time the analysis of the grouped data (see Table 6, row 4) gave a slope of 0.168. It is a matter of conjecture which value is 'best'; present evidence is that the the slope of the best-fit regression line relating maximal lifespan to body weight in mammals generally has a slope of 0.15 - 0.17.

Maximal lifespan in male and female mammals. The slope and inter-cepts for the regressions lines for maximal lifespan as a function of body weight in male and female mammals are essentially the same (see Table 3, rows 1 and 2, columns 7 and 8). Snyder and Moore (13) reported a similar finding, drawing on a smaller sample. This result suggests that there are no systematic differences in maximal lifespan as between male and female mammals in a sample drawn from about 70 species and 10 orders. It may be, however, that in any given population a larger pro-portion of females than males actually achieve the maximal lifespan, but the data analyzed here do not speak to this point. Whether females have a greater maximal lifespan than males, or vice versa, within specific orders, can be reliably determined only by drawing on a larger data base than that analyzed here.

Maximal lifespan in aquatic mammals, artiodactyls, carnivores, and rodents. Fig. 4 shows that, by and large, captive rodents, artiodactyls and carnivores have similar maximal lifespans to those of captive mam-mals generally (see Table 3, rows 3, 4, and 6). Aquatic mammals in the wild have maximal lifespans at least as large as those for (captive) mammals generally (see Table 4, row 4). This inference is tempered by the very small sample size and by the fact that maximal lifespans in these species are estimates based on indirect criteria (e.g., ear-plug laminations or the state of the dental pulp).

The slopes for the regression lines of maximal lifespan on body weight in artiodactyls, carnivores, marsupials, primates and rodents as calculated from the aggregated data set (see Table 6, rows 5-14) are equal to or higher than those obtained from the individual data sets (see Table 3), but the differences are not statistically significant.

Western (8) has reported the results of maximal lifespan studies in artiodactyls, carnivores and primates and Economos (7) gives results for carnivores, rodents and ungulates (see Table 8, rows 12,13,14). All of the results reported here are based on larger sample sizes than those drawn on in these earlier studies.

Maximal lifespan in captive mammals as a function of organ weight. We find that brain weight accounts for only about 60% of the variance in lifespan, whereas Sacher (5) reports that brain weight accounts for some 70% of the variance (see Table 4, row 2; Table 6, row 7). In a substan-tially smaller sample, we see that about 75% of the variance in maximal lifespan in captive mammals is accounted for by variation in kidney weight (see Table 4, row 2).

Mean and maximal lifespan in captive mammals. Fig 5. shows that the slope of the regression line for mean lifespan is quite similar to the slope for the best-fit line for maximal lifespan (see Table 2, row 10) and equation (6) above). The slopes for the regression lines for mean and maximal lifespan are 0.185 ± 0.038 and 0.163 ± 0.022 in artiodactyls; 0.162 ± 0.031 and 0.170 ± 0.021 in carnivores; 0.188 ± 0.033 and 0.195 ± 0.029 in primates; 0.103 ± 0.025 and 0.127 ± 0.030 in rodents respectively (see Table 5, column 7 and Table 3, column 8). None of these slopes for mean and maximal lifespan within an order are significantly different.

The slope (0.127) of the regression line for mean lifespan as a function of body weight obtained here is lower than the value (0.17) obtained by Blueweiss et al. in a smaller sample (compare row 10, Table 2 with row 3, Table 6).

The ratio of maximal to mean lifespans, as estimated from the ratios of the intercepts, are 4.1, 2.7, 5.4 and 3.3 for artiodactyls, carnivores, primates and rodents, respectively.

Maximal lifespan in bats, birds and primates. On the basis of existing evidence, it is clear from Fig. 5 that bats (in the wild) are the longest lived mammals over their whole weight range (i.e., for body weights less than one kg)(see Table 6, row 11). Data for bats have often been excluded from lifespan studies on the grounds that these animals engage in torpor and hibernation. However, tropical bats, which, in general, neither enter torpor nor hibernate (22) are also very long-lived. Captive primates on average have shorter maximal lifespans than bats over their common weight range, but greater maximal lifespans than non-flying mammals of similar size.

Birds are shorter-lived on average than bats over their common weight range and have longevities similar to those of primates over their shared weight range. Apart from bats and primates, birds in the sample studied have greater maximal lifespans than mammals of similar size. Because of the large standard error (0.063), the slope of the bat line is not significantly different from the slopes for the other groups (see Table 6, row 11).

The reader who compares our plot of maximal lifespan in birds and mammals (Fig. 4) with the plot of Lindstedt and Calder (31) will note that their regression line for maximal lifespan in mammals is parallel and rather close to the bird line. Our regression for maximal lifespan in mammals generally is significantly lower than the bird line and has a noticeably smaller slope. There are two reasons for this discrepancy. First, these workers (31) use the value of 15.7 for the weight-coefficient in Sacher's equation (12) for maximal lifespan as a function of body weight. The correct value is 11.6, which is 26% lower (see Table 6, row 1 and Table 1 and Fig. 1 in the more recent paper by Lindstedt and Calder[45]). Second, like Economos[6,7], these authors draw on Sacher's earlier work rather than on his recent and more extensive studies. The slope Sacher obtained in his first study (12) of maximal lifespan as a function of body weight in 63 species of mammals was 0.198, but in his second study (5) of 239 species he obtained a slope of 0.172.

As an aside we recall that it has been argued (45) that lifespan can be expected to scale with body weight as do frequencies (e.g, heart rate), which in several cases seem to vary as about the negative one-quarter power of body weight. Several remarks are in order. First, our empirical results do not support any such contention. Maximal lifespan in captive mammals generally does not scale even approximately as the one-quarter power of body weight. Second, since maximal lifespan is by definition a single-valued quantity for any one species, the concept of frequency is inapplicable. Finally, the data bases on which the inverse one-quarter power rule for frequencies are based appear to have neglected the possible influence of activity cycles. The study of the scaling of biological frequencies with body weight would perhaps benefit from a critical re-examination of the data from this standpoint (46).

<u>Maximal lifespan in wild and captive mammals.</u> The regression line shown in Fig. 4 suggests that mammals in the wild, and more specifically aquatic mammals, may have maximal lifespans not very different from those expected for (captive) terrestrial mammals (see Table 4, rows 3,4). It is true, however, that the data base on which this inference is based is small and the lifespan evidence itself is circumstantial.

GENERAL DISCUSSION

The data base assembled here is quite heterogeneous. The data of Flower (14), summarized in Table 2 (rows 1,2), cover the widest weight range (column 4), have the smallest number of points deviating by more than 100% from the regression lines calculated for FDS (column 12) and show the highest correlation ceofficient (for the RDS). The Anonymous data set (Table 2, rows 3,4,,10) covers the largest number of species, exhibits the greatest mean percent deviation from the calculated regression line and shows the greatest asymmetry. The data of Crandall (24) have the smallest weight range of the five large (N > 150) data bases and show the least asymmetry (see Table 2, row 5). The data of Jones (25) cover the greatest number of orders but show the lowest correlation coefficient for maximal lifespan as calculated from a RDS (see Table 2,row 6, columns 1,9). The data set of Eisenberg (26) shows the greatest symmmetry of points about the regression line (see Table 2, row 7, column 11). We emphasize again that only two (i.e.,(14,23)) or possibly three (i.e., (14,23,25)) of the data sets are independent of one another. The remaining data sets overlap to an indeterminate degree.

It is interesting to find that significant numbers of the values for maximal lifespan deviate from the regression lines by more than 100%, and always fall below the lines. This finding may reflect an inherent dispersion in maximal lifespans in captive mammals at constant body weight. On average, bats, and over part of their weight range, primates and possibly aquatic mammals, have substantially greater lifespans than other mammals of similar body weight. But when we delete the lifespan data for these three groups from the data set of Crandall (24) we find that the mean percent deviation is essentially unaffected, and the asymmetric distribution of points actually worsens (compare rows 5 and 9, Table 2). Thus, the asymmetric distribution does not seem to be attributable simply to inter-group variation. On the other hand, the mean percent deviations from the regression lines for individual orders are mostly smaller than the deviations for the mammalian lines generally, and the asymmetry smaller, suggesting that intergroup variation may make some contribution to the global asymmetry (compare columns 10,11 in Table 3 with those in Table 4).

We think it more plausible, in the absence of other evidence, to assume that the asymmetric distribution of data points results chiefly from some species thriving very much better in captivity than others. The typically high, but very variable values for infant mortality in zoos seems to point in this direction (Anonymous (23)). Since survivorship curves are skewed to the right, the probability of reporting a low value of maximal lifespan is greater than that of reporting a high value. Whatever the correct interpretation our findings mean that there is a systematic skewness in the maximal lifespan data which thus far has gone unreported. However, this skewness apparently has only a rather small effect on the intercept and slope of the regression lines (see Fig. 1 and compare rows 1 and 2, and rows 3 and 4 in Table 2 and rows 1 and 2 in Table 6).

Parenthetically, we observe that because of the low correlation coefficients, the slopes and intercepts which we find would change if we adopted an analytical method other than regression analysis (e.g., reduced major axis analysis). However, there is no reason to anticipate that the inter-relationships among the various regression lines would be significantly altered by doing the calculations in another way. We are chiefly interested in the pattern of relationships among different orders of mammals, and in the best-fit line for mammals generally. Gender does not seem to introduce a systematic bias into the data, a finding in keeping with our earlier studies of organ scaling in mammals (42,43,44) and with a mammalian lifespan study of Snyder and Moore (13).

It is perhaps surprising, but also reassuring, to find that maximal lifespan seems to reflect the same underlying phenomenon as mean lifespan. There is considerable skepticism as to whether mean lifespan is a meaningful statistic, due to the possibly capricious effects of disease and animal husbandry. Based solely on the regression characteristics, we do not see compelling grounds for regarding mean lifespan as fundamentally different from maximal lifespan. To a rough approximation, our results suggest that maximal lifespan in captive mammals is simply a multiple of mean lifespan. A reasonable inference is that maximal lifespan measures a fundamental life-history characteristic of a species and not just the aberrant characteristics of a few resilient members of a species, as has sometimes been suggested. The relationship between mean and maximal lifespan is one worthy of further study.

Synder and Moore (13) put forward the conjecture that maximal lifespan in wild mammals may not be very dissimilar to that found in captive mammals. Our findings, in a small sample dominated by aquatic species (for which values of maximal lifespan in captivity are unknown), seem to support this (see Table 4, rows 3,4).

One of the motivations for undertaking this study was to re-examine the question of the dependence of maximal lifespan on organ weight. Unlike Sacher (5,12), we do not find empirically that brain weight necessarily accounts for significantly more of the variance than does body weight (compare row 1, column 9, Table 4 with row 2, Table 2). Moreover, as Economos (6,7) has already emphasized, there is nothing special about brain weight as a variate. Kidney, liver or adrenal weights explain as much of the variance as brain or body weight (compare Table 4, row 2, and Table 8, rows 9,10 with Table 2, rows 1 - 9). In general, there is little theoretical reason to expect that organ weight will explain more of the variance in maximal lifespan than body weight.

CONCLUSIONS

Many species of bats and primates have a substantially longer lifespan than other mammals of comparable body size. In the case of bats this positive difference in maximal lifespan is not explicable in terms of greater brain weight (22). Birds have maximal lifespans akin to those of primates of similar size, but less than those of like-sized bats. By-and-large, birds are longer lived than mammals of comparable size. Again, this difference in maximal lifespan is not generally explicable in terms of greater brain size. Birds weighing more than 100 grams have smaller brains, on average, than mammals of comparable size (50). (The size of birds ranges from about 2 g for the Bee hummingbird to less than 200 kg for ostriches, giving a pWR of about 5 (51). Thus, approximately 60% of the avian size range, on a logarithmic scale, is above 100 grams). Brain size may be an important determinant of maximal lifespan, but neither the scaling data nor the supporting arguments have made a convincing case for it.

A plausible conjecture is that maximal lifespan in all species reflects a cellular function (e.g., one mediated by repair systems). The genetic substrate for "longevity-assurance" would presumably be distributed throughout all the cells of any organ, with the degree of expression no doubt varying from tissue to tissue and from species to species. But if the amount of cellular substrate actually expressed varies quantitatively with lifespan, on average, as seems reasonable, then a component of the variance in lifespan would automatically be associated with variance in body weight. But many factors, such as reproductive strategy, stability of food supply, and predator pressure may influence the selection of a particular value for mean or maximal lifespan in any given species. We see no reason at present to expect that these broadly ecological influences will have any significant coupling to body weight. (The fact that body weight accounts for only about 50% of the variance in maximal lifespan seems to point in this direction). There is the likelihood that many factors apparently correlated with maximal lifespan merely reflect joint correlations with body weight and have little, if anything, to do with aging per se. Thus factors well correlated with maximal life span but poorly correlated with body weight may be especially attractive for further investigation. The influence of such body-weight independent "longevity-assurance" factors may be mediated chiefly by subtle systemic changes in the neuroendocrine system (53,54).

ACKNOWLEDGEMENTS

We thank Dr. G. Martin for his constructive comments on a draft of this paper, and Ms. Doris Ringer for preparation of the manuscript. We are grateful to Mr. T. J. Hsiao for assistance with a portion of the data processing.

This work was supported in part by USPHS Grant No. 2 PO1 AG-01751 from the National Institutes of Health to Dr. George M. Martin.

REFERENCES

1. K. Y. Hall, R. W. Hart, A. K. Benirschke and R. L. Walford, Correlation between ultraviolet-induced DNA repair in primate lymphocytes and fibroblasts and species maximum achievable life span. Mech. Ageing Dev. 24 (1984) 163 - 173.
2. L. L. Pashko, and A. G. Schwartz, Inverse correlation between species life span and specific cytochrome P-448 content of cultured fibroblasts. J. Gerontolgy 37 (1982) 38-41
3. J. M. Tolmasoff, T. Ono, and R. G. Cutler, Superoxide dismutase: correlation with life-span and specific metabolic rate in primate species. P.N.A.S. 77 (1980) 2777-2781.
4. D. Rohme, Evidence for a relationship between longevity of mammalian species and life spans of normal fibroblasts in vitro and erythrocytes in vivo. P.N.A.S. 78 (1981) 5009-5013.
5. G. A. Sacher, Maturation and longevity in relation to cranial capacity in hominid evolution. R.H. Tuttle (ed.), Primate Functional

Morphology and Evolution. Mouton, The Hague, 1975.

6. A. C. Economos, Brain-life span conjecture: a reevaluation of the evidence. _Gerontology_ 26(1980) 82-89.
7. A. C. Economos, Taxonomic differences in the mammalian life span-body weight relationship and the problem of brain weight. _Gerontolgy_ 26 (1980) 90-98.
8. D. Western, Size, life history and ecology in mammals. _Afr. J. Ecol._ 17 (1979) 185-204.
9. L. Blueweiss, H. Fox, V. Kudzma, D. Nakashima, R. Peters, and S. Sams, Relationships between body size and some life history parameters. _Oecologia (Berl.)_ 37 (1978) 257 - 272.
10. M. J. Boddington, An absolute metabolic scope for activity. _J. theor. Biol._ 75 (1978) 443 - 449.
11. M. Rockstein, J. A. Chesky, M. L. Sussman, Comparative biology and evolution of aging. C. E. Finch, L. Hayflick (eds.) _Handbook of the Biology of Aging._ Van Nostrand Reinhold, New York, 1977.
12. G.A. Sacher, Relation of lifespan to brain weight and body weight in mammals. G. A. W. Wolstenholme and M. O'Connor (eds.) _Ciba Foundation Colloquia on Ageing._ Vol 5. _The Lifespan of Animals._ Churchill, London, 1959.
13. R. L. Snyder and S. C. Moore, Longevity of captive mammals in Philadelphia Zoo. _International Zoo Yearbook._ 8 (1968) 175-182.
14. S.S. Flower, Contributions to our knowledge of the duration of life in vertebrate animals. V. Mammals. _Proc. Zool Soc. Lond._ (1931) 145-234.
15. M.A. Hofman, On the presumed coevolution of brain size and longevity in hominids. _J. Human Evol._ 13 (1984) 371-376.
16. M. A. Hofman, Energy metabolism, brain size and longevity in mammals. _Quart. Rev. Biol._ 58 (1983) 495-512.
17. R. G. Cutler, Evolutionary biology of aging and longevity in mammalian species. J. E. Johnson, Jr. (ed.) _Aging and Cell Function._ Plenum Press, New York, 1984.
18. D. Western and J. Ssemakula, Life history patterns in birds and mammals and their evolutionary interpretation. _Oecologia (Berl.)_ 54 (1982) 281-290.
19. G. A. Sacher, Longevity and aging in vertebrate evolution. _Bioscience_ 28 (1978) 497-501.
20. R. S. Mallouk, Longevity in vertebrates is proportional to relative brain weight. _Fed. Proc._ 34 (1975) 2102-2103.
21. H. Zepelin and A. Rechtschaffen, Mammalian sleep, longevity and energy metabolism. _Brain Behav. Evol._ 10 (1974) 425-470.
22. K.D. Jürgens and J. Prothero, Scaling of maximal lifespan in mammals. Bats. (In Preparation)
23. Anonymous, Longevity Survey: length of life of mammals in captivity at the London Zoo and Whipsnade Park. _International Zoo Yearbook_ 11 (1960) 288-299.
24. L. S. Crandall, _The Management of Wild Mammals in Captivty._ University of Chicago Press. Chicago. 1964.
25. M. L. Jones, Longevity of mammals in captivity. _International Zoo News._ Apr/May (1979) 16-26.
26. J. F. Eisenberg, _The Mammalian Radiations: An Analysis of Trends in Evolution, Adaptation and Behavior._ University of Chicago Press. Chicago. 1981.
27. M.L. Jones, Longevity of captive mammals. _Zool. Garten N. F. Jena_ 52 (1982) 113-128.
28. J. Rearden (ed.) Alaska Mammals. _Alaska Geographic_ 8 (1981).
29. S. Ohsumi, Examination of age determination of the fin whale. _Sci. Rep. Whales Res.Inst., Tokyo_ No. 18 (1964) 49-88.
30. D. E. Sergeant, The biology of the pilot or pothead whale _Globicephala melaena_ (Traill) in Newfoundland waters. _Bull. Fisheries Res. Board Can._ No.132 (1962).

31. S. L. Lindstedt and W. A. Calder, Body size and longevity in birds. Condor 78 (1976) 91-145.

32. J. Mannard, A. Lindsay, J. Sundsten and J. Prothero, A plotted-to-tabular data conversion program for microcomputers. Int. J. Bio-Medical Computing 13 (1982) 369-373.

33. R. M. Nowak and J. L. Paradiso, Walker's Mammals of the World, 4th ed., Vols. I and II, John Hopkins University Press, Baltimore, 1983.

34. L. Boitani and S. Bartoli, Simon and Schuster's Guide to Mammals. Simon and Schuster. New York. 1982.

35. J. Dorst and P. Dandelot, A Field Guide to the Larger Mammals of Africa. Collins. London. 1980.

36. J. O. Whitaker, Jr., The Audubon Society Field Guide to North American Mammals. Alfred A. Knopf. New York. 1980.

37. G. Crile and D. P. Quiring, A record of the body weight and certain organ and gland weights of 3690 animals. Ohio J. Sci. 40 (1940) 219-259.

38. R. D. Martin, Department of Anthropology, University College, London. (personal communication).

39. G. B. Corbet and J. E. Hill, A World List of Mammalian Species. British Museum of Natural History, Comstock Publ., London, 1980.

40. J. H. Honacki, K. E. Kinman and J.W. Koeppl (eds.). Mammal Species of the World: a Taxonomic and Geographic Reference. Allen Press, Lawrence, KA, 1982.

41. A. L. Edwards, An introduction to Linear Regression and Correlation. W. H. Freeman. San Francisco. 1976.

42. J. Prothero, Organ scaling in mammals: the kidneys. Comp. Biochem. Physiol. 77A (1984) 133-138.

43. J. W. Prothero, Organ scaling in mammals: the liver. Comp. Biochem. Physiol. 71A (1982) 567-577.

44. J. Prothero, Heart Weight as a function of body weight in mammals. Growth 43 (1979) 139-150.

45. S. L. Lindstedt and W. A. Calder,III, Body size, physiological time and longevity of homeothermic animals. Quart. Rev. Biol. 56 (1981) 1-16.

46. J. Prothero, Scaling of standard energy metabolism in mammals: I. Neglect of circadian rhythms. J. theor. Biol. 106 (1984) 1-8.

47. R. D. Martin and P.H. Harvey, Brain size allometry: ontogeny and phylogeny. W. L. Jungers (ed.) Size and Scaling in Primate Biology. Plenum Press. New York. 1985.

48. G. A. Sacher, On longevity regarded as an organized behavior: the role of brain structure. R. Kastenbaum (ed.) Contributions to the Psychobiology of Aging. Springer. New York. 1965.

49. G. A. Sacher and E. F. Staffeldt, Relation of gestation time to brain weight for placental mammals: implications for the theory of vertebrate growth. Am. Naturalist 108 (1974) 593-615.

50. R. D. Martin, Relative brain size and basal metabolic rate in terrestrial vertebrates. Nature 293 (1981) 57-60.

51. G. L. Wood, Animal Facts and Feats. Sterling. New York. 1979.

52. G. C. Williams, Pleiotropy, natural selection, and the evolution of senescence. Evolution 11 (1957) 398-411.

53. G. A. Sacher, Evolutionary theory in gerontology. Perspectives Biol. Med. 25 (1982) 339-353.

54. C. E. Finch, The regulation of physiological changes during mammalian aging. Quart. Rev. Biol. 51 (1976) 49-83.

55. R. R. Sokal and F. J. Rohlf Biometry: The Principles and Practice of Statistics in Biological Research. 2nd ed., W. H. Freeman, New York, 1981.

WHY SHOULD SENESCENCE EVOLVE?

AN ANSWER BASED ON A SIMPLE DEMOGRAPHIC MODEL

Henry R. Hirsch

Department of Physiology and Biophysics
University of Kentucky
Lexington, KY

INTRODUCTION

Why age? Many single-celled organisms do not undergo either individual or clonal senescence. Moreover there are multicellular organisms which show no aging because lost cells, subcellular organelles, and smaller constituents are continually replaced. It would appear that evolution has simultaneously progressed in two divergent directions. On the one hand, highly evolved species tend, in general, to live longer than primitive ones. On the other hand, most higher forms, at least in the animal kingdom, exhibit aging. Other things being equal, it is clear that long life confers selective advantage on a species. It is much less obvious that aging does so.

According to an old saying, nothing is certain but death and taxes. The omission of senescence from this brief list reflects well upon the wisdom of the author of the maxim. Since thermal noise is ubiquitous, all patterns and structures are subject to eventual destruction, as are the plans and templates from which such structures can be repaired. Death appears to be the inevitable end of all life. However there is no law, thermodynamic or otherwise, which requires senescence to be universal.

Almost 100 years ago, August Weismann (1889) speculated on the causes of "normal death - senility so-called," i.e. what we now call "senescence." Weismann considered that such death "is not a primary necessity but that it has been acquired secondarily as an adaptation." He believed that "life is endowed with a fixed duration, not because it is contrary to its nature to be unlimited but because the unlimited existence of individuals would be a luxury without any corresponding advantage." Essentially the same view will be adopted in the present study, although no recourse will be made to the position that senescence has adaptive value. A very simple demographic model will be used to show that a hypothetical population displaying senescence can have selective advantage over one which is subject only to random accidental death. Thus it is possible that senescent organisms evolved from more primitive ancestors which did not age. The distinction between the evolution of senescence and the evolution of longevity will be emphasized.

The demographic model which will be investigated here was originally proposed in a more picturesque form by Medawar (1952). He considered a population of 1000 glass test tubes in use in a laboratory. Ten percent, or 100, were broken by accident each month, and these were regularly replaced. Once the population had achieved a stable distribution, there were 100 test tubes aged 0–1 month, 90 aged 1–2 months, 81 aged 2–3 months, and so on. There were very few that were very old. Medawar introduced senescence into this population by specifying that, after a certain age, as a result of some intrinsic shortcoming, the test tubes would suddenly fall to pieces. He argued that this disintegration would, if it occurred at a sufficiently great age, have little effect on the population as a whole because so few old test tubes would remain to be affected. Moreover, the disaster which would befall a small number of old individuals could be compensated by giving a small advantage, such as a modest percentage increase in the replacement rate, to the large number of young individuals in the population.

Williams (1957) placed Medawar's model in a more specifically genetic context. He assumed that senescence is an unfavorable character and that its development is opposed by selection. However he accepted Medawar's postulate that senescence might evolve as a result of processes that are favorable in early life but have cumulative bad effects later on. He presented evidence and arguments to show that these processes are mediated by the action of pleiotropic genes which are responsible for vigor in youth at the price of vigor at more advanced ages.

A footnote in Medawar's (1952) essay suggests that he investigated some of the mathematically accessible consequences of his "sudden-death" test-tube model. Unfortunately, as Wallace (1967) pointed out, none of this work has been reported. Wallace himself presented equations which describe several special cases of a demographic model in which senescence is compensated by an early advantage to the population. However Wallace did not employ a criterion by which a given degree of senescence may be balanced or "titrated" against a particular level of early improvement in the life history of an organism. Therefore the results of his calculations reflect changes in the longevity of the model population as well as changes in its degree of senescence.

This difficulty was circumvented in two later papers (Hirsch, 1980; Hirsch, 1982) by adjusting the parameters of the longevity function or survival curve such that its mean value is maintained constant for all degrees of senescence. The same method will be used here and will be supplemented by calculations in which the survival-curve parameters are adjusted to achieve constancy of the average age at death rather than constancy of the mean longevity.

Gompertzian and other qualitatively equivalent survival functions were employed by Hirsch (1980, 1982) to calculate the rate of natural increase of various model populations. In all cases in which biologically reasonable parameter values were chosen, there was a net selective advantage associated with the introduction of senescence, appropriately titrated against youthful survival, relative to a population in which the death rate was independent of age.

In the present work, the survival curve takes the exact form proposed by Medawar (1952). Senescence is represented by sudden death at a particular age. At that age, the death rate, previously constant, reaches an infinitely high peak, and the survival curve, previously a

declining exponential, drops vertically to zero. This survival function is not as good an approximation to longevity data in natural populations as the Gompertizian and other curves employed earlier (Hirsch,
1980; Hirsch, 1982). However it is more convenient to use when the
effects of senescence must be distinguished from those of longevity,
and it is of historic interest in view of the continuing influence of
Medawar's (1952) essay. Furthermore, the sudden-death model has the
important didactic advantage that the equations which describe it can
be solved straightforwardly by elementary mathematical methods rather
than with the use of Laplace transform techniques and machine
computation.

The research reported here consists of a more detailed
quantitative exploration of Medawar's (1952) ideas. The evolutionary
advantage of a population is evaluated by calculating its rate of
natural increase. Other parameters of interest, such as the
reproductive fraction, the generation time, the mean longevity, and the
average age at death are also obtained. Senescent populations are
compared to a nonsenescent reference population in which death takes
place only as a result of randomly occurring accidents. Results show
that a reduction in mortality at a early age can compensate for the
sudden death of the whole population at an advanced age because so few
individuals in the nonsenscent population survive to reproduce in old
age.

METHODS

Various hypothetical senescent and nonsenescent populations will
be compared below in order to examine the consequences of sudden-death
senescence. Numerical values of the rate of natural increase and of
other quantities which describe these populations will be obtained.
It is convenient for these purposes to express the following postulates
and results in analytic form:

Maternity Function

The demographic model presented here is completely characterized
by a birth-rate or maternity function and a survival or longevity function. It is assumed that the life history of each population which is
described is reflected in the mathematical properties of these two functions.

The maternity function, $m(t)$, represents the probability per unit
age interval that an organism reproduces between ages t and $(t + dt)$.
Constant and exponentially increasing and decreasing maternity functions were treated by Hirsch (1980), and a quasi-human function was
also examined (Hirsch, 1980). Here attention will be restricted to the
constant maternity function

$$m(t) = m, \tag{1}$$

where m is constant.

In addition to mathematical simplicity, this choice has the virtue
that it focuses attention on the survival curve. With the use of the
constant maternity function, it becomes completely clear that any
influence of senescence upon selective advantage is entirely independent of the timing of reproduction.

In much of what follows, the value of the constant m will be set equal to one. This is the same as choosing the unit of time to be the inverse of the rate of reproduction. For example, if the organism is a cell which divides daily, the time unit is one day.

Longevity Function

The longevity or survival function represents the probability that an organism survives to and dies at age t. The general form of the longevity function describing sudden-death senescence is

$$l(t) = e^{-\mu_0 t}, \quad t \leq T,$$

$$= 0, \quad t > T, \tag{2}$$

where μ_0 is the presenescent death rate and T is the time of senescence, that is, the time at which sudden death occurs. Both μ_0 and T are positive constants.

By definition, the age-specific death rate is

$$\mu(t) = -\frac{1}{l(t)} \frac{dl(t)}{dt}. \tag{3}$$

With the use of eqns. (2),

$$\mu(t) = \mu_0 + u_0(t - T), \quad t \leq T,$$

$$= 0, \quad t > T, \tag{4}$$

where $u_0(t - T)$ is a unit impulse function, i.e., a pulse or "spike" of unit area that is infinitely high but infinitesimally narrow. The unit impulse function is mathematically equivalent to the Dirac delta function.

As illustrated in Fig. 1(a), the longevity function falls exponentially from unity at the rate μ_0 until the time of senescence, T. At time T, sudden death strikes those organisms which remain alive. In terms of Medawar's example, the test tubes spontaneously disintegrate. The longevity function drops to zero. The death-rate function, Fig. 1(b), shows the same thing in a different way. The death rate remains constant until an instant at time T when it becomes infinite, reflecting the complete annihilation of the population.

A nonaging population, i.e., one for which $T \to \infty$, may be treated as a special case of eqns. (2) and (4). Since the unit impulse function in eqn. (4) occurs at infinite age, it operates on a population of zero size, has no effect, and may, in the absence of senescence, be omitted.

Rate of Natural Increase

The rate of natural increase, r, is used here as the measure of selective advantage. The value of r is the rate at which a population increases when it is growing exponentially and its age distribution is stable. The use of r selection to represent selective advantage is reasonable but is by no means mandatory. Medawar himself (1952) preferred Fisher's (1958) reproductive value. However Hamilton (1966) and Charlesworth (1980) argued against this choice and in favor of the rate of natural increase or its derivative with respect to age-specific survival.

Kirkwood (1981) discussed the merits of r selection relative to K selection. In K selection, the carrying capacity or equilibrium population size, K, is maximized for species under intense competition in stable environments. Kirkwood elected to use r selection and to represent the effects of competition implicity by their influence on birth and death rates. The same approach was adopted by Hirsch (1980, 1982) and will be used here.

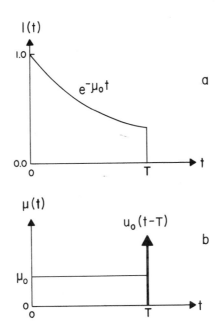

Fig. 1 (a) Longevity function, $l(t)$, and (b) death rate, $\mu(t)$, as functions of age, t. Sudden death, represented by a vertical drop in $l(t)$ and by a unit impulse, $u_0(t-T)$ in $\mu(t)$, occurs at time T. Prior to T, the death rate has the constant value μ_0.

The rate of natural increase can be calcuated with the use of the well established characteristic equation

$$\int_0^\infty e^{-st}l(t)m(t)dt = 1 .$$ (5)

Values of s for which eqn. (5) is valid are called its solutions or roots. The largest real root is r, the rate of natural increase. A modern derivation of eqn. (5) together with a brief description of its history has been presented by Hirsch (1980).

With the substitutions of eqn. (1) to represent the maternity function and eqns. (2) to represent the longevity function, integration of the characteristic equation (5) yields

$$\frac{m}{s'}\left[1 - e^{-s'T}\right] = 1 , \tag{6}$$

where

$$s' = s + \mu_0 . \tag{7.1}$$

Note that the upper limit of integration in eqn. (5) becomes T, since $l(t) = 0$ when $t > T$.

After the maternity rate, m, and the time of senescence, T, have been specified, eqn. (6) can be solved numerically for s'. Fortunately the solution of eqn. (6) and all of the other numerical calculations described here can be handled conveniently on an inexpensive pocket calculator which has a 32-step or larger key program.

Once eqn. (6) has been solved for s', the rate of natural increase, r, is immediately obtainable for any value of the presenescent death rate, μ_0. From eqn. (7.1), since $r = s$,

$$r = s' - \mu_0 . \tag{7.2}$$

An increment in the presenescent death rate is reflected in an exactly equal decrement in the rate of natural increase of the population.

Reproductive Fraction

The reproductive fraction, R, (sometimes called the net reproductive rate) is defined as the number of offspring per parent. If the function on the left-hand side of eqn. (5) is designated F(s),

$$R = \lim_{s \to 0} F(s) \tag{8.1}$$

$$= \int_0^\infty l(t)m(t)dt . \tag{8.2}$$

With the help of eqns. (1) and (2),

$$R = \frac{m}{\mu_0}\left[1 - e^{-\mu_0 T}\right]. \tag{9}$$

Generation Time

The generation time, T_g, is defined by the relation

$$R = e^{rT_g} , \tag{10}$$

or, solving for T_g,

$$T_g = \frac{\ln R}{r} \tag{11}$$

Mean Longevity

The mean of the longevity function, $\bar{t}$, is the average age of the living organisms. It is calculated from the definition of the mean in the usual way:

$$\bar{t} = \frac{\int_0^\infty t l(t)dt}{\int_0^\infty l(t)dt} .$$

(12)

The result of performing the indicated integrations with the use of eqns. (2) is

$$\bar{t} = \frac{1}{\mu_0}\left[1 - \frac{\mu_0 T}{e^{\mu_0 T} - 1}\right].$$

(13)

Average Age at Death

A general formula for the average age of an organism at death is

$$\bar{t}_d = \frac{\int_0^\infty t\mu(t)l(t)dt}{\int_0^\infty \mu(t)l(t)dt} .$$

(14)

Given the longevity and death-rate functions specified in eqns. (2) and (4) respectively,

$$\bar{t}_d = \frac{1}{\mu_0}\left[1 - e^{-\mu_0 T}\right].$$

(15)

Eqns. (14) and (15) are derived in the appendix.

Comparison of eqns. (9) and (15) reveals a simple relation between the reproductive fraction and the average age at death:

$$R = m\bar{t}_d .$$

(16)

RESULTS: EFFECTS OF SENESCENCE

The hypothetical populations which will be presented in order to assess the effects of senescence are special cases of the demographic model described by the equations which appear in the preceding section. The populations are characterized by the values of the parameters μ_0 and T, which appear in the longevity function.

Case 1: A Nonsenescent Reference Population

In the absence of sudden-death senescence, $T \to \infty$, and eqn. (6) reduces to $s' = m$. From eqn. (7.2), $r = m - \mu_0$; the rate of natural increase is equal to the difference between the birth rate and the death rate.

The value of m, in the interest of convenience, will be set equal to one for the nonsenescent population and for each of the senescent populations to be treated below. In the nonsenescent population the value of μ_0 will also be set equal to one so that the rate of natural increase is zero.

The nonsenescent population so specified will serve as a reference against which senescent populations can be compared. Populations to which senescence brings selective advantage will have positive r values; populations to which senescence is a disadvantage will have negative r values.

Case 2: Senescent Populations Having the Same Presenescent Death Rate as the Reference Population

Values of the rate of natural increase and other variables of interest are shown in Table 1 for the nonsenescent reference population (last row) and for senescent populations having the same presenescent death rate as the reference population. The rates of natural increase are also displayed in Fig. 2 to facilitate comparison with r-value results which will be obtained for other populations.

As Williams (1957) noted, senescence is an unfavorable character; if T is finite, the values of r which appear in Table 1 are negative. However the essence of Medawar's (1952) argument is borne out. The r values differ very little from zero if $T > 4$. Senescence has little effect on selective advantage if it is sufficiently delayed. The rate of natural increase becomes markedly negative only if sudden death takes place at an early age.

The decline in the rate of natural increase which accompanies sudden-death senescence is the result, in part, of a reduction in the reproductive fraction, R, and, in part of a shortening of the generation time, T_g. Inspection of eqn. (11) shows that smaller values of T_g are associated with larger values of r if $R > 1$ and $r > 0$, but result in more negative values of r if $R < 1$ and $r < 0$. If a population is expanding, faster turnover causes faster growth, but, by the same token, if it is declining, faster turnover hastens its demise.

It should be noted that the effect of sudden death upon the rate of natural increase in these populations cannot be attributed solely to senescence. A reduction in the value of T is associated with corresponding reductions in the average age at death, $\bar{t}_d$, and the mean longevity, $\bar{t}$. Thus the introduction of sudden death in the nonsenescent reference population has two effects: (1) It causes senescence by producing a dramatic increase in the death rate at time T, and (2) it reduces longevity by eliminating the oldest part of the population. Both of these effects contribute to the selective disadvantage associated with sudden death.

Case 3: Senescent Populations in which there is No Presenescent Death

The question arises as to what extent early selective advantage can compensate for the disadvantage of sudden death. If early advantage is to be represented by a change in the longevity function, the maximum advantage is secured by reducing the presenescent death rate, μ_0, to zero. The longevity function is then of the rectangular form associated with a maximally senescent organism.

Table 1. Cases 1 and 2: Values of Variables Describing Populations for which the Presenescent Death Rate Has the Value 1.

T: time at which sudden death occurs
r: rate of natural increase
Tg: generation time
R: reproductive fraction
$\bar{t}_d$: average age at death
$\bar{t}$: mean longevity

T	r	Tg	R = $\bar{t}_d$	$\bar{t}$
.5	−3.51	.266	.393	.229
.693	−2.00	.347	.500	.307
.75	−1.73	.369	.528	.329
1.00	−1.00	.459	.632	.418
1.20	−0.686	.522	.699	.483
1.50	−0.417	.605	.777	.569
2.0	−0.203	.716	.856	.687
3.0	−0.059	.858	.950	.843
4.0	−0.020	.932	.982	.925
5.0	−0.007	.968	.993	.966
∞	0.0	1.000	1.000	1.000

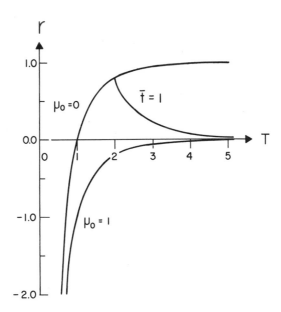

Fig. 2 Rate of natural increase, r, as a function of time of senescence, T, under the indicated conditions. In the nonsenescent population or if $\bar{t}_d$ = 1, r = 0. μ_0: presenescent death rate. $\bar{t}$: mean longevity, $\bar{t}_d$ average age at death.

Table 2. Case 3: Values of Variables Describing Populations for which the Presenescent Death Rate is Zero. Symbols are defined in the caption to Table 1.

T	r	T_g	$R = \bar{t}_d$	$\bar{t}$
.5	−2.51	.276	.5	.25
.693	−1.00	.367	.693	.347
.75	−0.73	.392	.75	.375
1.00	0.00	.500	1.00	.500
1.20	0.314	.581	1.20	.600
1.50	0.583	.696	1.50	.750
2.0	0.797	.870	2.00	1.000
2.412	0.880	1.000	2.412	1.206
3.0	0.940	1.167	3.00	1.500
4.0	0.980	1.414	4.00	2.000
5.0	0.993	1.621	5.00	2.500

As shown in Table 2 and in Fig. 2, rates of natural increase for populations in which $\mu_0 = 0$ are greater by one unit than the corresponding values given in Table 1 for populations in which $\mu_0 = 1$. Thus $r > 0$ for $T > 1$. The action of a pleiotropic gene which would eliminate death until age T in exchange for certain death at age T would lead to selective advantage if $T > 1$.

This improvement is largely due to an increase in the reproductive fraction. In the range $2.412 > T > 1.0$, a reduction in the generation time relative to that of the reference population also contributes to the improvement in the rate of natural increase. For $T > 2.412$, an increase in generation time above that of the reference population partially offsets the effect of the increase in the reproductive fraction.

Here, as in case 2, it is impossible to distinguish the influence of senescence from that of longevity upon changes in the rates of natural increase. Rectangularizing the survival curve by lowering the presenescent death rate to zero produces a greater degree of senescence in case 3 than in cases 1 and 2. However the lower death rate, which leads to greater selective advantage, is also associated with values of the average age at death and of the mean longevity which are greater than in case 2.

Case 4: Senescent Populations Having the Same Mean Longevity as the Reference Population

The mean of the longevity function which describes the survival of a population is equal to the mean age of a living individual in the population. By appropriate adjustment or "titration" of the presenescent death rate, it is possible to specify senescent populations which differ in the time at which sudden death takes place but which have the same mean longevity as the reference population. This is accomplished by setting $\bar{t} = 1$ in eqn. (13) and solving numerically to obtain μ_0 for any desired value of T.

The results, which appear in Table 3, show that, as senescence occurs at progressively earlier ages, the presenescent death rate must

Table 3.   Cases 1 and 4: Values of Variables
            Describing Populations for which the Mean
            Longevity Has the Value 1.

μ_0: Presenescent death rate
Other symbols are defined in the caption to
Table 1.

T	μ_0	r	Tg	$R = \bar{t}_d$
2.0	0.000	.797	.870	2.000
2.2	.249	.595	.886	1.694
2.4	.424	.455	.901	1.506
2.6	.550	.354	.914	1.383
2.8	.645	.280	.925	1.296
3.0	.716	.224	.935	1.233
3.5	.833	.133	.955	1.135
4.0	.898	.081	.969	1.083
4.5	.936	.051	.979	1.051
5.0	.960	.032	.985	1.032
∞	1.00	0.00	1.00	1.00

be correspondingly reduced to maintain the value of the mean longevity
equal to one age unit. When T = 2, the presenescent death rate is
zero, and the longevity function is rectangular. No further reduction
in T is possible.

The lower the age at which sudden death occurs, the greater the
rate of natural increase, and the more nearly rectangular the survival
curve becomes. This improvement is due to a substantial increase in
the reproductive fraction and to an accompanying modest decrease in the
generation time.

The improvement in the rate of natural increase cannot be attributed to a gain in longevity, since the mean longevity is the same for
all populations considered, that is, for sudden death at any age
greater than 2. Thus the same result that was demonstrated earlier
(Hirsch, 1980; Hirsch, 1982) is also obtained here: Senescence leads
to selective advantage if titrated against an improvement in the
presenescent death rate in such a way that there is no effect on the
mean longevity. Moreover, the greater the degree of senescence, the
greater the advantage.

Case 5: Senescent Populations Having the Same Average Age at Death as the Reference Population

The mean of the longevity function measures the average age of a
living organism. In the reference population, the mean longevity is
the same as the average age at death. Both have the value 1. However
it is evident that this coincidence is not general. For example, in
the case of a rectangular survival curve describing sudden death at age
2, the average age at death is also 2, but the mean longevity is 1.

This difference suggests that it would be worthwhile to titrate
the presenescent death rate against the age of sudden death in such a
way that the average age of death retains the value, unity, which it

has in the reference population. Values of μ_0 can be obtained by
setting $\bar{t}_d = 1$ in eqn. (15) and solving it numerically. Results,
shown in Table 4, indicate that the presenescent death rate for any
specified value of T is higher than the corresponding entry in Table
3. Presenescent death rates in populations in which the average age at
death is held constant are higher than in populations in which the mean
longevity is held constant but lower than in the nonsenescent reference
population.

Note that if $\bar{t}_d = 1$ and $m = 1$, eqns. (6) and (15) have exactly
the same form. If eqn. (6) were solved for s' and eqn. (15) were
solved for μ_0, the results would be identical. Stated more simply,
$s' = \mu_0$. From eqn. (7.2), $r = s' - \mu_0 = 0$. Thus the rate of
natural increase is zero for all populations having the same average
age at death as the reference population. Selective advantage relative
to the reference population is neither positive nor negative but remains
neutral.

Since $R = \bar{t}_d = 1$ [eqn. (16)], the reproductive fraction, like r,
is independent of T. In view of the relation between r, R, and T_g
given in eqn. (11), it might be anticipated that the generation time,
T_g, would be similarly constant, but this is not the case. Substitution of the values $r = 0$ and $R = 1$ in eqn. (11) yields an indeterminate
"0/0" form. A straightforward calculation presented in the appendix
establishes this fact more rigorously and shows that $T_g = \bar{t}$.

Table 4. Cases 1 and 5: Values of Variables
Describing Populations for which the
Average Age at Death has the Value 1.
For all T, $r = 0$ and $R = 1$ (See text).

μ_0: Presenescent death rate
Other symbols are defined in the caption
to Table 1.

T	μ_0	$T_g = \bar{t}$
1.0	0.0	.500
1.1	.176	.532
1.2	.314	.562
1.6	.642	.665
2.0	.797	.745
3.0	.940	.873
4.0	.980	.939
5.0	.993	.972
∞	1.00	1.00

Since the generation time is equal to the mean longevity, it can be
calculated with the use of eqn. (13). Results given in Table 4 show
that sudden-death senescence reduces the values of both of these
quantities.

DISCUSSION

The foregoing demographic model demonstrates that a senescent
population may evolve from an "immortal" one if the disadvantage of

senescence is sufficiently compensated by an early advantage, such as a diminution in the presenescent death rate. To determine whether the model has any basis in reality, it is necessary to ask whether senescence has, in fact, evolved.

There can be little doubt that longevity has evolved under the influence of natural selection. Although there is a great deal of scatter in the data, many observations, e.g., those summarized by Cutler (1978), support the thesis that more highly evolved species tend to have longer lives. However the longevity of a population is easier to ascertain than its level of senescence. Longevity can be character-ized by a single number, such as the maximum lifespan, the average age at death, or the mean of the survival curve. To demonstrate senescence requires the collection of sufficient data to construct the entire survival curve. This rather arduous task has been accomplished for very few living species and is virtually impossible for extinct species.

If survival curves, or what is equivalent, death-rate functions, were available for many species on the evolutionary ladder, their shapes could be examined to determine the point or points at which aging first appeared or whether, indeed, it had always existed. Exponentially declining survival curves and flat death-rate functions would signify nonsenescent populations. Aging would reveal itself through more rectangular survival curves and rising death-rate functions.

Although not much information of this sort exists, the little that is available supports the concept that natural selection has favored senescence as well as longevity. Sonneborn (1978) and Smith-Sonneborn (1985) noted that bacteria and certain other single-celled organisms are nonsenescent, while some unicellular organisms are known to age. Strehler (1977) reviewed evidence indicating that there are single-celled organisms which age and a few primitive multicellular organisms which do not. However, aging appears to be universal in highly evolved metazoa, and there are some survival data which indicate that the degree of senescence is greater in more highly evolved forms (Johnson, 1963). All of this suggests that senscence has evolved in parallel with longevity.

Sacher (1978) stated that the evolution of senescence and the evolution of longevity are diametrically opposed hypotheses. The populations examined in the demographic model presented here show that there is no reason, in principle, why such a conflict must exist. Sacher's argument appears to be based on the proposition that a nonsencenscent organism is "potentially perfect." In the demographic model, the nonsenescent organism is subject to random destruction which cannot be repaired. It is not perfect but is potentially immortal only in the sense that its probability of death is independent of age. Senescence compensated by a reduction in the presenescent death rate may have selective advantage whether or not it is accompanied by an increase in longevity. Senescence and longevity may both be favored by natural selection.

SUMMARY

The demographic model of senescence described here provides an answer to the question, "Why should senescence evolve?" Most generally stated, the answer is that senescence should be expected to evolve if its negative effect on the rate of natural increase of a nonsenescent population is sufficiently offset by the early appearance of an advantageous characteristic. This is a nonadaptive point of view in the sense discussed by Kirkwood (1985) and by Kirkwood and Cremer (1982). It corresponds more closely to Medawar's (1952) position than to Weisman's (1889).

The demographically based model in which senescence is represented by sudden death supplies an explanation which is simple and credible for the evolution of senescence. It supports the following specific conclusions:

1. The introduction of sudden death (case 2) in a nonsenescent population otherwise subject only to randomly occurring death (case 1) is, by itself, disadvantageous from the standpoint of natural selection.

2. However the population may enjoy a net selective advantage if the disadvantage of sudden-death senescence is compensated by an appropriate improvement early in its life history, e.g., by a reduction in its presenescent death rate.

3. In the most extreme example possible, in which the presenescent death rate is zero and the survival curve is rectangular (case 3), the early improvement is associated with an increase in the degree of sensescence of the population, in its mean longevity, and in its average age at death. Thus natural selection can simultaneously favor both senescence and longevity.

4. Among populations in which the age of sudden death is balanced against the presenescent death rate in such a way that mean longevity is held constant (case 4), sudden-death senescence provides selective advantage relative to a nonsenescent population (case 1). Up to the point at which the survival curve becomes rectangular, the earlier the age at which sudden-death occurs, the greater the selective advantage. Similar conclusions were reached earlier with respect to forms of senescence which take effect more gradually than the sudden-death mechanism postulated here.

5. Populations in which the age of sudden death is balanced against the presenescent death rate in such a way that the average age at death is held constant (case 5) are selectively neutral with respect to a nonsenescent population (case 1).

Thus a reduction in mortality at an early age can compensate for the sudden death of the whole population at an advanced age because so few individuals in the nonsenescent population survive to reproduce when old. Senescence, even in the drastic form in which no individual lives beyond a fixed age is favored by evolution when it is accompanied by an enhancement of the rate of natural increase of the population.

ACKNOWLEDGEMENT

Of all the scientists with whom I have been personally acquainted, Dr. Howard J. Curtis, late Chairman of the Biology Department of the Brookhaven National Laboratory, is the one whom I most admire. In 1971, when I was a beginner in gerontology, Dr. Curtis gave me indispensable

help and encouragement by allowing me to spend my sabbatical leave
working and studying with him. He was full of suggestions for research
projects, some of which continue to influence my efforts to this day,
and he was infinitely tolerant of my ignorance. His devotion to his
family, to his community, to science, and to Brookhaven was evident.
This paper is dedicated to his memory.

REFERENCES

Charlesworth, B., 1980, "Evolution in Age-Structured Populations,"
    Cambridge University Press, Cambridge.
Cutler, R. G., 1978, Evolutionary biology of senescence, in: "The
    Biology of Aging," J. A. Behnke, C. E. Finch, and G. B. Moment,
    eds., Plenum, New York.
Fisher, R. A., 1958, "The Genetical Theory of Natural Selection," Dover,
    New York.
Hamilton, W. D., 1966, The moulding of senescence by natural selection,
    J. theor. Biol., 12:12.
Hirsch, H. R., 1980, Evolution of senescence: Influence of age-dependent
    death rates on the natural increase of a hypothetical
    population, J. theor. Biol., 86:149.
Hirsch, H. R., 1982, Evolution of senescence: Natural increase of
    populations displaying Gompertz- or power-law death rates and
    constant or age-dependent maternity rates, J. theor. Biol.,
    98:321.
Johnson, H. A., 1963, Redundancy and biological aging, Science, 141:910.
Kirkwood, T. B. L., 1981, Repair and its evolution: Survival versus
    reproduction, in: "Physiological Ecology: An Evolutionary
    Approach to Resource Use," C. R. Townsend and P. Calow, eds.,
    Blackwell, Oxford.
Kirkwood, T. B. L., 1985, Comparative and evolutionary aspects of
    longevity, in: "Handbook of the Biology of Aging, 2nd ed.,"
    C. E. Finch and E. L. Schneider, eds., van Nostrand Reinhold,
    New York.
Kirkwood, T. B. L., and Cremer, T., 1982, Cytogerontology since 1881:
    A reappraisal of August Weismann and a review of modern progress,
    Hum. Genet., 60:101.
Medawar, P. B., 1952, "An Unsolved Problem of Biology," H. K. Lewis,
    London.
Sacher, G. A., 1978, Longevity and aging in vertebrate evolution,
    BioScience, 28:497.
Smith-Sonneborn, J., 1985, Aging in unicellular organisms, in: "Hand-
    book of the Biology of Aging, 2nd ed.," C. E. Finch and E. L.
    Schneider, eds., van Nostrand Reinhold, New York.
Sonneborn, T. M., 1978, The origin, nature, and causes of aging, in:
    "The Biology of Aging," J. A. Behnke, C. E. Finch, and G. B.
    Moment, eds., Plenum, New York.
Strehler, B. L., 1977, "Time, Cells, and Aging, 2nd ed.," Academic,
    New York.
Wallace, D. C., 1967, The inevitability of growing old, J. chron. Dis.,
    20:475.
Weismann, A., 1889, The duration of life, in: "Essays Upon Heredity and
    Kindred Biological Problems," A. Weismann, Oxford University
    Press, Oxford.
Williams, G. C., 1957, Pleiotropy, natural selection, and the evolution
    of senescence, Evolution, 11:398.

APPENDIX: AVERAGE AGE AT DEATH

Based on the definition of an average in integral notation, the average age of a population at death is

$$\bar{t}_d = \frac{\int t\,dn}{\int dn} , \tag{A1}$$

where dn is the number of individuals dying in a brief age interval dt, i.e., $n(t)$ is the number having ages between (t and $t + dt$). Since $n(t)$ is proportional to $l(t)$,

$$\bar{t}_d = \frac{\int t\,dl}{\int dl} . \tag{A2}$$

From the definition of the death rate given in eqn. (3), $dl(t) = -\mu(t)l(t)dt$. With this substitution, eqn. (A2) assumes the form which appears in eqn. (14). Eqn. (15) is obtained from eqn. (14) by replacing $l(t)$ and $\mu(t)$ with the functions specified in eqns. (2) and (4) respectively and performing the indicated integrations.

Generation time, $\bar{t}_d = 1$

As stated in the main text, the generation time calculated with the use of eqn. (11) is indeterminate if the average age at death is held to the value $\bar{t}_d = 1$ which applies to the nonsenescent population. To show that this is true, let $r = s' - \mu_0$ as in eqn. (7.2). Then, by substitution in eqn. (11)

$$T_g = \frac{\ln R}{s' - \mu_0} . \tag{A3}$$

It was demonstrated in connection with case 5 that, if $\bar{t}_d = 1$, $\mu_0 \to s'$ and $R \to 1$. Then $s' - \mu_0 \to 0$, $\ln R \to 0$, and eqn. (A3) is indeterminate in the limit $\mu_0 \to s'$. It can be evaluated by application of L'Hospital's rule:

$$T_g = \lim_{\mu_0 \to s'} \frac{\dfrac{d (\ln R)}{d\mu_0}}{\dfrac{d (s' - \mu_0)}{d\mu_0}} \tag{A4}$$

$$= - \lim_{\mu_0 \to s'} \frac{dR/d\mu_0}{R} . \tag{A5}$$

A result which is identical to eqn. (13) can be obtained by applying eqn. (A5) to the function which appears in eqn. (9). Thus $T_g = \bar{t}$.

MUTANT GENES THAT EXTEND LIFE SPAN

Thomas E. Johnson, David B. Friedman, Paul A. Fitzpatrick, and
William L. Conley

Molecular Biology and Biochemistry
University of California
Irvine, California 92717

INTRODUCTION

One way to gain an understanding of any biological process is through
the use of mutant analysis and selective breeding to generate stocks which
have genetic alterations in that process. We have taken just such an
approach in the analysis of aging.

The genetic approach has the advantage of being holistic and
independent of prior assumptions about the exact nature of the events
determining aging, or more exactly organismic life span. Unfortunately,
previous attempts to analyze senescence and death with genetic techniques
have been largely unsuccessful. More recently, several groups have
identified genotypes that have extended life spans (Johnson and Wood, 1982;
Johnson, 1986; Luckinbill, et al. 1984; Rose, 1984a; Munkres and Furtek,
1984; Leffelaar and Grigliatti, 1984) Many of these studies are described
within this volume. Most of these groups have identified strains that are
longer-lived than wild type. Long-lived stocks must be altered in those
events which are rate-limiting in specifying length of life. Such stocks
may, therefore, have genetically specified alterations in the basic aging
rate. Our searches for aging specific mutants have concentrated on
identifying long-lived stocks in the nematode *Caenorhabditis elegans*.
Several long-lived stocks have been produced both by mutant screening and by
selective breeding. These stocks have both mean and maximum life spans more
than 60% longer than wild type strains.

C. elegans is uniquely suited for such a genetic analysis for three
reasons: (1) its short life span, (2) its well developed and convenient
genetics, and (3) its self-fertilizing, hermaphroditic mode of reproduction.
This hermaphroditic life style leads to complete inbreeding in both
laboratory and wild populations. This is important because life span is a
quantitative trait that is quite prone to inbreeding depression in most
organisms. However, in *C. elegans* measures of life span accurately reflect
the underlying genotype, free of the disruptive effects of heterosis.

C. elegans is a nonparasitic, free-living nematode. It can be grown
on petri plates and fed *E. coli* (Brenner, 1974). It has a 3-day life cycle
and a 20-day life span at $20^{o}C$ under standard laboratory conditions
(Johnson, 1984; Johnson and Simpson, 1985). Genetic analysis of *C. elegans*

is quite sophisticated. Over 400 mutants are currently available on all six linkage groups. Existing mutations affect behavior, development, morphology, and enzymatic processes. Both temperature-sensitive and suppressible allelles are available; duplication and deletion stocks for much of the genome and balancers for several linkage groups also are available. New mutants can be induced at high frequency, made homozygous by allowing hermaphrodites to self fertilize, and analyzed in crosses using spontaneous males.

Transposon mediated mutagenesis has facilitated the molecular cloning of genes from *C. elegans* (Greenwald, 1985; Moerman et al., 1986). In short, this organism has most of the classical and molecular genetic tools needed to facilitate a genetic analysis. These tools need only be applied to aging.

QUANTITATIVE GENETIC STUDIES

Characterization of life span as a genetic marker

Since life span of individuals and of genotypes is of central significance in the study of senescence processes, we have developed techniques in which accurate life span analyses can be performed simultaneously on a number of different genotypes. At any one time as many as 2500 different genotypes may be under assay in our laboratory. Thus, over the last 5 years, we have assayed over 1/4 million animals. Four easily scored parameters (lack of movement, lack of response, lack of osmotic turgor and visible tissue degeneration) were chosen as objective criteria of death (Johnson & Wood, 1982). These assays, combined with controlled environmental conditions, enable us to generate internally consistent survival curves.

Computer-aided recording of data using interactive programs accessed directly from the laboratory and the development and use of programs for the statistical analysis of survival have aided us in performing many assays simultaneously. When coupled with the short life span, these methods allow life expectancy to be analyzed by classical and molecular genetic techniques. Nevertheless, assay of life span is tedious and involves about two months per assay to complete.

A frequent complication in life span experiments is variation between identical genotypes assayed at different times: such variation is not seen when samples are assayed at the same time. We control for this variation between experiments by using duplicates or triplicates of each genotype as internal controls of consistency. All experiments also include wild type and appropriate mutant controls for statistical comparison. The failure of a test of internal consistency signals the presence of disturbing factors and the need for additional analysis. Since life span is quite sensitive to environmental fluctuations, internal controls are important for data validity and are incorporated routinely in all our data analyses. Our succeses in identifying and mapping mutant loci stem largely from our care in experimental design and data reduction, as well as from the unique biology of *C. elegans* .

Advantages of *C. elegans* for quantitative studies of life span

In hermaphrodites of *C. elegans* there is no heterosis effect on length of life. Analyses of the F1 from a cross between N2 males and Berg BO hermaphrodites (two common laboratory strains) confirmed this fact for these genotypes (Johnson and Wood, 1982). Crosses between these strains also reveals a lack of heterosis for other life-history traits (Johnson, in preparation). These results have been replicated in two other experiments and suggest that hermaphrodite life span is specified by genetic loci that do not display dominance. Male life span, on the other hand, does have a significant dominant genetic component. A consequence of these findings is that hermaphrodites can be assayed for life span and the results easily interpreted without the disruptive effects of inbreeding or heterosis that are seen in other organisms (Lints, 1978).

A second unique advantage of *C. elegans* is the fact that all visible and morphological mutants were derived in one genetic background (the N2). Most mutants have also been extensively backcrossed to N2 to eliminate both linked and unlinked mutations. Third, *C. elegans* stocks do not accumulate modifier or suppressor mutations in the laboratory because stocks are cryogenically preserved in a nongrowing state and are easily recovered later without genetic alteration.

The major import of all of these facts for aging research is that long-lived stocks can be generated, knowing that long life is not due to hybrid vigor and that the long life phenotype will be maintained during subsequent genetic and biochemical analyses.

Life Spans of Existing Mutant Stocks

Behavioral, morphological, and temperature-sensitive developmental mutants have been analyzed and found to have mean life spans that range from about 0.3 to 1.5 that of wild type controls (Figure 1). Two phenotypically uncoordinated (Unc) stocks that live longer than wild type may warrant more study. Since decreased rate of food intake has been shown to extend life span, under certain conditions, the long life in these strains may result from the ingestion of less bacteria than wild type; this will be checked.

A surprisingly large number of existing morphological, behavioral and developmental mutants have almost normal life spans. Stocks with normal life spans have been useful as markers for mapping a major locus specifying length of life (Fitzpatrick and Johnson, in preparation).

The situation in Caenorhabditis is different from that typically observed in Drosophila where few, if any, morphologically mutant lines have normal life spans (Baker, Jacobson, and Mokrynski, 1985). This difference may result from the presence of tightly linked, sublethal recessive loci in Drosophila (Mukai et al., 1972) which are made homozygous in the same crosses used to make recessive mutants homozygous. These sublethal recessive loci could also be responsible for the differences between the two species in the effects of inbreeding on quantitative traits (Johnson and Wood, 1982; Rose, 1984b; Johnson, submitted).

In at least one case in *C. elegans*, a short life span trait has been genetically separated from the visible marker (temperature sensitive sterility) by backcrossing to wild type (Johnson, 1984). Thus for *fem-2(b245)*, shorter life span is not a pleiotropic effect of the marker in question but rather is due to a separate locus, still present in the genetic background of these mutant stocks. Other stocks that are short-lived may harbor similar, genetically separable loci producing shortened life span.

Morphological, behavioral and temperature-sensitive developmental mutations may have shorter life spans than typical for wild type but longer life span is only rarely found. Thus, life span extensions longer than 20% over the wild may serve as a distinctive signal for mutational events in genes involved more directly in the specification of life span.

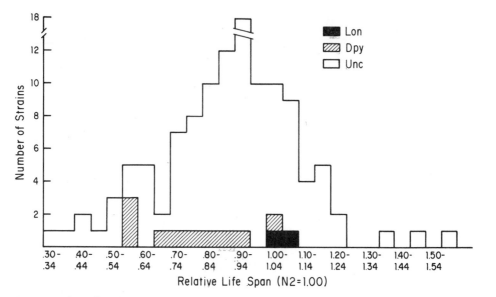

Fig. 1. Distribution of mean life spans for 114 morphological and behavioral
mutants: Unc, uncoordinated behavior, Lon, longer than wild type,
Dpy, shorter, squatter than wild type. For more information see
Brenner (1974).

Heritability of Life Span

Genetic variability in life span has been exploited by analysis of
recombinant inbred lines derived from Bristol (N2) and Bergerac BO crosses.
Three different approaches established that heritability of life span is
about 40% in this genetic background (Johnson and Wood, 1982). Based on
these first estimates, we established a series of recombinant inbred
(RI) lines between N2 and Bergerac BO; these lines had a three-fold
variation in mean and maximum life span (Johnson and Wood, 1982; Johnson,
1983). These RI's also displayed significant variation in other life-
history traits and both phenotypic and genetic correlations between
these various traits and life span have been determined (Johnson, 1986;
Foltz and Johnson, submitted).

Significant positive phenotypic and genetic correlations between total
fecundity or early-age fecundity and life span were observed (Figure 2).
There were negative genetic correlations between late-life fecundity and
life span, but no significant relationship between the loci specifying life
span and those determining development or behavior (Foltz and Johnson,
submitted). These findings are different from the negative covariances
between early-life fecundity and life span predicted by theoretical models
of the evolution of life-history traits (Charlesworth, 1980) and observed in
Drosophila by two different groups (Luckinbill et al., 1984; Rose, 1984a).
One reason for the differences between *C. elegans* and Drosophila may be that
in Drosophila experiments that select for longer fecundity indirectly select
for hybrid vigor.

Alternatively, *C. elegans* may be subject to inbreeding depression, as
demonstrated by Rose (1984b) in previous studies in Drosophila. These
multivariate analyses have been replicated twice with essentially similar
results.

We also observe significant genetic covariance between male and
hermaphrodite mean life spans (data not shown). This observation is

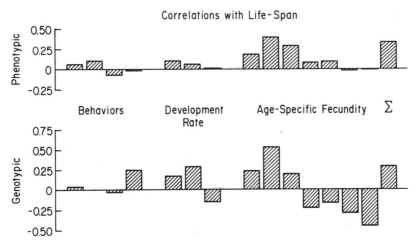

Fig. 2. Phenotypic and genetic correlations between life span and 4
components of behavior, 3 measures of rate of development (Johnson,
1986), or age-specific fecundity (Johnson, unpublished data).
Statistical significance for phenotypic correlations is P < .05 for
r $\geq$ .17 and p < .01 for r $\geq$ .23; for genetic correlations P < .05
where r $\geq$ .48.

consistent with the notion that the loci specifying hermaphrodite life
span also function to specify life span in the male.

Correlation between a Biomarker of Aging and Mean Life Span

The simplest definition for a biomarker of aging is a character that
displays age-dependent changes that are correlated with chronological age.
Many have assumed that such a biomarker is more than this and also has
predictive capability for remaining life. There are very few cases is which
such predictive capabilities have been shown (Schneider et al., 1981;
Ingram, 1983). Two biomarkers of aging (age-specific fecundity and age-
specific spontaneous movement) have been extensively analyzed in the RI
lines to estimate predictive capability. As mentioned above, age-specific
fecundity shows significant covariance with chronological age.
Spontaneous movement rate, a marker of total motor activity, is correlated
with chronological age and decreases linearly throughout life (Bolanowski et
al., 1981; Johnson, submitted). A high correlation between the expected age
of zero movement (the X-intercept of the regression of spontaneous movement
rate on age) and both mean and maximum life span, was also observed. Across
six genotypes that displayed an almost 3 fold variation in mean life span,
the X-intercept of the rate of decrease in movement was an accurate
predictor of mean life span of the stock (Johnson, submitted). Even within
genotypes, the rate of decrease in movement is positively correlated with
individual life span and reached levels of significance in several instances
(Keller and Johnson, unpublished).

Localization of Major Genes Affecting Life Span

The recombinant inbred lines segregate genetic factors specifying
life-history traits (life span, developmental rate, etc.) as well as 300 or
more restriction fragment length polymorphisms (RFLP's) generated by
the insertion of the Tc1 transposable element in one of the progenitor
strains (Bergerac BO) but not the other (N2) (Emmons et al., 1983). Many
RFLP's have been localized on the standard genetic map and can be used as
molecular markers for that region of the genome (Files, Carr and Hirsh,

1983; Rose et al., 1982). Using cloned unique sequences homologous to an RFLP, we have determined whether the Bristol or the Bergerac RFLP is present in each RI line, thereby ascertaining the strain of origin, not only of the sequence containing the RFLP, but also the origin of a larger surrounding genomic region, expected to be about 7×10^6 base pairs. (These calculations are based on the expectation that each RI has undergone, on the average, 2 rounds of detectable recombination during the inbreeding process, that the genetic map of the worm totals about 300 map units, and that the genome size is 8×10^7 base pairs.) This region is roughly equal to 1/2 of a chromosome in length. If there are only one or two major genes specifying life span and other life-history traits or if clusters of genes are present within one or a few chromosome regions, this technique will detect those regions as positions where long-lived RI lines tend to have one RFLP and short-lived lines the other. These analyses suggest that none of the three regions examined contain major loci involved in the specification of length of life (Johnson, 1986). Quantitative genetic estimates also suggest that each of the six linkage groups contain genes affecting length of life (Johnson, 1986).

MOLECULAR STUDIES LEADING TO PHYSIOLOGICAL CORRELATES OF AGING

Cytosine Methylation

Klass et al. (1983) reported a 10,000-fold increase in the amount of 5-methyl cytosine (m^5C) present in the DNA of aging nematodes. Simpson, Johnson and Hammen (1986) extracted DNA using an SDS/protease K procedure, purified the DNA by banding on CsCl (Klass did not use highly purified DNA) and acid hydrolyzed the purified DNA yielding free bases which we analyzed by HPLC (high performance liquid chromatography) using a reverse phase, ion-pairing column (Altex Ultrasphere C_{18}, 5 micron) and monitoring at 254 nm. We observed low amounts of a peak eluting near authentic m^5C; 254/280 UV absorbance ratios of this peak led us to doubt that the peak in question was actually m^5C. UV spectral comparisons with authentic m^5C show clearly that the peak was not m^5C. Our conclusions are also based on isoschizomer analysis of genomic DNA sequences digested with MspI and HpaII and probed with the moderately repetitive transposable element of C. elegans, Tc1. MspI and HpaII differ in their ability to cut m^5C and have been used in a variety of studies to analyze cytosine methylation. No differences in digestion patterns were seen. We conclude that C. elegans does not contain m^5C at any age.

DNA Repair

Loss of DNA repair capability has been frequently proposed as a possible mechanism driving the senescence process (Hart and Setlow, 1974). In conjunction with Hartman we initiated a series of studies into the effects of altered DNA repair capability on life span. Three approaches have been used. First, we have determined mean life spans of unirradiated wild type control nematodes (N2) and of seven repair-defective mutants (Hartman and Herman, 1982); these data suggest that several rad mutants have near normal life span. Furthermore, when these mutants were irradiated with ^{137}Cs gamma irradiation several of the stocks displayed longer life spans than controls of the same genotype (Johnson and Etebar, manuscript in preparation). Such studies have been previously used to suggest that stimulation of DNA repair capability by irradiation results in prolonging life. Our results show that DNA repair is not a causal determinant of length of life.

Second, Hartman is assaying excision repair capability on four RI lines which display a three-fold variation in mean life span. These studies are not yet complete. Third, sensitivity to irradiation among these four RI

96

strains show no significant differences either among themselves or when compared with wild type (Simpson, Johnson, and Hartman, in preparation). This again suggests that altered DNA repair is not a part of the mechanism causing variation in life span in *C. elegans*.

Search for protein markers of life span by PAGE 2D gel electrophoresis

Larval development of the nematode is punctuated by four larval molts. Of the roughly 800 spots resolvable by PAGE 2D gels, 113 display changes during larval development (Johnson and Hirsh, 1979). We asked if any variation in resolvable adult proteins could be detected; if so, such changes could be used as simple biological markers of senescence (Johnson and McCaffrey, 1985). Nematodes were labeled by growth on ^{35}S labeled *E. coli* as a food source for 5 hours at 20°C, were washed free of exogenous label, and were chased for 30 minutes with excess unlabelled bacteria. Gels received 5×10^{5} cpm/gel and were examined by fluorography after a 2 to 3 week exposure. The temperature sensitive mutant strain (DH26) was used in all of these studies since progeny production could be effectively blocked by growth at high temperatures which simplified the maintenance of synchronous stocks. The mean life span of DH26 under these conditions was approximately 15 days. Samples were taken at days 4, 7, 14, 19 and 21. In older samples (19 and 21 days) only 300 spots could be resolved as compared to the 800 spots in young worms, but this was entirely due to problems in labeling older worms to high levels of specific activity.

These experiments gave high reproducibility but failed to reveal qualitative changes in any major spots that could be consistently detected over the life span of the nematode, a situation quite unlike development. We conclude that no major changes in gene expression occur throughout adult life. Our data also revealed that there was no significant spreading of spots in the isoelectric focusing dimension as might be expected if significant misincorporation of amino acids occurs late in life as predicted by several "error-catastrophe" models of senescence. We would not have detected the qualitative modulations in protein synthetic spectrum in these experiments such as reported by Fleming et al. (1986).

ANALYSIS OF SINGLE GENE MUTANTS THAT PROLONG LIFE

age-1

We have studied the long-lived mutants isolated by Klass (1983). Klass dismissed these mutants as uninteresting because they displayed a decreased rate of food ingestion. Decreased food ingestion has been shown to cause a prolongation of life span in *C. elegans* (Friedman and Johnson, submitted) and in a wide variety of metazoans. In multiple repeats of assays similar to those used by Klass, we find that these mutants take up normal amounts of food and have normal pharyngeal pump rates (Johnson, 1986; Friedman and Johnson, submitted). The locus conferring long life in MK542 and MK546 (termed *age-1*) is separable from a gene, *unc-31*, that results in uncoordinated movement (Johnson, 1986). MK546, MK542, and MK31 (long-lived mutants isolated by Klass) all contain an allele of *unc-31*. Klass acknowledges (personal communication) that MK542 and MK546 could be duplicate isolates of the same initial mutational event but the fact that these strains are subtly but clearly different argues against such genetic identity.

Complementation analysis of the age locus could not readily be performed in the original strains since the males were sterile. *age* reisolates from a backcross to wild type are male-fertile and have enabled us to perform complementation tests for life span as well as to map the *age-1* locus. Our conclusions are that MK546 and MK542 contain alleles

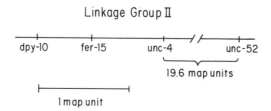

Fig. 3. A simple genetic map of chromosome II. The *age-1* gene is tightly
    linked to *fer-15*.

(perhaps identical) of a major gene termed, *age-1* (Friedman and Johnson,
submitted). The *age-1* locus is associated with decreased hermaphrodite
fecundity (termed Hef) (Friedman and Johnson, submitted). The Hef
phenotype co-segregates with the Age phenotype and both are tightly
linked to a temperature-sensitive mutant, *fer-15* (Figure 3).

The *age-1* locus has been more precisely mapped to linkage group II,
using its tight linkage to *fer-15*. Three point crosses with *dpy-10* and *unc-4* are underway. The *age-1* locus has been tentatively assigned a position
almost midway between *dpy-10* and *unc-4* (Figure 3) to the right and separable
from *fer-15* (Fitzpatrick and Johnson, unpublished). Deficiency mapping,
using existing deficiencies covering this area, is underway and has
confirmed both this map position and the association of the *fer-15* locus
with the Hef and Age phenotype of *age-1* (Friedman, Shoemaker and Johnson,
unpublished).

Genetic Dissection of Organismic Aging

The finding that blocking larval development results in the
lengthening of organismic life span (Johnson et al., 1984) can
be interpreted to mean that the process of development and the process of
organismic senescence are either coupled or are sequential with development
preceding senescence. Organismic senescence has been broken into three
components: life expectancy, general motor senescence and reproductive
senescence. Common genetic controls of these processes have been detected in
the studies described above. It is also clear that each of these processes
is also specified by genes that are not pleiotropic and do not affect the
other processes (Johnson, submitted).

We are hopeful that the continued study of the genetic basis of
senescence in *C. elegans* will lead to significant insights into the
molecular and physiological mechanisms that limit life span.

ACKNOWLEDGEMENTS

We thank P.M. Cuccaro, and M. Keller for excellent technical help, and
R. H. Davis, N. L. Foltz, M. E. Cruzen, and J. E. Shoemaker for useful
discussions or for permission to cite unpublished data. Supported by grants
from the National Institute of Health (AG05720), the National Science
Foundation (8208652), and a Charles A. Dana Award from the American
Federation for Aging Research. Some stocks were supplied by and are
available through the Caenorhabditis Genetics Center, which is supported by
contract NO1-AG-9-2113 between the NIH and the curators of the University of
Missouri.

REFERENCES

Baker, G. T. III., Jacobson, M., and Mokrynski, G., 1985, Aging in Drosophila, in: "Handbook of Cell Biology of Aging," V.J. Cristofalo, ed., CRC Press., Inc., Boca Raton, FL. pp. 511.

Bolanowski, M. A., Russell, R. L., and Jacobson, L. A., 1981, Quantitative measures of aging in the nematode *Caenorhabditis elegans*. I. Population and longitudinal studies of two behavioral parameters, Mech. Ageing. Dev., 15:279.

Brenner, S., 1974, The genetics of *Caenorhabditis elegans*, Genetics, 77:71.

Charlesworth, B., 1980, Evolution in age-structured populations, Cambridge University Press, Cambridge, U. K.

Emmons, S. W., Yesner, L., Ruan, K. S., and Katzenberg, D., 1983, Evidence for a transposon in *Caenorhabditis elegans*, Cell, 32:55.

Fleming, J. E., Melnikoff, P. S., Latter, G. I., and Bensch, K. G., 1986, Age dependent changes in the expression of Drosophila mitochondrial proteins, Mech. Ageing Dev., 34:63.

Files, J. G., Carr, S., and Hirsh, D., 1983, Actin gene family of *Caenorhabditis elegans*, J. Mol. Biol., 164: 355.

Greenwald, I., 1985, *lin-12*, a nematode homeotic gene, is homologous to a set of mammalian proteins that includes epidermal growth factor, Cell, 43:583.

Hart, R. W., and Setlow, R. B., 1974, Correlation between deoxyribonucleic acid excision repair and lifespan in a number of species, Proc. Natl. Acad. Sci. USA, 71:2169.

Hartman, P. S., and Herman, R. K., 1982, Radiation-sensitive mutants of *Caenorhabditis elegans*, Genetics, 102:159.

Ingram, D. K., 1983, Toward the behavioral assessment of biological aging in the laboratory mouse: concepts, terminology, and objectives, Exp. Ag. Res., 9:225.

Johnson, K., and Hirsh, D., 1979, Patterns of proteins synthesized during development of *Caenorhabditis elegans*, Dev. Biol., 70:241.

Johnson, T. E., 1983, *Caenorhabditis elegans*: a genetic model for understanding the aging process, in "Intervention in the Aging Process. Part B: Basic Research and Preclinical Screening," W. Regelson and F. M. Sinex, eds., Alan R. Liss, NY, 1983, p. 287.

Johnson, T. E., 1984, Analysis of the biological basis of aging in the nematode, with special emphasis on *Caenorhabditis elegans*, in: "Invertebrate Models in Aging Research," D. H. Mitchell and T. E. Johnson, eds., CRC, Boca Raton, FL. pp. 59.

Johnson, T. E., 1986, Molecular and genetic analyses of a multivariate system specifying behavior and life span. Behav. Genet. 16:221.

Johnson, T. E., and McCaffrey, G., 1985, Programmed aging or error catastrophe? An examination by two-dimensional polyacrylamide gel electrophoresis. Mech. Ageing. Dev., 30:285.

Johnson, T. E., Mitchell, D. H., Kline, S., Kemal, R., and Foy, J., 1984, Arresting development arrests aging in the nematode *Caenorhabditis elegans*, Mech. Ageing Dev., 28:23.

Johnson, T. E. and Simpson, V. J., 1985, Aging studies in *Caenorhabditis elegans* and other nematodes, in: "Handbook of Cell Biology of Aging," V. Cristolfalo, ed., CRC, Boca Raton, FL., pp. 481.

Johnson, T. E., and Wood, W. B., 1982, Genetic analysis of life-span in *Caenorhabditis elegans*, Proc. Natl. Acad. Sci. USA. 79:6603.

Klass, M. R., 1983, A method for the isolation of longevity mutants in the nematode *Caenorhabditis elegans* and initial results, Mech. Ageing Dev., 22:279.

Klass, M. R., Nguyen, P. N., and Dechavigny, A., 1983, Age-correlated changes in the DNA template in the nematode *Caenorhabditis elegans*, Mech. Ageing Dev., 22:253.

Leffelaar, D., and Grigliatti, T. A., 1984, A mutation in Drosophila that appears to accelerate aging, Develop. Genet., 4:199.

Lints, F. A., 1978, "Genetics and Ageing", Interdisciplinary Topics in Gerontology, Vol. 14, Karger, Basel.

Luckinbill, L. S., Arking, R., Clare, M. J., Cirocco, W., and Buck, S., 1984, Selection for delayed senescence in *Drosophila melanogaster*, Evolution, 38:996.

Moerman, D. G., Benian, G. M., and Waterston, R. H., 1986, Molecular cloning of the muscle gene *unc-22* in *Caenorhabditis elegans* by Tc1 transposon tagging, Proc. Natl. Acad. Sci. USA., 83:2579.

Mukai, T., Chigusa, S. I., Mettler, L. E. and Crow, J. F., 1972, Mutation rate and dominance of genes affecting viability in *Drosophila melanogaster*, Genetics, 72:335.

Munkres, K. D., and Furtek, C. A., 1984, Selection of conidial longevity mutants of *Neurospora crassa*, Mech. Ageing Dev., 25:47.

Rose, A. M., Baillie, D. L., Candido, E. P., Beckenbach, K. A., and Nelson, D., 1982, The linkage mapping of cloned restriction fragment length differences in *Caenorabditis elegans*, MGG., 188:286.

Rose, M. R., 1984a, Laboratory evolution of postponed senescence in *Drosophila melanogaster*, Evolution, 38:1004.

Rose, M. R., 1984b, Genetic covariation in Drosophila life history: untangling the data, Am. Nat., 123:565.

Schneider, E. L., Reff, M. E., Finch, C. E., and Weksler, M., 1981, Introduction, in "Biological Markers of Aging," M. E. Reff and E. L. Schneider, eds., USDHHS, NIH Publication No. 82-2221, p. 235.

Simpson, V. J., Johnson, T. E., and Hammen, R. F., 1986, *Caenorhabditis elegans* does not contain 5-methylcytosine at any time during development or aging. 1986, Nuc. Acids Res.: 14, 6711.

LONGEVITY IN THE PROTOZOA

Joan Smith-Sonneborn

Department of Zoology and Physiology
University of Wyoming
Laramie, Wyoming 82071

With respect to the evolution of longevity, two fundamental questions
are considered. 1) When did senescence arise? and 2) What role did sex
and DNA repair play in lifespan duration?

Bacteria and haploid protozoa are apparently immortal; they seem
capable of unlimited proliferation potential. Loss of the ability to
multiply forever was seen first in eucaryotic protozoa. The protozoa
therefore, may well be the guardian of the secret to the origin of senescence. Aging in the protozoa will be examined to discover the biological
events coincident with the emergence of senescence.

When the minimal biological requirements for senescence are known the
period of evolution with these requisites can be identified as a minimum
estimate of the time of evolution of the senescence phenomenon. Prokaryotes
have been dated 3.5 billion years old, eucaryotes 1.2-1.4 billion years
old. Since protozoans are the first eucaryotes, and aging is seen in some
of the protozoa, aging may have arisen a billion years ago.

VENTURE CAPITAL THEORY OF AGING

Senescence appeared after recombination, sex, multiple chromosomes,
diploidy, and meiosis. The appearance of senescence coincided with the
appearance of specialization of nuclei within a single cell (the germ line
micronuclei and somatic line macronuclei in ciliates) or cell specialization (into the reproductive and somatic cell types of colonial flagellates
such as Volvox). Senescence could not emerge in any organism until it
could separate its immortal part from its disposable part. The importance
of the "disposable soma" was already recognized by Kirkwood and Cremer
(1985).

If there were only one infinite unit, and it lost that attribute, by
definition, it would cease to exist. The option for senescence therefore,
originated with the ability to retain more than one representative of the
immortal part in the same organism. Once there was a redundant copy of
the immortal unit, the organism had the option to keep separate accounts,
an immortal reserve and a venture capital account. The redundant unit was
a second nucleus in ciliates, and spare cells in colonial flagellates.

As Weismann (1891) so clearly states, "Let us now consider how it happened that the multicellular animals and plants, which arose from unicellular forms of life came to lose this power of living forever. The answer to this question is closely bound up with the principle of division of labour...the first multicellular organism was probably a cluster of similar cells, but these units soon lost their original homogeneity...the single group would come to be divided into two groups of cells, which may be called somatic or reproductive. As these changes took place, the power of reproducing large parts of the organism was lost, while the power of reproducing the whole individual became concentrated in the reproductive cells alone. But it does not therefore follow that the somatic cells were compelled to lose the power of unlimited cell reproduction." Weismann appreciated the significance of division of labor in the onset of senescence at a time when senescence in ciliates first was observed (Maupas, 1888). However, the fact that aging in ciliates could occur implies that the nucleus is the fundamental unit of immortality since only the nucleus was used for division of labor. If aging arose with the appearance of a second nucleus within an organism, then there should be transitional organisms in which both nuclei have equal potency, and some in which one nucleus is immortal. Likewise in colonial flagellates, there should be colonies in which all cells can multiply indefinitely, and those in which only certain cells can multiply without limit.

Clonal aging and colonial aging will be reviewed from this perspective. Clonal aging refers to the limited proliferation potential of a cell after fertilization. As the number of cell divisions from the previous mating increases, the probability that a cell will give rise to two viable daughters decreases. Life is measured by the number of days or fissions from fertilization to death of a given number of cell isolates used as representatives of the clone. Clonal aging has been documented in certain species of Paramecium, Euplotes, Stylonychia, Tokophrya, Spathidium, and can be induced by inbreeding in Tetrahymena (Williams, 1980; see, reviews by Nanney, 1974; Smith-Sonneborn, 1981). Colonial aging refers to the programmed cell death seen in particular cell types within a colony of flagellates.

COLONIAL FLAGELLATES AND AGING

Within some colonies of protozoa, some cells are set aside which do not divide and are discarded. These members age and die. Colonial green flagellates are algae whose colony is composed of chlamydomonad building blocks (Coleman, 1979; Weise, 1976). The only diploid cell is the zygote, formed when two gametic cells fuse. Meiosis occurs at zygote germination, and the haploid product undergoes cleavage divisions to form a colony. In most genera, all cells can form daughter cells, but some show differentiation of a proportion of generative cells (gonidia) with unlimited proliferation potential, and those which never again divide (somatic cells).

After daughter colony formation is complete, the young colonies escape from the parent colony matrix which undergoes gradual dissolution. Vegetative reproduction is accomplished by 2^n successive divisions in each of the cells of the colony capable of reproduction; the maximum value of n is a species-specific characteristic. Some clones must outbreed, others are self-fertile. Fertilization does not appear to be a requisite for species survival (Coleman, 1979).

In certain Volvox colonies, more than 99 percent of the cells are somatic and undergo synchronous programmed senescence and cell death every generation (Hagen and Kochert, 1980). A small number of reproductive cells survive to produce the next generation. The potential reproductive cells are set aside at a particular stage by unequal cell division (Kochert, 1968; Starr, 1969). The electrophoretic pattern of polypeptides changes at the onset of senescent characteristics in somatic cells (Hagen and Kochert, 1980).

In the terminally differentiated somatic cells of the colonial green algae Volvox carteri, there are age-related disorganizations of chloroplast structure, decreases in cytoplasmic ribosomes, and accumulations of cytoplasmic lipid bodies. Since these changes are typical of those noted in starved cells, there may be an inability to take up or utilize nutrients which causes or contributes to senescence in terminally differentiated somatic cells (Pommerville and Kochert, 1981).

The colonial green flagellates provide a model system for regulation of cell proliferation potential. There are mutants in Volvox which fail to segregate replicating and nonreplicating cells. The array of mutants suggests that proliferative capacity involves several regulatory genes (Sessoms and Huskey, 1973).

THE CILIATE GENETIC COMPLEX

In general, ciliates contain two kinds of nuclei, the micronuclei or germline and the macronuclear somatic line nuclei. The micronuclei and macronuclei have different functions at different times in the life cycle, i.e., during the sexual and asexual cycle.

During the sexual cycle the micronuclei undergo meiosis to produce gametes which eventually differentiate the new micro- and macronuclei for the progeny cells. During the asexual cycle, the micronucleus undergoes mitosis, exhibits very little transcriptional activity and functions as the repository of genetic information, while the macronucleus dictates the metabolic cell functions. The macronucleus therefore, would be assumed to be the sole regulator of asexual cell function and duration of life. Despite the minimal transcriptional activity of the micronucleus during vegetative growth, the presence of micronuclei is correlated with cell growth.

The proportion of the micronuclear genome retained in the somatic macronucleus differs in different ciliated protozoans. Both Paramecium tetraurelia and certain Tetrahymena retain most of their micronuclear genome in their macronucleus (Cummings, 1975; Doerder and Debault, 1975). Chromosome polytenization and chromosome diminution followed by rapid synthesis is observed in lower ciliates (Kovaleva and Raikov, 1978) and in some hypotrichs (Ammermann, 1965, 1970; Ammermann et al., 1974; Bostock and Prescott, 1972; Lauth et al., 1976; Lawn et al., 1977; Lipps et al., 1978; Riewe and Lipps, 1977). There are strains of Paramecium bursaria in which amplification of certain chromosome segments and chromosome resorption or condensation were observed in the macronucleus (Schwartz and Meister, 1975). Therefore, the strategy for macronuclear development from the synkaryon (zygote nucleus) varies with species and generalizations from one species to another could be at best misleading, at most they could be totally inaccurate.

Differences are found in the molecular composition and conformation of micro- and macronuclei (Yao and Gorovsky, 1974; Yao and Gall, 1979). The transcriptionally active macronucleus of Tetrahymena has acetylated histones, whereas the transcriptionally inactive micronucleus does not (Gorovsky et al., 1973). Z DNA is an alternative conformation of the DNA double helix in which the Watson-Crick base pairing is preserved but the molecular form is a left-handed helix quite distinct from the right-handed

B DNA helix (Wang et al., 1979). The Z DNA conformation may be related both to specific organization of the chromosome and genetic activity (Nordheim et al., 1981). In Tetrahymena the tandemly repeated hexanucleotide C4A2 is present in a set of macronuclear DNA restriction fragments that differ from the set in the micronucleus (Yao and Gall, 1979). Differences in the micro- and macronucleus then include: (1) the presence of acetylated histones, (2) the conformation of the DNA, and (3) a different association of the C4A2 with micro- and macronuclear DNA. The micronucleus is the germ line. The macronucleus is the somatic line. We can ask if in ciliates, during the differentiation of the nucleus, the macronucleus lost the capacity for unlimited proliferation.

Loss of micronuclear function with age occurs in species of Tetrahymena, Paramecium, Stylonychia, Euplotes and Tokophyra (see reviews, Smith-Sonneborn, 1985a, b; Allen et al., 1984). Since the macronucleus determines the phenotype of the cells, we assume that there would be a loss of macronuclear immortality in any ciliate which requires fertilization for survival. Ciliates having a limited lifespan include representatives from all the species cited above, which also show micronuclear age-dependent deterioration. In contrast to the limited proliferation potential of these ciliates, certain micronucleated and amicronucleated strains of Tetrahymena show an apparent indefinite capacity for cell proliferation.

The rule seems to be that if one nucleus retains the ability to replicate indefinitely, the other can lose that capacity and the species can still survive. If both lose the capacity for indefinite replication, the reserve nucleus must be activated or escape from the deteriorating unit before the damage is devastating to the next generation. Selection would operate to maintain the organism long enough for reproduction and adjust the lifestyle to favor mating at an appropriate age. Mutations that assured a program for a limited period of fruitful fertilization, followed by aging and death were selected (or there was not selection against these combinations) and fertilization ceased to be optional and became obligatory (Sonneborn, 1978).

LIFESPAN, SEX AND REPAIR

Unicellular Organisms

Aging in Paramecium was characterized in different species (Jennings, 1945; Sonneborn, 1954). The most short-lived Paramecium is also the most inbred. Paramecium tetraurelia lives about 50 days, while the longest-lived Paramecium, Paramecium multimicronucleatum , lives at least 2500 days (Sonneborn, 1957).

Outbreeding organisms may require a lower mutation rate than inbreeders to achieve comparable genetic variety (Nanney, 1974) and their repair systems may be evolutionarily adjusted for their respective genetic strategies (Sonneborn, 1978). The life styles of the ciliates is adjusted to favor their breeding preference.

Outbreeders tend to mate with "strangers" and therefore tend to accumulate genetic variety. To favor outbreeding, these organisms have multiple mating types (increasing the chance that a stranger will be of a different mating type and therefore will be suitable as a sexual partner), long immaturity periods (to allow spatial separation between closely related individuals before mating can occur), and inability to undergo self-fertilization (discouraging homozygosity). Inbreeders can undergo self-fertilization, have only two mating types, and have short immaturity periods. Spontaneous recessive mutations quickly become homozygous after autogamy, and if nonadaptive in that genetic and environmental background, the possessor of that mutation may die or be overpowered by neighbors, reducing genetic variety (Sonneborn, 1957). The transition from optional to obligate fertilization would have occurred when the macronucleus could no longer support an indefinite replication or when a life-sustaining repair could take place only during fertilization. Repair of double-stranded DNA breaks, which may require a redundant chromosome, are repaired during meiosis or whenever homologous chromosomes could pair. It has been argued that sex is required to provide for recombinational repair and is the primary function of the process (Bernstein et al., 1985). Such a view underestimates a major role of sex and meiosis, i.e., for independent assortment of chromosomes and the contribution from the mate to allow mutations on separate chromosomes to come within a common nucleus. Mutations that are detrimental alone, may be beneficial in combination with other mutations. For example, a change in a flanking promotion sequence may be lethal without co-evolution of a recognition change for that sequence. Gene expression changes would have an opportunity then to be maintained both in the immortal or mortal nuclei or cells of multicellular species. Diploidy allows the maintenance of regulatory mutations, masked until expressed at an advantageous time. Independent assortment and recombinational repair may be critical components in the maintenance of sex in evolution.

There is evidence that levels of DNA damage can change with age and alter longevity. In Paramecium tetraurelia, an age-dependent increase in UV sensitivity occurs with advanced clonal age (Smith-Sonneborn, 1971). Also, UV-irradiation reduced lifespan of P. tetraurelia but not when the damage was enzymatically repaired by subjection to photoreactivation repair (Smith-Sonneborn, 1979). Photoreactivation is effective in removal of UV-induced lesions in human skin cells (D'Ambrosio et al., 1981a, b) and in Paramecium (Sutherland et al., 1968). In Paramecium, the cumulative effect of two cycles of irradiation followed by photoreactivation repair resulted in significant extension in mean and maximal lifespan. Those cells pretreated with UV and then photoreactivated responded to UV-irradiation like younger cells (Smith-Sonneborn, 1979). Photoreactivation alone induced no beneficial response. It is not known whether the beneficial effect of UV and photoreactivation represents a decelerated rate of aging, or if an age-clock was reset with respect to this age-correlated trait (decreased sensitivity to UV, relative to clonal age). If the UV-induced damage exceeds the capacity of cells to repair the damage, reduced lifespan results. If the damage does not saturate the repair system, increased repair capacity also might facilitate correction of some age-correlated damage. Should some age-related damage be repaired, the clock would be reset to some extent, but if the repair of new damage is facilitated, the rate of aging may be retarded. For example, it may be possible that the UV-induced damage can trigger repair of kinds of DNA damage which enhance mutagenesis. Recent studies show that apurinic sites in the DNA molecule may result in mutations when DNA replicates (Schaaper and Loeb, 1981). Removal of apurinic sites could lead to reduction of subsequent mutations associated with those lesions (Schaaper et al., 1980). Our studies indicate that DNA polymerase activity does not decline with age (Williams and Smith-Sonneborn, 1980). Loss of capacity to repair DNA with age could not be attributed therefore, to loss of activity of that enzyme. Increase in other age-related loss of function of repair enzymes could be involved, or the UV could alter DNA conformation, and therefore gene expression, in a manner which decreases DNA damage or creates greater accessibility of the DNA to repair. Evidence for increased repair after radiation is found in Paramecium (Smith-Sonneborn, 1979), in insects (Ducoff, 1976) and in some mammals (Calkins and Greenlaw, 1971). The amount of UV dosage was found to be correlated with longevity (Smith-Sonneborn, 1979). UV treatment in procaryotes is known to initiate complex induction processes accumulating in the repression of a group of metabolically diverse but coordinated functions that could provide increased survival (Witkin, 1976).

Multicellular Organisms

DNA damage and repair have been correlated with longevity in mammals (Hart and Setlow, 1974; Hart et al., 1978), though some exceptions have been noted (Kato et al., 1980). The emphasis of future studies should try to understand the apparent paradoxes and enigmas associated with the relationship between DNA repair and lifespan since herein may reside the clues to understanding a major regulation of cell lifespan. For example, there may be no specific DNA repair enzymes but rather several species of DNA polymerases whose functions overlap in a variety of conditions (Mosbaugh and Linn, 1984). Enzymes used in repair besides polymerases also may be involved in the fundamental recombination process in germ line and in somatic cells. If so, in adult multicellular organisms, a major role for recombination is the somatic recombination required to form antibodies. Both excision and rejoining of DNA are required to fashion the different antibodies required for immunity to new foreign invaders. A relationship between the immune system, aging and repair has already been observed. Lymphocytes from short-lived mice lost repair capability more quickly than long-lived strains (Licastro and Walford, 1985) and lifespan and repair capacity are linked to the major histocompatibility locus in mice (Walford and Bergmann, 1979). In addition, repair ability segregates with the H2 locus in mice (Hall et al., 1981). Most previous studies have focused on repair in cells when normal DNA synthesis was blocked or inhibited. Since the replicative polymerase can be involved also in large gap repair (Mosbaugh and Linn, 1984), a major component of the repair pathway, the replicative polymerase should be included in our concept of repair capacity.

Accurate repair, it seems, can depend on such variables as the replicative state of the cell (Krauss and Linn, 1986), enzyme activation (Busbee et al., in press) and gap size (Mosbaugh and Linn, 1986). Evidence is emerging to change our concepts of all of these variables which could influence DNA repair. For example, repair has been induced when non-dividing cells are stimulated to divide (Licastro and Walford, 1985) and when mice cells undergo transformation (LaBelle and Linn, 1984), though the mechanisms responsible for stimulation of repair are not understood. Likewise, in the protozoan Paramecium a cycle of UV damage and photoreactivation repair increased their lifespan by 27% (Smith-Sonneborn, 1979).

SUMMARY

In ciliates there are examples of cells which have different proliferation potential in the macronucleus. Those species with limited macronuclear proliferation potential require sex to activate the reserve nucleus. In terms of the capital investment theory, some ciliates invested in their spare nucleus without loss of their original potential, while others accumulated debts and needed the reserve account to maintain life. Other cells neglected maintenance of their reserve account and failed unless their venture capital account was not a self-sustaining venture. Sex provided access to the reserve account and had to occur before deterioration of the reserve account. The question is not when cellular immortality was lost, but rather when immortality was partitioned from a mortal segment. The separation provided the option both for senescence and evolution in multicellular organisms.

In colonial flagellates, separation of cells with infinite and finite cell lifespan potential occurred in some species, while in others the separation did not involve loss of immortality. In colonial flagellates, sex did not become an obligate stage. The immortal cells are haploid and could not accumulate damage and live (in contrast with the diploids in the ciliated protozoans).

The present theory predicts that differences between species or cells with infinite versus finite lifespan potential may reveal differences in the critical determinants of longevity.

Senescence could arise as an accident, as well as a design of nuclear differentiation. Cells therefore may have a much greater reserve for totipotency than would be predicted if they were assumed to lose immortality simply by the act of differentiation.

REFERENCES

Allen, S. L., Ervin, P. R., McLaren, N. C., and Brand, R. E., 1984, The 5S ribosomal RNA gene clusters in Tetrahymena thermophila: strain differences, chromosomal localization, and loss during micronuclear aging, Mol. Gen. Genet., 197:244.

Ammermann, D., 1965, Cytologische und genetische Untersuchungen an dem Ciliaten Stylonychia mytilus Ehrenberg, Arch. Protistenkd., 108:109.

Ammermann, D., 1970, The micronucleus of the ciliate (Stylonychia mytilus, its nucleic acid synthesis and function, Exp. Cell Res., 61:6.

Ammermann, D., Steinbruck, G., Berger, L. V., and Henning, W., 1974, Development of the macronucleus in the ciliated protozoan Stylonychia mytilus, Chromosoma, 45:401.

Bernstein, H., Byerly, H. C., Hopf, F. A., and Michod, R. E., 1985, Genetic damage, mutation, and the evolution of sex, Science, 229:1277.

Bostock, C. J., and Prescott, D. M., 1972, Evidence of gene diminution during formation of the macronucleus in the protozoan, Stylonychia, Proc. Nat. Acad. Sci., USA 69:139.

Busbee, D. L., Joe, C. O., Sylvia, V. L., Norman, J. D., and Ragsdale-Robinson, S. S. (in press), DNA polymerase alpha must be phosphorylated in order to bind DNA template/primer, Proc. Nat. Acad. Sci., USA.

Calkins, J., and Greenlaw, R. H., 1971, Activated repair of skin: a damage-induced radiation repair system, Radiology, 100:389.

Coleman, A., 1979, Sexuality in colonial green flagellates, in "Biochemistry and Physiology of Protozoa." 2nd ed., M. Levandowsky and S. H. Hutner, eds., Academic Press, New York.

Cummings, D. J., 1975, Studies on macronuclear DNA from Paramecium aurelia, Chromosoma, 53:191.

D'Ambrosio, S. M., Slazinski, L., Whetstone, J. W., and Lowney, E., 1981a, Excision repair of UV-induced pyrimidine dimers in human skin in vitro, J. Invest. Derm., 77:311.

D'Ambrosio, S. M., Whetstone, J. W., Slazinski, L., and Lowney, E., 1981b, Photorepair of pyrimidine dimers in human skin in vivo, Photochem. Photobiol., 34:461.

Doerder, F. P., and Debault, L. E., 1975, Cytofluorimetric analysis of nuclear DNA during meiosis, fertilization and macronuclear development in the ciliate Tetrahymena pyriformis syngen, J. Cell Sci., 17:471.

Ducoff, H. I., 1976, Radiation-induced increase in life span of insects, in: "Biological and Environmental Effects of Low Level Radiation, Vol. 1," pp. 103-109, International Atomic Energy Agency, Vienna.

Gorovsky, M. A., Pleger, G. L., Keevert, J. B., and Johmann, C. A., 1973, Studies on histone fraction F2A1 in macro- and micronuclei of Tetrahymena pyriformis, J. Cell Biol., 57:773.

Hagen, G., and Kochert, G., 1980, Protein synthesis in a new system for the study of senescence, Exp. Cell Res., 127:451.

Hall, K. Y., Bergmann, K., and Walford, R. L., 1981, DNA repair H-2 and aging in NZB and CBA mice, Tissue Antigens, 16:104.

Hart, R. W., Hall, K. Y., and Daniel, B., 1978, DNA repair and mutagenesis in mammalian cells, Photochem. Photobiol., 28:131.

Hart, R. W., and Setlow, R. B., 1974, Correlation between deoxyribonucleic acid and excision-repair in a number of mammalian species, Proc. Nat. Acad. Sci., USA, 71:2169.

Jennings, H. S., 1945, Paramecium bursaria: life history, V. Some relations of external conditions, past or present, to aging and to mortality of exconjugants, with summary of conclusions on age and death, J. Exp. Zool., 99:15.

Kato, H., Horada, M., Tsuchiya, K., and Moriwaki, K., 1980, Absence of correlation between DNA repair in ultraviolet irradiated mammalian cells and lifespan of the donor species, Japan J. Genetics, 55:99.

Kirkwood, T. B., and Cremer, T., 1982), Cytogerontology since 1881: A reappraisal of August Weismann and a review of modern progress, Hum. Genet., 60:101-121.

Kochert, G. D., 1968, Differentiation of reproductive cells in Volvox cateri, J. Protozool., 15:438.

Kovaleva, V. G., and Raikov, I. B., 1978, Diminution and resynthesis of DNA during development and senescence of the diploid macronuclei of the ciliates Trachelonoema sulcata, Gymnostomata karyorelictida, Chromosoma, 67:177.

Krauss, S. W., and Linn, S., 1986, Studies of DNA polymerase alpha and tetra from cultured human cells in various replicative states, J. Cell Physiol., 126:99.

LaBelle, M., and Linn, S., 1984, DNA repair in cultured mouse cells of increasing population doubling level, Mut. Research., 132:51.

Lauth, M. F., Spear, B. B., Heumann, J. M., and Prescott, D. M., 1976, DNA of ciliated protozoa: DNA sequence diminution during macronuclear development of Oxytricha, Cell, 7:67.

Lawn, R. M., Herrick, G., Heumann, J. M., and Prescott, D. M., 1977, The gene-size molecules in Oxytricha, Cold Spring Harb. Symp. Quant. Biol., 42:483.

Licastro, F., and Walford, R. L., 1985, Proliferative potential and DNA repair in lymphocytes from short-lived and long-lived strains of mice, in relation to aging, Mech. Ageing Dev., 31:171.

Lipps, H. J., Nock, A., Riewe, M., and Steinbruck, G., 1978, Chromatin structure in the macronucleus of the ciliate Stylonychia mytilus, Nuc. Acid Res., 5:4699.

Maupas, E., 1888, Recherches expérimentales sur la multiplication des infusiores ciliés, Arch. Zool. Exper., (2) 6:165.

Mosbaugh, D. W., and Linn, S., 1984, Gap-filling DNA synthesis by HeLa DNA polymerase α in an in vitro base excision DNA repair scheme, J. Biol. Chem., 259:10247.

Nanney, D. L., 1974, Aging and long-term temporal regulation in ciliated protozoa. A critical review, Mech. Age. Dev., 3:81.

Nordheim, A., Pardue, M. L., Lafer, E. M., Moller, A., Stoller, B. D., and Rich, A., 1981, Antibodies to left-handed Z DNA bind to interband regions of Drosophila polytene chromosomes, Nature, Lond., 294:417.

Pommerville, J. C., and Kochert, G. D., 1981, Changes in somatic cell structure during senescence of Volvox carteri, Eur. J. Cell Biol., 24:236.

Riewe, M., and Lipps, H. J., 1977, Template activity of macronuclear and micronuclear chromatin of the ciliate Stylonychia mytilus, Cell Biol. Int. Rep., 1:517.

Schaaper, R. M., Kunkel, T. A., and Loeb, L. A., 1983, Infidelity of DNA synthesis associated with bypass of apurinic sites, Proc. Nat. Acad. Sci., USA 80:487.

Schaaper, R. M., and Loeb, L. A., 1981, Depurination causes mutations in SOS-induced cells, Proc. Nat. Acad. Sci., USA 78:1773.

Schwartz, V., and Meister, H., 1975, Einige quantitative Daten zum Problem des Alterns bei Paramecium, Arch. Protistenk. Biol., 117:85.

Sessoms, A. H., and Husky, R. J., 1973, Genetic control of development in Volvox, isolation and characterization of morphogenetic mutants. Proc. Nat. Acad. Sci., USA 70(5):1335.

Smith-Sonneborn, J., 1971, Age-correlated sensitivity in ultraviolet radiation in Paramecium, Radiat. Res., 46:64.

Smith-Sonneborn, J., 1979, DNA repair and longevity assurance in Parmecium tetraurelia, Science, 230:1115.

Smith-Sonneborn, J., 1981, Genetics and aging in protozoa, Int. Rev. Cyt., 73:319.

Smith-Sonneborn, J., 1985a, Aging in unicellular organisms, in: "Handbook of Biology, 2nd Edition," C. E. Finch and E. L. Schneider, eds., Van Nostrand Press, New York.

Smith-Sonneborn, J., 1985b, Genome interaction in the pathology of aging, in: "Handbook of The Cell Biology of Aging," V. Cristofalo, ed., CRC Press, Boca Raton.

Sonneborn, T. M., 1954, The relation of autogamy to senescence and rejuvenescence in Paramecium aurelia., J. Protozool., 1:38.

Sonneborn, T. M., 1957, Breeding systems, reproductive methods, and species problems in Protozoa, in: "The Species Problem," E. Mayr, ed., American Association of the Advancement of Science, Washington, D.C.

Sonneborn, T. M., 1978, The origin, evolution, nature and causes of aging, in: "The Biology of Ageing," J. M. Behnke, C. E. Finch, and G. B. Moment, eds., Plenum Publishing, New York.

Starr, R. E., 1969, Structure, reproduction and differentiation in Volvox cateri, J. nagariensis lyengar, strains HK9 and 10, Arch. Protistenkd., 111:204.

Sutherland, B. M., Carrier, W. L., and Setlow, R. B., 1968, Photoreactivation in vivo of pyrimidine dimers in Paramecium, Biophys. J., 8:490.

Walford, R. L., and Bergmann, K., 1979, Influence of genes associated with main histocompatibility complex on deoxyribonucleic acid excision repair capacity and bleomycin sensitivity in mouse lymphocytes, Tissue Antigens, 14:336.

Wang, A. H.-J., Quigley, G. J., Kolpak, F. J., Crawford, J. L., Boom, J. H., von, Marel, G. van der, and Rich, A., 1979, Molecular structure of a left-handed double helical DNA fragment at atomic resolution, Nature, Lond., 282:680.

Weise, L., 1976, Genetic aspects of sexuality in Volvocales, in: "The Genetics of Algae," R. A. Lewin, ed., University of California Press, Berkeley.

Weismann, A., 1889, 1891, Essays upon heredity and kindred biological problems, Vol. 1, 1st ed., 1889, 2nd ed., 1891, Clarendon Press, Oxford.

Williams, D. B., 1980, Clonal aging in two species of Spathidium (Ciliophora: Gymnostomatida), J. Protozool., 27:212.

Williams, T., and Smith-Sonneborn, J., 1980, DNA polymerase activity in aged clones of P. tetraurelia, Exp. Gerontol., 15:353.

Witkin, E. M., 1976, Ultraviolet mutagenesis and inducible DNA repair in Escherichia coli, Bact. Rev., 40:869.

Woodhead, A. D., Setlow, R. B., and Grist, E., 1980, DNA repair and longevity in three species of cold-blooded vertebrates, Proc. Nat. Acad. Sci., USA, 15:301.

Yao, M. C., and Gorovsky, M. D., 1974, Comparison of the sequence of macro- and micronuclei on DNA of Tetrahymena pyriformis, Chromosoma, 48:1.

Yao, M. C., and Gall, J. G., 1979, Alteration of the Tetrahymena genome during nuclear differentiation, J. Protozool., 26:10.

THE HEREDITY-ENVIRONMENT CONTINUUM:

A SYSTEMS ANALYSIS

Barbara E. Wright and Margaret H. Butler

Department of Microbiology
University of Montana
Missoula, MT 59812

We hope to make four points in this metabolic and biochemical analysis of the heredity-environment continuum: first, that metabolic transitions such as differentiation and aging result from the interaction of multiple critical or rate-limiting events; second, that it is necessary to understand these complex interactions in vivo in order to have a rational basis for influencing them; third, that such an understanding must involve a dynamic systems analysis; and fourth, that such an analysis is possible with our present knowledge of biochemistry and computer technology.

One metabolic transition which can occur, and may in part be responsible for the aging process in mammals, is the accumulation of cholesterol. This area of metabolism therefore represents a good model for illustrating the kinds of rate-limiting events which could be involved.

Figure 1 summarizes a small fraction of what we know about cholesterol metabolism. All of these events and many more are involved in the synthesis and utilization of cholesterol. The important questions are: which ones are critical, and when, to cholesterol accumulation during the aging process? There are many possibilities; e.g., (1) an increase in the rate of availability of β-hydroxy-β-methylglutaryl-CoA (HMG-CoA) due either to an increased rate of synthesis from acetyl CoA or to a decreased rate of conversion to ketone bodies; (2) an increased rate of mevalonate synthesis due to increased levels of active HMG-CoA reductase, resulting from decreased levels of the phosphorylated kinase which converts it to the inactive form; and (3) a decrease in the rate of cholesterol oxidation or conversion to other metabolites. Enzymes and metabolites involved in reactions which are essential but not unique to cholesterol accumulation are just as important to consider as potential rate-controlling steps; e.g., the enzymes controlling the conversion of glycogen to acetyl CoA, amino acid and ATP availability, and the levels of nucleotides and tRNA.

Many correlations with age have been made with respect to enzyme activities, cholesterol synthesis and catabolism. The effect of diet on enzyme activities and cholesterol levels has also been studied. However, no clear picture has emerged to explain the rise in serum cholesterol

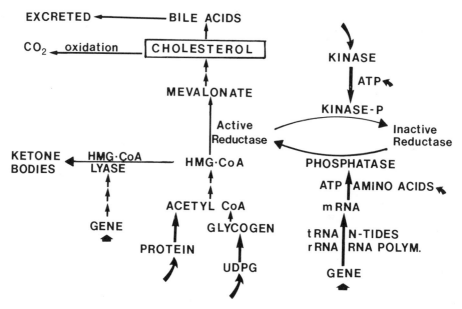

Fig. 1. Some of the reactions involved in cholesterol synthesis
and utilization.

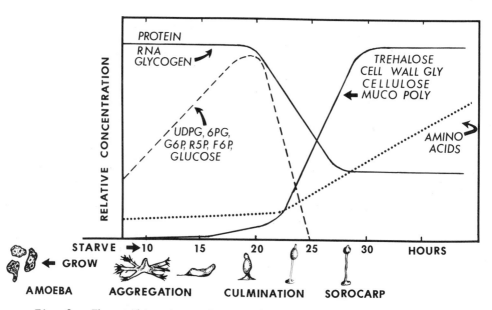

Fig. 2. The utilization and accumulation of carbohydrates during
differentiation and aging in D. discoideum.

levels. This is not surprising in view of the complexity of this metabolic system and the number of critical, interacting variables involved. Not only is this metabolic system intrinsically complex, but a different set of variables may be critical, or rate-controlling, at successive periods during the aging process. This problem might well benefit from a dynamic systems analysis which could be carried out, for example, in young, mature, and old rats. Before discussing a dynamic systems analysis approach, Figure 1 may be used to consider the genetic approach to understanding a problem such as cholesterol accumulation during aging.

Let us consider this area of metabolism in the context of two so-called "longevity" mutants--one that extends, and one that shortens the life span in rats. Let us assume that we have identified the gene product in both of these cases: one is a phosphatase catalyzing the conversion of inactive to active HMG-CoA reductase, and the other is HMG-CoA lyase, catalyzing the conversion of HMG-CoA to ketone bodies. Both mutations partially inactivate the enzyme involved. Decreased phosphatase activity will result in more inactive than active reductase and therefore a lower rate of cholesterol accumulation. This rat will have a longer life-span. Decreased lyase activity, on the other hand, will result in higher levels of HMG-CoA and consequently increased levels of cholesterol. This rat will have a shorter life span. Has the existence of these mutants contributed to our understanding of cholesterol accumulation? We think not. However, they do confirm what our in vitro studies have already told us about the essential role of these two enzymes in this area of metabolism. In other words, to understand why a clock ticks faster or slower when it is dropped, we must know what made it tick in the first place. At best, mutants can confirm which proteins are essential or not essential to cholesterol accumulation. They cannot tell us which gene products control this metabolic transition during the normal aging process. A dynamic systems analysis can provide such information.

Genes which are essential but not unique, like those coding for glycogen phosphorylase or tRNA, are as critical to cholesterol metabolism as the two unique genes indicated above. It should also be noted that the metabolites unique to cholesterol synthesis, like HMG-CoA, as well as those essential but not unique to cholesterol metabolism, like ATP and the amino acids, are as critical as the genes. However, since they are not gene products they cannot be selectively removed by mutation to prove that they are essential. These circumstances tend to bestow an unjustified importance upon genes in controlling metabolic events.

We would now like to apply our dynamic systems analysis in a microbial model system, Dictyostelium discoideum. This work will illustrate the usefulness of such an approach in the discovery of rate-controlling steps which regulate complex metabolic transitions during aging. The fascinating life cycle of this cellular slime mold is depicted along the time axis of Figure 2. In the presence of external nutrients, the organism grows and multiplies as free-living single amoebae. Under starvation conditions, growth ceases and the amoebae aggregate to form a multicelullar colony which differentiates through several distinctive stages to form a sorocarp composed of stalk cells, which die, and spore cells, which will give rise to amoebe under appropriate conditions. During differentiation there is no net loss of carbohydrate. At aggregation most of the carbohydrate material is present as glycogen and RNA-pentose. In the middle of differentiation there occurs a transient accumulation of metabolites such as glucose-6-phosphate (G6P), 6-phosphogluconate (6PG), and UDP-glucose (UDPG). At the end of the aging process there is a decrease in glycogen and RNA and a comparable increase in new polysaccharide end products (trehalose, cellulose-glycogen wall complex and mucopolysaccharide). Protein serves as the energy source in this system, and amino acids accumulate about three-fold at the end of development[1].

As in the case of cholesterol metabolism, the literature documents countless correlates at the enzyme and mRNA level with the process of differentiation and aging in D. discoideum. However, most of these data have not yet been linked mechanistically to events essential to the metabolic changes which occur. Thus, although thousands of proteins and mRNAs change in concentration, very few have been identified as relevant. In fact, it has been estimated that about 90% of these changes are not essential, and a number of mutants lacking specific "developmentally regulated enzymes" differentiate and age normally[2]. Furthermore, among the many enzymes (thus far studied) which are essential to the accumulation of the new carbohydrate end products of development, very few (if any) arise de novo. Some change from an inactive to an active form. Some change from using a soluble to an insoluble substrate, and some change in concentration due to imbalances in their rates of synthesis and degradation. If control were primarily at the level of transcription and translation, it could not be analyzed with the help of kinetic models as the requisite dynamic data are not yet available in these areas of metabolism. Most of the reactions we have studied are primarily controlled by substrate-product-effector interactions. This is fortunate because we can therefore analyze those aspects of metabolism containing the rate-controlling steps of development and aging in this system. Energy metabolism clearly impinges upon the pathways of carbohydrate synthesis as well as upon the integrity and survival of the organism.

As indicated in Figure 2, starvation is an early environmental control essential to differentiation and, as will be shown, the rates of most reactions are limited by substrate availability throughout development. In considering the continuum of time and essential events preceding this differentiation and aging process, there is no one event or type of event which has unique importance. Events occurring during the initial 10 hours of starvation are as critical as those depicted in Figure 2. The composition and characteristics of growing amoebae are equally critical as are those cellular and environmental circumstances involved in the evolution of the amoebae as they are today. Nor is it meaningful to try to specify a particular moment in time when the process of aging begins.

The model in Figure 3 represents energy metabolism and carbohydrate metabolism in spore cells and stalk cells of Dictyostelium[3,4,5,6]. There are a great many inter-dependent pathways in this complex network. Ninety percent of the parameters composing this model are experimental data. These data are of four kinds: first, evidence for the existence of all the reactions and metabolic compartments indicated in this biochemical network; second, the concentrations over the course of differentiation and aging of all the metabolites shown; third, reaction rates or fluxes determined in vivo with isotope tracers (all of the reactions depicted by solid arrows have been so determined); and fourth, enzyme kinetic mechanisms and constants (all enzymes catalyzing the numbered reactions which are encircled have been purified and kinetically characterized). The model integrates and simulates approximately 45 established reactions and flux patterns, 100 metabolite accumulation profiles for normal and perturbed differentiation, 20 enzyme mechanisms,

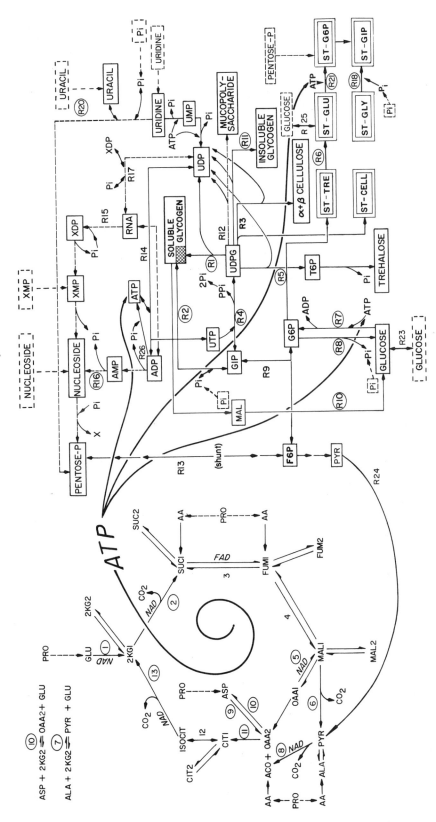

Fig. 3 A kinetic model of energy and carbohydrate metabolism in D. discoideum. See text for details.

and 60 kinetic constants. The differential equations describing each
reaction are solved simultaneously, and output from the model consists of
reaction rates and metabolite concentrations as a function of time. This
output must be consistent with experimental data obtained during the
differentiation and aging process. The double boxes represent
metabolites in stalk cells which become very permeable as they are dying
but still retain a vestigial type of metabolism. The broken boxes on the
edges of the model represent exogenous metabolites with which the
organism and the model have been perturbed to test the model under new
conditions. The thicker the web of interdependent pathways, the more
constrained and stronger the model becomes.

Enzyme activities as a function of time are input to the model.
They are calculated as the only unknown in each reaction because of the
poor correlation between enzyme activity determined in vitro and activity
in vivo. Consider the following simple initial velocity rate expression:

$$\text{Rate} = V = V_{max} \ (A/(Ka+A))$$

$$V = Vv(t) \ (A/(Ka+A))$$

Knowing V, A and Ka, we calculate Vmax and call it Vv. Since Vv can
change with time during a metabolic transition we call the expression
Vv(t) an "enzyme activation function."

The preparation of cell extracts destroys cellular organization and
creates various artifacts. Enzyme activity is then measured under non-
physiological conditions of pH and protein concentration as well as in
the absence of products and effectors which may modify enzyme activity in
vivo. For all these reasons, the conditions under which enzyme activity
is determined in vitro may have little relevance to circumstances
existing in vivo. By contrast, the other factors in an enzyme kinetic
expression (e.g. flux determined in vivo and kinetic constants) are
relatively reliable data to use as input for a kinetic model purporting
to simulate metabolism in vivo. Therefore, for each reaction in our
models of metabolism in vivo, we have experimentally determined the
cellular levels of substrates, products and effectors, the relative sizes
of metabolic compartments, the velocity of the reaction with isotope
tracers, and the enzyme kinetic mechanism and constants. The value which
will represent V_{max}, is then calculated as the only unknown in the
appropriate enzyme kinetic expression.

We believe this model does in fact reflect many aspects of
metabolism in vivo because predictive value has frequently been
demonstrated. This, of course, is the ultimate test of any model. Of
the many predictions made thus far, about 35, or 90% of those tested,
have been substantiated. These predictions have been concerned with the
flux and turnover of metabolites in vivo, the activity patterns of
enzymes both in vivo and in vitro, the kinetic mechanisms and constants
of specific reactions, the presence of enzyme inhibition in vivo, the
effects of external metabolites or altered enzyme activities on
respiration or on metabolite accumulation patterns, permeability
patterns, intra- and inter-cellular compartmentation of metabolites and
of enzymes[2,5,6]. Some of the predictions have been substantiated
unknowingly in other laboratories; for example, the existence of two
metabolic pools of glucose and the effect of glycogen phosphorylase
activity on the concentrations of trehalose, cellulose, G6P and UDPG[1].

In the model, reaction rates controlled in part by substrate-product-effector levels are those in which the levels of the metabolites are below the Km values of the relevant enzymes. Many of these relationships (which are also predictions based on in vitro kinetic constants and metabolite levels from tracer studies[2,6]) have been confirmed by perturbing the system with exogenous rate-limiting or inhibiting metabolites and measuring the resultant changes in levels of the intermediate and end products. As an illustration of the complex relationships involved, the level of UDPG is simultaneously controlled by the activity of UDPG pyrophosphorylase, the concentration and rate of availability of UTP and especially G1P, the inhibition of the enzyme by UDPG (an inhibitor at cellular levels), and the activity of six enzymes competing for UDPG. These predicted relationships can be substantiated by changing enzyme activities and the rate of G1P availability in the model as well as by perturbation experiments with exogenous glucose. To summarize, rate-controlling metabolites and enzymes are discovered through a combination of studies to determine enzyme kinetic mechanisms and constants, measure cellular metabolite levels, determine flux and metabolic compartments in vivo with (^{14}C)-tracer analyses, perturb the organism and model with external metabolites and fluxes, and to alter enzyme mechanisms, activities, and kinetic constants in the model to determine those conditions most compatible with the data. In Figure 3, there are more than 160 enzymes, substrates, products, and allosteric effectors controlling the rates of the reactions depicted.

The model simulates the rate of turnover and net utilization or accumulation of all the metabolites shown. Although the rates of turnover of average protein[7], UDPG pyrophosphorylase[8] and glycogen phosphorylase[9] are known, these cannot be modelled until dynamic data are available pertaining to the mechanisms involved.

This model simulates the period of time (900 min) between aggregation and sorocarp formation. In the future, data may justify extension of the model to include aging of the mature sorocarps or extension backwards in time to simulate the 10 hour period between the cessation of growth and aggregation of the amoebae. As we are currently involved in finalizing the model of the citric acid cycle, the rest of this presentation will deal with specific aspects of energy metabolism.

As mentioned, total carbohydrate levels remain constant during development. However, about 50% of the cellular protein in amoebae is degraded over the course of differentiation and aging in this system (Figure 2). An amino acid analysis of Dictyostelium protein was carried out at three stages: aggregation, culmination, and sorocarp. The results are given in Table I. The percent concentration of each amino acid in average protein is given. The similarities of these values at the three stages indicates an "even" use of the available protein; i.e., comparable oxidation rates of individual amino acids during development and aging. Knowing the pathways by which each amino acid is converted to one or more citric acid cycle intermediate(s)[12], the flux of each amino acid into specific intermediates can be calculated (see Figure 4). Total flux into the cycle must equal approximately 0.5 umoles/min/ml packed cell volume (pcv) since this is the cycle flux based on O_2 consumption, net protein degradation, or NH_3 production. In a system using only amino acids as the source of cycle intermediates, more amino acids are converted to four- and five-carbon intermediates than to acetyl-CoA. For the citrate synthase reaction to operate and maintain steady state levels of cycle intermediates, the flux of acetyl-CoA into the cycle must equal that of oxaloacetate. Therefore a pathway is required which converts "excess" four- or five-carbon intermediates to acetyl-CoA.

Table I. Amino Acid Analysis of Cellular Protein During Aging and the
TCA Cycle Intermediates to Which They are Converted

TCA Intermediate(s)	Amino Acid	Percent of Total Protein		
		Aggregation	Culmination	Sorocarp
Pyruvate	Alanine	6.88	6.75	6.71
α–Ketoglutarate	Arginine	4.18	4.19	4.25
Oxaloacetate	Aspartate/			
	Asparagine	11.50	11.72	11.90
Pyruvate	Cysteine	1.37	1.34	1.33
α–Ketoglutarate	Glutamate/			
	Glutamine	10.67	10.72	10.44
Pyruvate	Glycine	7.36	7.18	7.26
α–Ketoglutararte	Histidine	1.95	1.92	1.92
Succinate, Acetyl CoA	Isoleucine	6.33	6.78	6.17
Acetyl CoA	Leucine	8.23	8.14	7.99
Acetyl CoA	Lysine	7.77	7.81	7.80
Succinate	Methionine	1.22	1.95	1.93
Fumarate, Acetyl CoA	Phenylalanine	4.75	4.39	4.56
α–Ketoglutarate	Proline	3.77	3.99	4.05
Pyruvate	Serine	7.15	7.14	7.14
Succinate	Threonine	5.99	5.97	6.05
Acetyl CoA	Tryptophan	0.00	0.00	0.00
Fumarate, Acetyl CoA	Tyrosine	3.72	3.62	3.63
Succinate	Valine	7.13	6.87	6.86

The pathway for converting citric acid cycle intermediates to
acetyl-CoA involves malic enzyme. In this reaction, malate is
decarboxylated to yield pyruvate which is in turn decarboxylated to form
acetyl-CoA via the pyruvate dehydrogenase complex (PDHC). This pathway
has been shown to occur in Dictyostelium, and both of these enzymes have
been purified and kinetically characterized[10,13].

Malic enzyme was shown to be allosteric, being positively affected
by aspartate, glutamate, succinate, and fumarate. Thus, amino acid
production from protein degradation stimulates a reaction essential to
their efficient utilization for energy. The PDHC was shown to proceed
via a multi-site ping pong kinetic mechanism. No effectors were found
that significantly altered the activity of PDHC; however, the products
AcCoA and NADH were inhibitory, indicating that the ratios of
(AcCoA)/(CoA) and (NADH)/(NAD) found in the cell are important to this
reaction.

Knowing the essential role of malic enzyme and PDHC in this system,
knowing the cycle flux and the fluxes into the cycle from amino acids,
the flux map in Fig. 4 emerges. The relative concentrations of
intramitochondrial and extramitochondrial pools (labeled 1 and 2,
respectively) and the fluxes between them were determined from a specific
radioactivity tracer analysis of this system under steady state
conditions[3,4]. Since pyruvate is formed at a rate of 0.09 mM/min (based
on pcv) from amino acids, it must be formed at the rate of 0.218 mM/min
from malate. In vitro the rate of the reaction catalyzed by malic enzyme

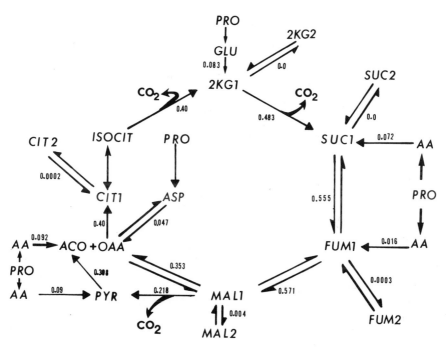

Fig. 4. A flux map of the citric acid cycle in D. discoideum.
See text for details.

was examined in crude cell extracts and estimated to be 0.86 mM/min, or 4 times that required based on this flux map (Figure 4). Thus, the activity of malic enzyme does not appear to be rate limiting to cycle flux, if one considers the in vitro determination as being valid.

As indicated in Figure 4, acetyl-CoA must be formed at the rate of 0.308 mM/min from pyruvate in order to equal the rate at which oxaloacetate is formed (0.4 mM/min). In vitro studies estimated the rate of the reaction to be 0.5 mM/min in crude extracts (or 1.7 times that required based on the flux map). Significantly, the reaction in crude extracts was completely dependent upon CoA, NAD, and thiamine pyrophosphate, suggesting that pyruvate was converted to CO_2 only via the reaction catalyzed by PDHC. The relatively low in vitro activity of PDHC when compared to other enzymes in the citric acid cycle suggested that PDHC may play a rate-limiting role to cycle flux. It was therefore of interest to examine the rate of this reaction in vivo. Cells were exposed to tracer $(1-^{14}C)$ alanine, and at various time intervals cellular (^{14}C)-pyruvate was isolated and its specific radioactivity determined. With this information and the rate of $^{14}CO_2$ production the rate in vivo of this reaction was estimated to be 0.33 µmoles/min/ml pcv which is remarkably close to the value of 0.308 calculated completely independently for the flux map of the citric acid cycle (Figure 4). This agreement is a convincing confirmation of the flux of this reaction in vivo.

The rate equation expressing the kinetic mechanism for PDHC used in the model is shown in Figure 5. Knowing the reaction rate (V), the kinetic constants, and the relevant substrate and product concentrations, the enzyme activity Vv may be calculated. A value of 83 mM/min was obtained: two orders of magnitude greater than the activity of the enzyme in vitro (0.5 mM/min) as determined in the crude cell extracts. This discrepancy suggests at least two possible explanations: (1) only 0.6% of the enzyme complex existing in vivo was recovered in vitro, or (2) one or more of the parameter values used in the calculation were incorrect. Because of the stability of the enzyme, and its behavior during purification, it seems unlikely that such a small fraction was recovered in vitro and therefore the second possiblity is more likely. As discussed previously, we assume that enzyme kinetic mechanisms and constants are reliable data for use in a model. The mitochondrial pyruvate and acetyl CoA concentrations were determined by tracer analysis[3,4] and are also considered to be reliable. The most suspect values are the CoA, NAD and NADH concentrations used in the calculation. As mitochondrial levels are not yet available, cellular levels were used. If the NAD level in the model is raised to its Km value, the calculated Vv value falls to 16 (Fig. 5). Further experimentation may clarify the basis for the differences between the in vitro and calculated in vivo enzyme activities, and hopefully will eventually provide a convincing picture of the circumstances and rate-limiting steps operative in the intact cell.

Having considered this kind of in-depth analysis in the energy metabolism of Dictyostelium, let us return for a moment to cholesterol metabolism (Figure 1). Perhaps energy metabolism, which is not unique to cholesterol synthesis, is the most important factor controlling its accumulation. Starvation is known to have a striking positive effect on longevity in rats, and ATP is critical in the interconversion of the active and inactive reductase. Under conditions of nutritional stress, levels of acetyl CoA may be limited due to the demands of pathways more essential to viability. Hence, cholesterol accumulation suffers, resulting in an increased life span.

$$V = \frac{V_v (PYR)(CoA)(NAD)}{\begin{aligned}&(KmNAD)(PYR)(CoA) + (KmCoA)(PYR)(NAD) + (KmPYR)(CoA)(NAD) + (PYR)(CoA)(NAD)\\&+ (KmPYR)(KiCoA)(KiNAD)(KmCO_2)(AcCoA)(NADH) / (KiAcCoA)(KmNADH)(KiCO_2)\\&+ (KmNAD)(PYR)(CoA)(NADH) / (KiNADH) + (KmCoA)(PYR)(NAD)(AcCoA) / (KiAcCoA)\\&+ (KmPYR)(KiCoA)(KiNAD)(KmCO_2)(PYR)(AcCoA)(NADH) / (KiPYR)(KiAcCoA)(KmNADH)(KiCO_2)\end{aligned}}$$

(cellular NAD level) MODEL V_v	= 83	mM/min pcv
(5X cellular NAD level at Km) MODEL V_v	= 16	mM/min pcv
in vitro activity	= 0.5	mM/min pcv

Fig. 5. The pyruvate dehydrogenase mechanism, and calculated enzyme activity values.

We believe that differentiation and aging result from a complex
interaction of many cellular components, structures, and environmental
influences. An explanation of the aging process must be sought at a
similar level of complexity. This requires an integrative systems
analysis. The organism ages as a whole and must therefore be analyzed as
a dynamic, in vivo system. Only after the system has been described at a
realistic level of complexity can we begin to unravel the critical and
multiple rate-controlling steps involved. At that point, we will have a
rational basis for influencing the process.

Acknowledgement: This work was supported by the Public Health Service
Grant AG03884 from the National Institutes of Health.

References

1. B. E. Wright and P. J. Kelly, Kinetic models of metabolism in intact
   cells, tissues and organisms, Curr. Topics Cell. Reg. 19:103-158
   B. Horecker and E. Stadtman, eds., Academic Press, New York,
   (1981).
2. D. J. Watts, Protein synthesis during development and
   differentiation in the cellular slime mold Dictyostelium
   discoideum, Biochem. J. 220:1-14 (1984).
3. P. J. Kelly, J. K. Kelleher, and B. E. Wright, The Tricarboxylic
   acid cycle in Dictyostelium discoideum. Metabolite
   concentrations, oxygen uptake and ^{14}C-amino acid labeling
   patterns, Biochem. J. 184:581-588 (1979).
4. P. J. Kelly, J. K. Kelleher, and B. E. Wright, The tricarboxylic
   acid cycle in Dictyostelium discoideum. A model of the cycle at
   preculmination and aggregation, Biochem. J. 184:589-597 (1979).
5. B. E. Wright, D. A. Thomas, and D. J. Ingalls, Metabolic compartments
   in Dictyostelium discoideum, J. Biol. Chem. 257:7587-7594 (1982).
6. Y. Y. Chiew, J. M. Reimers, and B. E. Wright, Steady state models of
   spore cell metabolism in Dictyostelium discoideum, J. Biol. Chem.
   260:15325-15331 (1985).
7. B. E. Wright and M. L. Anderson, Protein and amino acid turnover
   during differentiation in the slime mold. II. Incorporation of
   ^{35}S methionine into the amino acid pool and into protein,
   Biochem. Biophys. Acta 43:67-78 (1960).
8. G. L. Gustafson, W. Y. Kong, and B. E. Wright, Analysis of uridine
   diphosphate-glucose pyrophosphorylase synthesis during
   differentation in Dictyostelium discoideum, J. Biol. Chem.
   248:5188-5196 (1973).
9. D. A. Thomas and B. E. Wright, Glycogen phosphorylase in
   Dictyostelium discoideum. II. Synthesis and degradation during
   differentiation, J. Biol. Chem. 251:1258-1263 (1976).
10. J. K. Kelleher, P. J. Kelly, and B. E. Wright, Amino acid catabolism
    and malic enzyme in differentiating Dictyostelium discoideum,
    J. Bacteriol. 138:467-474 (1979).
11. J. U. Liddel and B. E. Wright, The effect of glucose on respiration
    of the differentiating slime mold, Devel. Biol. 3:265-276 (1961).
12. T. N. Palmer and M. C. Sugden, The stochiometry of the citric acid
    cycle, Trends Biochem. Sci. 8:161-162 (1983).
13. M. H. Butler, G. P. Mell, and B. E. Wright, The pyruvate
    dehydrogenase complex in Dictyostelium discoideum, Curr. Topics
    Cell. Reg. 26:337-346 (1985).
14. M. Satre and J. Martin, ^{31}P-nuclear magnetic resonance analysis of
    the intracellular pH in the slime mold Dictyostelium discoideum,
    Biochem. and Biophys. Res. Comm. 132:140-146 (1985).

THE PROXIMATE AND ULTIMATE CONTROL OF AGING IN <u>DROSOPHILA</u> AND HUMANS

Alan R. Templeton[1], J. Spencer Johnston[2] and Charles F. Sing[3]

[1]Department of Biology, Washington University, St. Louis, MO 63301; [2]Department of Entomology, Texas A&M University College Station, Texas 77843-2475; and [3]Department of Human Genetics, University of Michigan, Ann Arbor, MI 48109-0618

Debates concerning the relative merits of reductionistic versus holistic approaches are commonplace in biology, and aging research is no exception. Although such debates commonly dwell on the issue of which approach is "superior," it is far more fruitful to acknowledge that both approaches offer unique perspectives on aging, and hence these approaches are complementary rather than antagonistic. There are three basic levels of control of aging: 1) the proximate causes leading to aging in particular cell lines or tissues, 2) the regulatory processes that integrate the cell and tissue specific patterns into an individual life history, and 3) the evolutionary forces (ultimate causes) that select upon life history traits to determine the characteristic aging pattern of the species or population. To understand the control of aging at all of these levels, or even just the first two, requires the simultaneous use of reductionistic and holistic studies.

The central thesis of this paper is that modern genetics provides a tool that makes an integrated holistic/reductionistic research program feasible. Before elaborating this thesis, we must first make some general comments concerning the genetics of aging. Our primary assumption is that there is no such thing as a gene for aging. Rather, there are genes that control a variety of biological functions, and aging effects occur as a secondary effect or consequence of their primary biological functions. This assumption arises from theoretical studies on the ultimate, evolutionary causes of aging. In most evolutionary models of aging, senescence is not regarded as being directly adaptive. Rather, senescence arises as an indirect consequence of other evolutionary phenomena. For example, the two most common models for the evolution of senescence are 1) that late acting deleterious mutations will accumulate precisely because their senescent effects have minimal impact on fitness (Medawar, 1957), and 2) that senscence arises because selection favors some gene with beneficial effects early in life, but that as a pleiotropic consequence, reduces fitness later in life (Williams, 1957). Thus, we should not be searching for a special category of "aging genes." Rather, we should focus on the aging effects associated with genes controlling a variety of biochemical, physiological, and developmental functions.

We already have an extensive, albeit incomplete, store of knowledge concerning the genetic control of many basic biochemical, physiological and developmental processes. Recent advances in molecular genetics are making it easier to study genes that control specific functions. The basic research program that will be illustrated in this paper is as follows. By studying the phenotypic effects (including aging effects) of an inherited syndrome, it is often possible to use the accumulated background knowledge to identify a class of candidate loci that are likely to be involved in the direct control of the phenotypic effects being investigated. Recombinant DNA techniques then can be used to study genetic variation at the candidate loci. Next, one can directly test for associations between the genetic variation detectable at the molecular level with the phenotypic effects observed at the biochemical, physiological, or developmental levels. If relevant genetic variation is discovered at this step, the research program can be extended to the population and ecological levels to study the evolutionary or adaptive significance of the relevant genetic variation. In this manner, both the proximate and ultimate causes of aging effects can be studied in a research program that integrates reductionistic and holistic approaches. In this paper, we will present two examples of such integrated research programs: one dealing with _Drosophila_ and one with humans.

ABNORMAL ABDOMEN IN DROSOPHILA MERCATORUM

Natural populations of _Drosophila_ _mercatorum_ from the Island of Hawaii are polymorphic for a trait known as abnormal abdomen (_aa_) (Templeton and Rankin, 1978). As the name implies, the trait can be recognized from morphological effects. Flies with _aa_ tend to retain juvenile abdominal cuticle as adults, resulting in a disruption of the normal pigmentation, segmentation, and bristle patterns on the adult abdomen. However, the morphological effects are not very penetrant, and under field conditions are rarely expressed. More importantly, _aa_ has many effects on aging in both the larval and adult phases (Templeton, 1982, 1983). In particular, _aa_ prolongs the larval developmental stage by up 40%, but speeds up adult reproductive maturity to 2 days after eclosion versus about 4 to 5 days in most non-_aa_ flies. These early maturing female flies also have increased ovarian output, but greatly decreased longevity under laboratory conditions. These morphological and life history effects are all temperature dependent, with higher temperatures accentuating the disparity between _aa_ and non-_aa_ lines.

This suite of temperature dependent phenotypes resembles similar suites of phenotypic effects in _Drosophila melanogaster_ that are associated with the bobbed syndrome. Fortunately, the molecular basis of the bobbed phenotypic syndrome is known; it is a deficiency in the number of 18S/28S ribosomal genes (Ritossa et al., 1966). In most _Drosophila_ species, the 18S/28S ribosomal genes exist as tandemly duplicated clusters on the X and Y chromosomes. Each duplicated unit consists of an 18S gene, a transcribed spacer, a 28S gene, and a non-transcribed spacer. About 200 to 250 copies of this basic unit are normally found on the X chromosome. Hence, the phenotypes associated with the _aa_ syndrome suggested that the 18S/28S rDNA cluster would be a reasonable candidate set of loci. This hypothesis was strengthened by Mendelian genetic studies that revealed that the _aa_ syndrome is controlled by two closely linked X-linked elements that map very near the centromere -- the same physical location of the rDNA cluster (Templeton et al.,1985). Moreover, _aa_ expression is normally limited to females, but male expression is Y-linked (Templeton et al.,1985). The Y chromosome has very few genes, but as noted earlier it does have a rDNA cluster. Hence, the phenotypic and Mendelian genetic studies strongly suggest that the underlying molecular cause of aa lies in the ribosomal DNA.

We therefore began investigating the molecular biology of rDNA in D. mercatorum and relating our findings to the presence or absence of aa. This work was facilitated by spontaneous mutations both to and from aa. Since this work has already been published (DeSalle et al.,1986; DeSalle and Templeton, 1986), we will only present the conclusions here. First, aa flies have normal to slightly more rDNA in the germline than non-aa flies. Hence, aa is not the molecular equivalent of bobbed, which represents a numerical, germline reduction in the amount of rDNA. However, diploid somatic cells of aa flies display increased levels of rDNA relative to the diploid somatic cells of non-aa flies. This increase is known as compensatory response and is normally found only in bobbed flies. Hence, although aa flies had plenty of germline rDNA, their diploid somatic cells were behaving as if there were a deficiency of rDNA.

Since the quantity of rDNA was normal, we investigated the qualitative nature of the rDNA present in aa flies through restriction endonuclease mapping. We discovered that all aa flies have at least a third of their X-linked 28S genes interrupted by a 5 kilobase insertion. This insert has a transposon-like structure, with long direct repeats on the ends and with 14 base pair long inverted terminal repeats at the ends of the direct repeats. However, there is no evidence for this element transposing in the present population. All copies seem to be confined to the X-linked rDNA. Northern analyses indicate that the insert disrupts normal transcription of the 18S/28S unit in which it is imbedded. Hence, this insert creates a functional deficiency of rDNA, although there is no quantitative deficiency of rDNA.

Further studies (DeSalle and Templeton, 1986) reveal that the presence of many inserted 28S genes is necessary but not sufficient for the expression of aa. The other necessary element for aa expression involves the control of under-replication of rDNA in the formation of polytene tissues (DeSalle and Templeton, 1986). The process of polytenization in Drosophila involves many rounds of endoreplication of nuclear DNA in certain somatic lineages (such as larval salivary glands and fat bodies). Hence, in general, the DNA of the fly is greatly over-replicated in these cells. However, there is heterogeneity within the genome in the amount of over-replication. In general, the rDNA is under-replicated relative to most single copy DNA during the process of polytenization. We discovered an X-linked genetic system that causes the preferential under-replication of inserted 18S/28S units. Hence, even if a fly has a large number of inserted 28S genes, compensatory response circumvents this functional deficiency in diploid, somatic cell lineages, and preferential under-replication of inserted 28S genes circumvents this functional deficiency in polytene, somatic cell lineages. Thus, the expression of aa requires two molecular events; 1) a third or more of the 28S genes must bear the insert, and 2) there must be no preferential under-replication of inserted 28S genes during the formation of polytene tissue. When these two molecular requirements are satisfied, a functional deficiency of ribosomal DNA can be induced in polytene tissues, thereby explaining the bobbed-like suite of phenotypic effects.

A ribosomal deficiency in critical larval tissues such as the fat body would be expected to slow down protein synthesis in general, and hence explain the overall slowdown in larval development. Moreoever, the proteins most effected by a ribosomal deficiency would be those that are normally synthesized very rapidly over a short developmental time period. One such protein is juvenile hormone esterase, a protein made by the larval fatbody that degrades juvenile hormone. This protein is usually made at the end of the larval period. The abdominal histoblasts are very sensitive to juvenile hormone titers in the pre-pupal and early pupal stages, and phenocopies of abnormal abdomen can be induced by topical application of juvenile hormone at this time (Templeton and Rankin, 1978). Studies on aa flies reveal a deficiency of juvenile hormone esterase during this critical time period (Templeton and Rankin, 1978); thereby providing a straightforward explanation for the morphological effects of aa. Polytene tissues are not as important in the adult, so no general slowdown in adult development is expected. However, the alterations in juvenile hormone metabolism induced by aa may explain the alterations in adult life history because juvenile hormone stimulates the production of egg specific proteins and ovarian maturation and output (Wilson et al.,1983). This hypothesis is currently being investigated.

We have now defined the molecular basis of aa and the effects this syndrome has on individual life history. To understand the ultimate causes of why this aging syndrome is polymorphic in natural populations, we must now turn to field studies. Our primary field site is located in the Kohala Mountains on the Island of Hawaii. This site was chosen for several reasons. First, the only repleta group Drosophila inhabiting this site are D. mercatorum and D. hydei, which are readily distinquishable. Hence, problems with sibling species that occur in mainland locations are avoided. Second, unlike the mainland, D. mercatorum has only one host plant in Hawaii, the cactus Opuntia megacantha. Thus, only one larval environment needs to be characterized and collecting sites for adults are readily identified and located. Third, the Kohala Mountains have an extremely steep rainfall gradient. This provides environmental diversity needed to uncover the selective importance of the aa syndrome. Fourth, the trade winds blow very strongly in this locality, and these winds greatly limit the opportunity for dispersal between cactus patches (Johnston and Templeton, 1982). Hence, if the environmental diversity does create selective differences in aa, the limited dispersal insures that local differences in the frequency of aa should evolve that reflect these selective differences.

Before studying the ultimate significance of the aging effects of aa in natural populations, it is first necessary to measure the age structure in nature and to discover the primary sources of adult mortality. Our previous work (Johnston and Templeton, 1982) indicates that one of the primary determinants of mortality in adult Drosophila is desiccation. We are able to determine the age of wild-caught adults (in days from eclosion) up to about 2 weeks of age by using the techniques described in Johnston and Ellison (1982). During normal weather years, when the top of the mountain is very humid and the bottom very dry, we observe dramatic shifts in age structure as a function of elevation (Johnston and Templeton, 1982). In the humid regions, flies are so long-lived, that most are too old to be reliably scored (i.e., greater than 2 weeks of age). As one descends into drier habitats, the age structure shifts towards younger flies such that at the bottom virtually all adult flies are less than one week old. Capture/recapture studies confirm this pattern. Under dry conditions, the daily mortality of adult flies is estimated to be 19% per day, which is consistent with very few flies living more than a week (Templeton and Johnston, 1982). In constrast, no detectable mortality over a three day period could be detected under the more humid conditions.

These results on the age structure of natural populations as a function of humidity have several important implications concerning the predicted fitness effects of the aa aging phenotypes. Under low humidity conditions, the decreased innate longevity of aa flies is virtually irrelevant because almost all flies are dead from desiccation long before these innate differences should have an impact. However, earlier sexual maturation and increased egg-laying capacity give aa flies a fecundity advantage over non-aa flies under desiccating conditions (Templeton and Johnston, 1982). As the humidity increases and the age structure of the population shifts towards older individuals, the early fecundity advantage of aa flies should be counteracted or even reversed by their decreased longevity relative to non-aa flies (Templeton and Johnston, 1982).

These predictions can be tested by taking advantage of the natural variation in humidity that occurs over space and time. As shown in Figure 1, a transect of study sites was established on the leeward side of the Kohala mountains, going from the upper elevational limits of the D. mercatorum range (site A, 1030 meters above sea level) to the lower elevational limit on the transect (site F, 795 m above sea level). In addition, a site at the base of Kohala, in the saddle between Kohala and the volcano Mauna Kea, was also studied (site IV, 670 m above sea level). In normal weather years (i.e., years close to the long term average in rainfall, and with humid conditions at the top of the mountain and dry at the bottom), the above fitness considerations lead to the prediction of a cline in the frequency of aa, with aa being more common at the bottom of the hill and rarer at the top. Moreover, the frequencies of aa at both sites F and IV should be high because the humidity at these sites is normally very similar and low. Table 1 presents the data on the frequency of X chromosomes that allow the expression of aa. As can be seen, in 1980 (a normal weather year), there is a statistically significant difference in the frequency of aa, with only about 25% of the X chromosomes supporting aa near the top of the hill, and almost 50% of the X's being aa at the bottom (Templeton and Johnston, 1982).

In 1981, the Island of Hawaii suffered a severe drought, and the humidity ecotone disappeared that year. It was dry throughout the entire range, and the age structure cline also disappeared, with almost all individuals being less than a week of age irrespective of their site of capture (Templeton and Johnston, 1982). The model now predicts that the cline in aa frequency should disappear, and in particular, that there should be an overall increase of aa frequencies at the high elevation sites to the frequencies normally seen at the lower elevations. As can be seen from Table 1, this is precisely what happened. There are now no significant differences in aa frequency between sites, and these frequencies are not significantly different from the low elevation frequencies of 1980 but are significantly different from the high elevation frequencies of 1980 (Templeton and Johnston, 1982).

Early in 1982, the El Chichon Volcano had an explosive eruption in Mexico. The resulting debris cloud reduced the incidence of solar radiation by 10% that spring in Hawaii. This apparently triggered one of the wettest, most humid springs and early summers in Hawaiian history. Once again, the humidity ecotone did not exist, but this time it was humid both at the top and bottom of the mountain. The aa-fitness theory of Templeton and Johnston (1982) predicts no cline in aa frequencies, but unlike 1981, the frequencies should now be low at all sites (around 25%). This is exactly what happened (Table 1). As in 1981, there are no significant differences in aa frequencies between

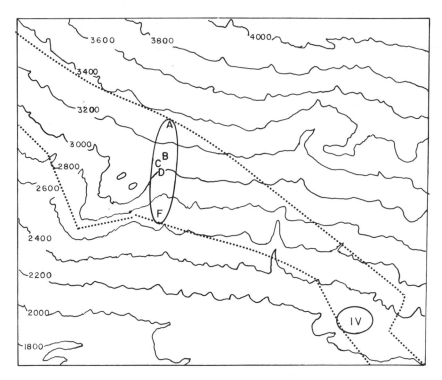

Fig. 1. Study sites on the leeward side of the Kohala mountains on the
         Island of Hawaii. The dotted line encloses the range of the
         cactus Opuntia megacantha, the host plant for D. mercatorum.
         Sites A through F represent a transect through the altitudinal
         range of the host plant on the side of Kohala. The contour lines
         indicate the altitude in feet above sea level. The distance
         between sites A and F is about two-thirds of a mile. An
         additional site, site IV, was established at the base of Kohala,
         in the saddle between Kohala and Mauna Kea.

Table 1. Changes in the Frequency of X-Chromosomes Allowing Expression
          of Abnormal Abdomen in Drosophila mercatorum as a Function of
          Site Location and Temporal Fluctuations in Weather

Year: Weather:		1980 Normal	1981 Drought	1982 Humid	1984 Normal[*]	1985 Normal[*]
Site	Altitude	Frequency of Abnormal Abdomen X-Chromosomes				
A	1030 m	-	-	0.285	0.111	0.222
B	950 m	0.275	0.486	0.250	0.291	0.265
C&D	920 m	-	0.380	0.213	0.334	0.429
F	795 m	-	0.406	-	0.540	0.367
IV	670 m	0.455	0.438	0.325	0.360	0.276

[*]Site IV was unusually humid due to an alteration in wind patterns.

128

sites, but unlike 1981, the aa frequencies are now significantly different from the 1980 low elevation frequencies (and the 1981 frequencies) and not significantly different from the 1980 high elevation frequencies.

In 1984 and 1985, the weather had reverted to an almost normal pattern. The one exception was the local humidity conditions at site IV. Sites A through F are located well on the side of Kohala, but site IV is located at the base of Kohala, in the saddle between Kohala and the volcano Mauna Kea. Usually, the trade winds blow humid air through the saddle, but shear off before reaching site IV. Hence, normally site IV is quite dry and has a similar humidity to site F. However, starting in 1984 and continuing into 1985, the winds blew further through the saddle, causing site IV to become much more humid than previously. As can be seen from Table 1, the expected cline in aa frequency was re-established in 1984 and 1985, with aa X chromosomes being rarer at the top and becoming increasingly common towards the bottom. The exception to this pattern was site IV, which had significantly lower aa frequencies than site F but which had frequencies homogeneous to the high altitude site B.

The abnormal abdomen system tracks the spatial and temporal heterogeneity in the natural environment in the manner predicted by the models given in Templeton and Johnston (1982). Therefore, we conclude that the ultimate causes that maintain this polymorhic aging syndrome relate to its adaptive advantages in the demographic environment imposed by desiccating environments. Note that aa does not represent a direct adaptation to desiccation itself, but rather it is favored because the early maturation and fecundity of aa females confers a fitness advantage under the age structure imposed by desiccation. Moreover, under this age structure, the decreased longevity of the aa flies has very little fitness impact. Hence, the abnormal abdomen complex provides an excellent example of Williams' (1957) "trade-off" model for the evolution of senescence that was mentioned earlier.

The above inferences are possible because the measured genotype approach allowed us to follow the evolutionary fate over space and time of specific genetic variants for which we had generated a priori evolutionary predictions based upon our knowledge of the variant's phenotypic significance. The measured genotype approach to the aa syndrome also clearly illustrates how reductionistic molecular studies can be integrated with holistic individual-level and ecological studies to simultaneously investigate both the proximate and ultimate causes of aging.

CHOLESTEROL METABOLISM IN HUMANS

We will now show how this same basic approach can be applied to a very different organism: the human. A primary determinant of longevity in humans in industrialized societies is well known: coronary heart disease. In the United States, coronary heart disease is responsible for 30% of all deaths and is by far the leading cause of death (Fiscal Year 1983 Fact Book, National Heart, Lung, and Blood Institute, NIH). Thus, the major phenotype associated with longevity in our society has already been identified. Moreover, this phenotype is definitely associated with a senescent process because the best predictor of coronary heart disease risk is age. In order to implement the research program outlined in the introduction, we need to identify candidate gene loci that may contribute to the development of coronary heart disease.

A number of genetic factors that determine the predisposition to develop heart disease have been identified. One is gender.

Epidemiological studies have identified sex as the second most important predictor of risk, with males being at higher risk than females. In this paper, we will focus on the third most important predictor of risk: serum cholesterol levels. There is an almost fourfold increase in the rate of coronary heart disease for males between 30 to 59 years of age with cholesterol levels higher than 300 mg/dl compared to the rates in males with cholesterol levels less than 175 mg/dl (Dawber, 1980). The lipid infiltration theory explains this association and has much supporting evidence (Sing et al., 1985). It is hypothesized that plasma cholesterol infiltrates the intima of the arterial wall following endothelial injury from high blood pressure, anoxia from smoking, or other trauma. Proliferation of cells in the injured region, accompanied by the accumulation of cholesterol esters, results in the development of a fatty plaque. Growth of this plaque in a major artery may eventually cause an occulsion that results in the restriction of oxygen and nutrition to the muscle of the heart.

Detailed studies of how cholesterol is involved in this process have focused upon cholesterol metabolism and the lipoprotein molecules that transport cholesterol in the blood stream. Lipids enter through the intestine primarily in the form of triglycerides. Since oil and water do not mix, the lipids must be solubilized before they can be transported via the blood stream. This is accomplished by a set of proteins known as apolipoproteins, which complex with the various lipids to form lipoproteins. The complex that transports the triglycerides from the intestine is known as a chylomicron, and chylomicrons are converted to chylomicron remnants by the action of lipoprotein lipase. These chylomicron remnants are taken up by the liver. The liver excretes very low density lipoprotein particles made up mostly of triglycerides and some cholesterol. After a series of metabolic steps, a cholesterol rich lipoprotein particle known as low-density lipoprotein (LDL) is formed. Most of the serum cholesterol is contained in the LDL particles, which are responsible for transporting cholesterol to the peripheral tissues. Elevated levels of LDL are associated with increased risk to coronary heart disease (Castelli et al., 1977). Cholesterol is removed from the serum by peripheral tissues through a receptor mediated pathway. The peripheral cells excrete the used lipids in the form of high-density lipoprotein (HDL), whose primary lipid is also cholesterol. Low levels of HDL are associated with increased risk to coronary heart disease, and indeed, HDL may be the strongest predictor of the disease, particularly in people over 50 (Castelli et al., 1977).

This brief outline of cholesterol metabolism and transport allows one set of candidate genes to be immediately identified: the apolipoprotein genes. These genes not only control the transport of cholesterol and other lipids, but they provide recognition entities for lipoprotein receptors and are necessary for many of the enzymatically determined steps in cholesterol metabolism. All the apolipoprotein genes in humans have now been cloned, so it is possible to study genetic variation at all of these genes using restriction fragment length polymorphisms.

Consequently, all of the elements are present for executing an integrated molecular, individual, and population level study on determinants of coronary heart disease in humans. The work of Templeton et al.(1987) represents one attempt at such a study. Templeton et al. (1987) analyzed the data described in Kessling et al.(1985) on the St. Mary's Hospital Metabolic Unit Patient Group in London. This group of patients consists of 89 unrelated, adult individuals of both sexes who were biased in favor of being normo- or hyperlipidaemic. DNA samples were obtained from all 89 individuals, followed by restriction enzyme digestion, Southern blotting, hybridization, and autoradiography. All individuals were probed with a cloned DNA fragment from the ApoA-I, C-III, A-IV region on chromosome 11, which contains three apolipoprotein loci. Three polymorphic restriction sites were detected by the enzymes XmnI, SstI, and PstI. All individuals were also measured for their fasting levels of serum triglyceride and HDL-cholesterol.

The three polymorphic restriction sites defined a total of 5 haplotypes in this DNA region (Templeton et al.,1987), as shown in Table 2. The primary phenotype used by Templeton et al.(1987) is the natural logarithm of the ratio of triglyceride to HDL-cholesterol levels, after adjustment for age and sex effects. This phenotype was chosen because it should be very sensitive to any genetic variation present in cholesterol metabolism. As noted above, triglycerides essentially represent the input into this metabolic pathway, while HDL represents the output. Hence, the ratio of triglyceride to HDL-cholesterol represents an input/output ratio for the entire metabolic pathway. The logarithm of this ratio is taken because the biochemical systems analysis theory of Savageau (1976) indicates that a logarithmic space is useful in describing the dynamics of a metabolic pathway.

The phenotypic effects associated with each haplotype were measured by the standard quantitative genetic measure of average excess. The average excess of a haplotype is simply the conditional mean phenotypic value of all individuals bearing the haplotype of interest, minus the overall population mean. Table 2 shows the average excess values associated with the 5 haplotypes present in this population. To see if there are any significant genetic effects on the phenotypes, Templeton et al.(1987) devised a permutational test of whether or not two average excesses are significantly different from one another. This test was applied to contrasts of the average excess associated with haplotype 1, the most common haplotype in the population (Table 2), versus the average excesses of the remaining four haplotypes. The significance levels are given in Table 2. As can be seen, statistically significant genetic variation affecting this lipid phenotype was observed. In particular, haplotype 2 has a significantly elevated average excess over that of haplotype 1. Using the known risk factors of coronary heart disease, individuals bearing this haplotype should be at increased risk for coronary heart disease and therefore should have decreased longevity relative to individuals not bearing this haplotype. These predictions will be tested in later, more extensive studies on human populations.

DISCUSSION

As illustrated by the abnormal abdomen and cholesterol examples, molecular genetics is providing a powerful tool for integrating molecular level studies with individual and population level studies. In both examples, the ability to study genetic variation at specific genes of known function allows us to construct a bridge between biochemical and molecular processes, physiological and developmental phenotypes, and population level assessments of fitness or disease risk factors that are related to the aging process. Hence, both examples illustrate that reductionistic and holistic approaches to aging research need not be antagonistic, but rather show that both approaches can be integrated to take advantage of the complementary information each approach provides.

Table 2. Haplotypes in the A-I, C-III, A-IV Genetic Region
and Their Average Excesses With Respect to the
Phenotype of Ln(Triglyceride/HDL-Cholesterol)

Haplotype	Frequency	Average Excess	Significance of A(1)-A(i)
010 (1)	0.694	-0.047	-
011 (2)	0.061	0.463	0.014*
000 (3)	0.106	-0.109	0.726
110 (4)	0.109	0.075	0.471
001 (5)	0.016	0.085	0.747

* Significant at the 5% level.

These two systems also vindicate the view that there are no "aging genes" _per se_. Instead, genes involved with the normal life processes of a functioning organism affect the aging process as a side effect of their primary function. With abnormal abdomen, we were studying genetic variation controlling the functional amount of ribosomal DNA in certain cell types. The ribosomal genes are not from a special class of "aging genes." They are simply genes controlling a fundamental biological process (production of ribosomes for protein synthesis) that has aging effects. Similarly, the apolipoprotein genes should not be regarded as aging genes, but simply as genes controlling a critical biochemical process that is essential for living systems at all ages (lipid metabolism) and that also happens to have aging effects. In this case, the aging effects are so strong that they are the major determinant of longevity in humans living in Western societies. In both cases, the research program was greatly facilitated by regarding the aging phenomena as secondary phenotypes and focusing on phenotypes more directly related to the direct action of the genes involved. Reductionistic and holistic approaches are more easily integrated when one deals with a more narrowly defined phenotype than "aging" or "longevity."

ACKNOWLEDGEMENT

This work was supported by National Institutes of Health grant R01 AG02246.

REFERENCES

Castelli, W. P., Doyle, J. P., and Gordon, T., 1977, HDL cholesterol and other lipids in coronary heart disease - the cooperative lipoprotein phenotyping study, Circulation, 55:767.

Dawber, T. R., 1980, "The Framingham Study," Harvard University Press, Cambridge.

DeSalle, R., Slightom, J., and Zimmer, E., 1986, The molecular through ecological genetics of abnormal abdomen. II. Ribosomal DNA polymorphism is associated with the abnormal abdomen syndrome in Drosophila mercatorum, Genetics, 112:861-875.

DeSalle, R., and Templeton, A. R., 1986, The molecular through ecological genetics of abnormal abdomen. III. Tissue-specific differential replication of ribosomal genes modulates the abnormal abdomen phenotype in <u>Drosophila</u> <u>mercatorum</u>, <u>Genetics</u>, 112:877-886.

Johnston, J. S., and Ellison, J. R., 1982, Exact age determination in laboratory and field-caught <u>Drosophila</u>, <u>J. Insect Physiol.</u>, 28:773-779.

Johnston, J. S., and Templeton, A. R., 1982, Dispersal and clines in Opuntia breeding <u>Drosophila</u> <u>mercatorum</u> and <u>D</u>. <u>hydei</u> at Kamuela, Hawaii, <u>in</u>: "Ecological Genetics and Evolution: The Cactus-Yeast-Drosophila Model System," J. S. F. Barker and W. T. Starmer, eds., Academic Press, New York.

Kessling, A. M., Horsthemke, B., and Humphries, S. E., 1985, A study of DNA polymorphisms around the human apolipoprotein AI gene in hyperlipidemic and normal individuals, <u>Clinical Genet.</u>, 28:296-306.

Medawar, P. B., 1957, "The Uniqueness of the Individual," Methuen, London.

Ritossa, F. M., Atwood, K. <u>D</u>., and Spiegelman, S., 1966, A molecular explanation of the bobbed mutants of <u>Drosophila</u> as partial deficiencies of ribosomal DNA, <u>Genetics</u>, 54:818-834.

Savageau, M., 1976, "Biochemical Systems Analysis: A Study of Function and Design in Molecular Biology," Addison-Wesley, Reading, MA.

Sing, C. F., Boerwinkle, E., Moll, P. P., and Davignon, J., 1985, Apolipoproteins and cardiovascular risk: genetics and epidemiology, <u>Ann. Biol. Clin.</u>, 43:407-417.

Templeton, A. R., 1982, The prophecies of parthenogenesis, <u>in</u>: "Evolution and Genetics of Life Histories," H. Dingle and J. P. Hegmann, eds., Springer-Verlag, New York.

Templeton, A. R., 1983, Natural and experimental parthenogenesis, <u>in</u>: "The Genetics and Biology of Drosophila, Vol. 3C," M. Ashburner, H. L. Carson, and J. N. Thompson, eds., Academic Press, London.

Templeton, A. R., Crease, T. J., and Shah, F., 1985, The molecular through ecological genetics of abnormal abdomen in <u>Drosophila</u> <u>mercatorum</u>. I. Basic genetics, <u>Genetics</u>, 111:805-818.

Templeton, A. R., and Johnston, J. S., 1982, Life history evolution under pleiotropy and K-selection in a natural population of <u>Drosophila</u> <u>mercatorum</u>, <u>in</u>: "Ecological Genetics and Evolution: The Cactus-Yeast-Drosophila Model System," J. S. F. Barker and W. T. Starmer, eds., Academic Press, New York.

Templeton, A. R. and Rankin, M. A., 1978, Genetic revolutions and control of insect populations, <u>in</u>: "The Screwworm Problem," R. H. Richardson, ed., University of Texas Press, Austin.

Templeton, A. R., Sing, C. F., Kessling, A., and Humphries, S., 1987, A cladistic analysis of phenotypic associations with haplotypes inferred from restriction endonuclease mapping. II. Associations of triglyceride and cholesterol levels with the apolipoprotein A-I, C-III, A-IV region in a human population, to be submitted to <u>Genetics</u>.

Williams, G. C., 1957, Pleiotropy, natural selection, and the evolution of senescence, <u>Evolution</u>, 11:398-411.

Wilson, T. G., Landers, M. H., and Happ, G. M., 1983, Precocene I and II inhibition of vitellogenic oocyte development in <u>Drosophila</u> <u>melanogaster</u>, <u>J. Insect Physiol.</u>, 29:249-254.

THE MANY GENETICS OF AGING

Gerald E. McClearn

Institute for the Study of Human Development
The Pennsylvania State University
University Park, PA

That genetic factors influence processes of aging appears to be a proposition well accepted in the gerontological literature. The evidence that has been put forth to demonstrate or document this influence is extremely varied. In one context, the difference in longevity among species may be cited; in another, a decline in efficiency of the DNA repair system will be discussed. The apparent classical Mendelian pattern of transmission of the Hutchinson-Gilford syndrome of progeria provides yet further evidence of hereditary factors in aging, as does the resemblance of relatives in longevity.

All of these, and many other diverse observations, do indeed constitute the corpus of knowledge in the area of "genetics of aging." The range of methods employed and of concepts engaged by these various studies is so great, however, that one might be excused for taking seriously the dictionary's observation that, though using singular verbs, "genetics" is really a plural noun. From the molecular composition of the gene itself, through the biochemistry and biophysics of its proximal action to the mathematics of the population and evolutionary geneticists and the statistics of the quantitative geneticists, a panorama spanning nearly the whole of biological science has been deployed in the attempt to understand the "genetics" of the processes of aging.

In order to help myself relate these different kinds of evidence to each other, and to provide a guide for thinking about research strategies and tactics, I have made use of the simple heuristic model which follows. It is proferred with considerable humility; first because none of the elements of the model are original to me, and secondly, because, like all models, it is only a partial representation. Some of the elements of the model are simplified to the point that specialists might regard them as simple-minded; these lapses of commission are matched by errors of omission in that other, perhaps fundamental considerations are left out entirely. However, I hope that the model might be of some use to others as I imagine it to have been to me.

Basic Mendelian genetics arose in the context of understanding intraspecific individual differences of a qualitative sort. For a period, it was unclear whether Mendelian rules were generally applicable or whether they were pertinent only to dichotomous, "abnormal" phenotypes. About two decades after the rediscovery of Mendelian rules in 1900, the accumulated data were convincing that these rules, indeed, were general ones, describing inheritance both in the plant and animal kingdoms. By a theoretical extension of Mendelian rules, quantitative, continuously distributed traits as well as dichotomous ones were brought into the explanatory framework. This extension, which can be characterized as quantitative genetic theory, provides a powerful approach to the understanding of individual differences in aging, constitutes a valuable framework for merging the sometimes compartmentalized genetic ideas from molecular, population, evolutionary, and physiological realms and serves as a useful heuristic blueprint for gerontological research.

A QUANTITATIVE GENETIC MODEL

A basic, although greatly oversimplified, representation of the causal matrix through which genes act upon complex phenotypes is given in Fig. 1. Genes are denoted by pairs of double helices, representing stretches of deoxyribonucleic acid (DNA), at the bottom of the figure. The genetic information encoded by the sequences of nucleotides in the DNA molecules is transcribed into ribonucleic acid (RNA) here represented by the single line at the point of the arrow originating at the DNA, and is translated by complex cellular mechanisms into polypeptides. These polypeptides constitute the array of structural, transport and catalytic proteins of the body. Their actions and interactions give rise to the anatomical, biochemical, immunological, physiological and other properties (represented by numbered boxes in the figure) of the organism. The interrelationships among these structures and functions may be extremely complicated, with such control features of complex systems as feedback inhibition, feedback activation, and so on. Ultimately, this intricate causal nexus gives rise to a complex phenotype here represented by the circle at the top of the figure.

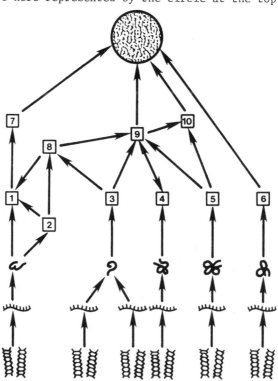

Fig. 1. A causation matrix, through which genes act upon complex phenotypes.

Several points may be drawn from this representation. First, it is obvious that a given gene can have a widespread effect through processes in which its primary products, the polypeptides, participate. This phenomenon is called <u>pleiotropy</u>. Second, a given phenotype may be influenced by many genes; this phenomenon might be labeled polygeny, or multiple factor inheritance. Third, there are no genes "for" a complex trait; genes determine polypeptides that enter into the processes of the organism; these processes eventuate in the phenotype of interest. Fourth, the complexities of the causal nexus will lead to correlations of varying magnitude among the differing phenotypes because of shared pathways of influence originating at the level of the genes. Finally, it will be apparent that what is called a phenotype is an arbitrary matter. Each of the elements of Fig. 1 can constitute a phenotype of primary interest, depending on the purpose of the study. That is to say, a molecular geneticist might be interested in the polypeptide as the phenotype; a physiological, pharmacological or nutritional geneticist might be concerned with metabolic products or organ functions; a quantitative geneticist might deal with a complex, continuously distributed phenotype, quite distal from the effects of any of its contributory genes. From the latter perspective, the legitimate phenotypes of the other levels of investigation become intermediate or mediating variables.

Figure 2 extends the model to include the effects of environmental factors which are here designated by wavy lines. These environmental influences are shown as impinging on the same causal pathways that mediate the influence of the genes. This depiction rests not only upon theoretical considerations, but also upon empirical results (DeFries et al., 1979) showing that environmental and genetic covariance matrices are very similar.

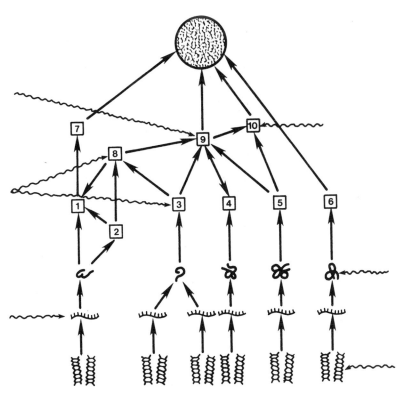

Fig. 2. An extension of the causation matrix, from Fig. 1, to include environmental factors, shown as the wavy lines.

It is important to note that environment has a sweeping definition in
this context. Briefly, environment is anything not coded in the DNA.
Thus, everything from the intimate cytoplasmic gradients of the fertilized
egg to peer group influences are comprehended in the environmental domain.
It is also apparent that there are environmental analogs of pleiotropy and
polygeny in this representation: single environmental factors can influence more than one phenotype and single phenotypes are influenced by more
than one environmental factor.

The picture presented by the foregoing matrix is obviously a static
one, a snapshot of a thin section through a continuous developmental
stream. The astounding progress in recent years of molecular researchers
on gene regulation make it reasonable to assume not only that different
genes are being expressed in different tissues, but also that, in any given
tissue, different genes are expressed at different parts of the developmental trajectory. Thus, a series of snapshots such as that of Fig. 3 probably
provides a more veridical model.

In the earliest frame, loci 2, 3, 4, 5 and 6 are shown to be operative,
but 1 is not. In the intermediate frame, 1, 2, 3, 4 and 6 are "on" and 5 is
"off"; and in the last frame 2 and 3 are "off," while 1, 4, 5 and 6 are
"on." This representation makes the important point that the genotype of an
individual is not a static conglomerate of alleles set at conception and
functioning totally in all parts of the organism throughout the rest of its
life. In any particular cell, only a small percentage of the genome will be
expressed, and in all parts of the body, that fraction of the genome that is
operative will change developmentally.

Of fundamental importance in this process are other genetic elements
described as regulatory genes. The function of these regulatory genes is,

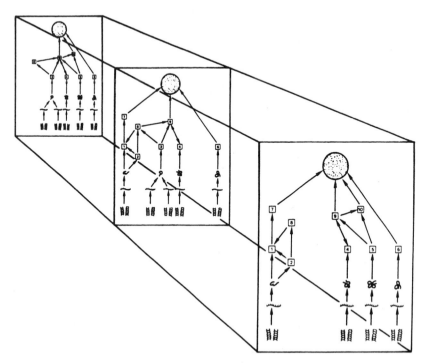

Fig. 3. The causation matrix throughout development, showing how
different genes may be expressed at different times in the
developmental trajectory.

in effect, the turning on and off of genes of the sort heretofore described (Eaves et al., 1986), which may be distinguished from the regulatory ones by the adjectives, "structural" or "producer." Most of what is known about the regulatory genes at present is at the molecular level of analysis, and in prokaryotes--the single celled organisms without nuclei that have been subjects of choice for much of molecular genetics research. The control of gene function of eukaryotes--organisms such as ourselves with cell nuclei--is one of the "cutting edges" of current molecular genetics.

Just as genetic factors can turn on and off, environmental factors may have differing onsets and offsets. It is probably most useful to think of differing onsets and differing durations because both genetic and environmental factors may have brief presence but lasting influence through structures or functions that persist, once established. The complexity of gene-environment interaction is suggested by the fact that some chemical environmental factors can also serve to activate or repress a regulator gene.

VITALITY AND AGING

To this point, the distal phenotype has been left undefined. For present purposes, it must obviously relate to aging. The problem of defining aging has proved to be quite refractory both theoretically and operationally. This presentation makes no pretense of comprehensive examination of all the issues, much less their resolution, but merely considers some facets of particular pertinence to the study of gerontological genetics.

Much theorizing concerning aging has invoked one or another variant of the idea that some attribute, defined by terms such as "vigor" or "vitality," declines as a function of chronological age. Ultimately, this vitality falls below some critical threshold value, and the individual succumbs. In its simplest form, this conception can be represented as in Fig. 4A. Many variants of this scheme are possible, of course. For example, it is not conceptually necessary that "vitality" declines linearly with chronological age. Indeed, the relationship need not even be monotonic, although in many discussions there is an implicit assumption that a monotonic function is descriptive of the population average function, at least after maturity has been reached.

Even brief consideration reveals that there are many difficulties with a concept such as that of vitality. Some few of these difficulties will be considered later. Whatever its shortcomings, however, a concept relating aging to declining vitality, even as simply represented in Fig. 4, can serve to support a further elaboration of the quantitative genetic perspective on aging. Therefore, I shall, for the time being at least, regard the distal phenotype of Figs. 1, 2 and 3 as "vitality."

The representation of Fig. 1 is a normative one. Each individual is a unique realization of this general schema. A fundamental reason for the variation among individuals is that many genes may exist in alternate forms or alleles. These different alleles may give rise to differing polypeptides with differing functional properties. Each individual organism of the species will have a different array of alleles for a large number of genes. Thus, excepting multiple identical births, parthenogenic groups in certain species and the very specialized laboratory inbred strains, every individual of a species is genetically unique. Each individual also experiences a unique environment. Individuality or variability must be regarded as systematic and quintessential to the attributes of living things and cannot be dismissed, as it is occasionally, as merely error term. The

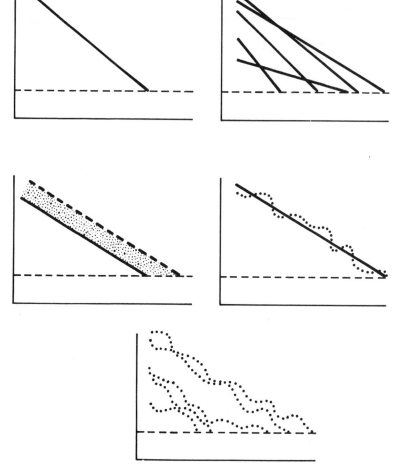

Fig. 4. A representation of the relationship of aging to declining
vitality. See text for a detailed explanation.

partitioning of this variability of phenotypes into genetic and environmental compartments, and then, by various designs, into more refined sub-
compartments of genetic (additive, dominance, epistatic or environmental
(shared, non-shared; common, general; long-term, short-term), is the prov-
ince of quantitative genetics. In fact, the research designs of quantitative genetics can be as informative about the environment as about genetics. It is thus appropriate to identify the general model with a more
comprehensive adjective, such as "differential."

THE DIFFERENTIAL MODEL AND AGING

The considerations presented above can now be more closely related
to the terms and concepts of aging research. First, in reference to the
schema of Figs. 1, 2 and 3, there are discernibly different routes from
the genetic and environmental causes to the phenotype of vitality, but
most of these have some degree of interlinkage. Gene pair number 6 is

shown as having a separate route of influence in order to illustrate the possibility, but all of the others are shown as interdependent to some extent. These different routes might represent domains that are reasonably congruent with current theories of aging--an immune system route, a free-radical route, a DNA repair system route--but we should not be surprised to find that measures in each of these domains covary with elements in other domains both cross-sectionally and longitudinally. In other words, we might expect pleiotropy and polygeny to frustrate the search for a single pacemaker of aging. The model leads us also to expect not only that individuals will differ overall in rate of aging because of unique genotype and environment, but also that individuals will differ in pattern of aging due to the particular combination of alleles and environmental agencies "driving" the different causal routes.

The wide individual differences that have been observed in any putative index of aging have inspired research and theorizing concerning "biological," "physiological" or "functional" age (see the recent excellent review and discussion by Ingram, 1983). Although many difficulties remain in elucidating and applying these concepts, there is little question but that some such notion must replace chronological age in any conceptualization that focuses upon individual differences.

The quantitative genetic study of change in phenotypes, as a complement to the molecular level of analysis, is at present a very scanty field of inquiry, though one which will undoubtedly come to be of great importance in the study of the genetics of development of whole organisms. Of special pertinence to the present topic is the observation that, just as the level of "vitality" of Figs. 1 and 2 could be regarded as an indicator of Biological Age, the processes underlying change in "vitality" (Fig. 3) represent Biological Aging. These dynamic measures of change can be the phenotypes of investigation just as well as a static measure, and the general polygenic, polyenvironmental, differential model is equally applicable to their analysis. We are then in a position to conceive of a genotypic vitality level, environmental deviations from that level, and a resultant phenotypic vitality. By extension to change over time, we may be able to develop concepts of a genotype-determined trajectory or reaction range around a trajectory, environmental deviations and the phenotypic changes we regard as aging.

Figure 4 gives a reprise of some of the notions just discussed. In Fig. 4A, a stylized aging function is shown for, say, human beings. The line is normative in that it is a representation of an entire species. Figure 4B amplifies by surrounding the repeated normative line of Fig. 4A, with genotypic age courses of individual human beings which the normative line typifies. We might expect that the population distribution of these functions would be approximately normal at any cross-sectional point of examination. However, the relative location of any individual might differ greatly from cross-section to cross-section. Figure 4C displays one of these individual genotypic functions as a solid line, with the impact of a long-term, persisting environmental deviation (such as, say, a strong cohort effect) shown by the shaded area resulting in a life course expectation indicated by the dashed line. Figure 4D now repeats this last line with relatively short-term environmental effects (resulting from infections, accidents, significant life events, favorable dietary opportunities, peer group interactions, marital disharmony and so on) resulting in the solid line representing the life course that would actually be observed. Finally, Fig. 4E shows the life courses of several individuals as we could measure them phenotypically, the resultants of the genotypic and long- and short-term environmental effects.

Clearly, those of us who are interested in applying quantitative genetic models to the aging process must consider phenotypes that represent the dynamic processes involved. Rather than static measures, we must be prepared to deal with equations describing the starting level, the shape and the rates of change of the longitudinal course of development. The phenotypes we will study may be intercepts and coefficients of perhaps many terms in perhaps complicated polynomials.

THE MEANING OF VITALITY

It is clear that "vitality" is a hypothetical construct that requires operational definition. At the population level, this is readily accomplished by the concept of probability of death. Much evidence is available to show that in many species, at least after a certain chronological age, the probability of death of a randomly chosen individual increases as chronological age increases. In application to a particular individual, however, such a probabilistic definition arises from translation of "vitality" to "resilience." This variant invokes notions of ability to recover from insults of some sort—accident, infection, or psychological trauma. These definitions are applicable to individual cases in theory, but the deliberate imposition of serious damage in a research context is ethically impossible, and observations on naturally occurring injury or harm are relatively inefficient from the point of view of analytical power. For differential genetic studies, then, the definition of vitality through consideration of its consequences is difficult.

A potentially powerful alternative approach is to attempt to define vitality in terms of its precedent variables—the scaffolding of Figs. 1, 2 and 3. Insofar as these figures constitute useful models of the real world, we might conclude immediately that no single variable will be all-revealing, and that we must perforce employ multivariable research strategies and tactics. Exploration of the multivariate causal nexus may proceed by the classic devices of experimental science, with manipulation of a specific element of the matrix and observations of change in another. Such research will necessarily be limited to a small part of the total matrix in any single experiment. To embrace a larger part of the causal pattern simultaneously will require the statistics of multivariable correlations, or the use of multiple outcome variables in manipulative research designs. By determining the degree to which the elements of the matrix vary together across individuals and across time, we can begin to identify the different causal routes from genes and environments to vitality, to locate the nodes of diverging influences that might be identified as pacemakers of converging influences that might be identified as rate-limiters (or rate-constrainers), and to estimate the extent to which aging is a monolithic process or a manifold aggregation requiring delineation and a differential taxonomy.

It may be useful to view the situation in terms of a Venn diagram relating observable variables or indicators to a latent variable or construct as shown in Fig. 5. Let us assume that the dashed circle encompasses all meaning of the concept of vitality. No one has ever measured vitality; they have simply been able to measure various correlates or operationally defined indicators of it--such as, for example, certain behaviors, immune system functioning, renal functioning, collagen cross-linkage, forced vital capacity, lipofuscin deposition, etc. Let us assume a number of these operational measures of vitality: A, B, C, D, and E, shown in Fig. 5 as closed circles. It may be seen that each of the measures taps some part of the vitality domain, and that none of them, singly or together, exhaustively assesses the total domain encompassed by the dashed circles. Furthermore, none of them measures only aspects of the domain; that is to say, some of the area of all of the closed circles lies outside the domain. Most measures are correlated (i.e., overlap) with others, but one (D) is completely independent. In one case (A and E), the correlation is only for elements outside the domain and is therefore meaningless with respect to vitality. Relating this representation to earlier ones, it can be imagined that the degree of overlap of the Venn circles represents the extent to which the various measures share membership in causal routes arising from genes and from environmental influence.

Inclusion of all of these empirical measures in an assessment of vitality would tap much, but not all, of the total meaning of the concept. Some parts of the domain would be "over measured" in that three of the measures overlap within the domain. However, the overall increase in comprehensiveness of measurement might make this duplication a very cheap price to pay.

One problem is, of course, that whereas we can apply multiple measures, we do not know, a priori, the structure of the domain or concept (the dashed circle) that we are measuring. Essentially, we need to build our abstract concept from the pattern of overlap of the various measures by induction. This may be accomplished mathematically by a variety of multivariate procedures which involve decomposition of the matrix of correlations or of covariances that exist among all the measures. With each

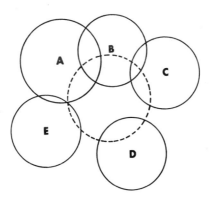

Fig. 5. Venn diagram relating the observable variables to vitality (see discussion in the text).

data value representing a point in n-dimensional space, certain analyses yield an estimate of the number of dimensions (or factors) that can be regarded as adequate for describing the space occupied by the data points. Such analyses provide an indication of the complexity of the domain and, thereby, an indication of the minimum number of variables that needs to be measured in order to guarantee adequate coverage. Another approach, principal component analysis, can be used effectively when the measures representing the domain tend to be intercorrelated. It will yield a linear composite score that accounts for a maximum proportion of the total variance of all the measures. The first principal component, not exactly the same as any of the original measures but drawing from several of them, can be used as a working definition of the phenomenon they were each individually intended to measure.

These brief examples may suffice to indicate the very great power of multivariate methodologies. Their judicious application in the context of longitudinal trajectories offers a potent array of developmental phenotypes for the gerontological genetics of the future. Useful progress can already be identified in the current and recent attempts to generate multivariate indices of biological age, and the eruption of applications of multivariate statistics in the field of behavioral genetics. Apparently adding new complexities, these methodologies instead offer ultimate promise of a more coherent view of aging processes and the many genetics thereunto pertaining.

ACKNOWLEDGEMENT

The debt I owe to John Nesselroade for help in thinking about these matters is enormous. He must be held blameless for any of the remaining flaws.

REFERENCES

DeFries, J. C., Kuse, A. R., and Vandenberb, S. G., 1979, Genetic correlations, environmental correlations and behavior, in: "Theoretical Advances in Behavior Genetics," J. R. Royce, ed., Sijthoff Noordhoff International, Alphen ann den Rijn, The Netherlands.

Eaves, L. J., Long, J., and Heath, A. C., 1986, A theory of developmental change in quantitative phenotypes applied to cognitive development, Behav. Genet., 16:143-162.

Ingram, D. K., 1983, Toward the behavioral assessment of biological aging in the laboratory mouse: Concepts, terminology and objectives, Exper. Aging Resch., 9:225-238.

LIFESPAN ENVIRONMENTAL INFLUENCES ON SPECIES

TYPICAL BEHAVIOR OF MERIONES UNGUICULATUS

MaryLou Cheal

Department of Psychology
Arizona State University
Tempe, Arizona 85287
University of Dayton Research Institute
P.O.Box 44
Higley, Arizona 85236

INTRODUCTION

There are many experiments in which effects of environment during development were studied. For instance, it is
well known that laboratory rodents that are housed in large
environments for a month or so during development will have
larger neocortical areas of the brain than those housed in
small cages (Diamond et al., 1965; Levine et al., 1967). More
recently, changes in brain size following enrichment have been
shown in rats over 900 days of age (Diamond et al., 1985).
Thus, it is known that brain plasticity is not limited to
developing animals. The present research project was planned
to further elucidate the effects of environmental influences on
life and death. That is, we wished to ask whether environmental changes affect growth and behavior throughout life and
whether they influence time of death. The gerbil, Meriones
unguiculatus, was chosen as a model because the gerbil is
small, active, relatively short-lived, and meets many of the
criteria of an animal model for aging research (Cheal, 1986).

An optimal study includes the comparison of animals maintained over the lifespan in a longitudinal study with animals
that are tested only once. Thus, the second group of animals
provides a cross-sectional study in which different animals are
tested for each age group. The effects of repeated testing
(one type of environmental influence) can thus be separated
from changes due to aging.

In the longitudinal study an enrichment experience was
given to half of the gerbils. In order to provide a natur-
alistic experience similar to what a feral gerbil would encounter, a miniature desert environment (8 feet by 30 inches) was
created within a dog run. The gerbils ran over stones, climbed
up on rocks, dug in the sand, and, on hot days, ran under the
water fall. A diagram of the apparatus has been published
(Cheal et al., 1986).

The gerbils were given a limited exposure to this environment for a number of practical reasons. Even in Arizona,
weather can be extreme: close to freezing on winter nights and
above 115° F (47° C) on summer afternoons. It would serve no
purpose to stress the gerbils' temperature regulation unduly.
Therefore, each group of gerbils that lived together was put
into the environment for just one hour each month. Since the
measurements were to be repeated, it was convenient to give the
enrichment experience after all of the measures were recorded
each month.

The gerbils received outdoor enrichment from two to 28
months of age. The gerbils were not put outside at younger
ages because pups have poor thermoregulatory mechanisms (McManus, 1971), and their size might have permitted escape through
the wire mesh. Enrichment was discontinued after 28 months of
age because older animals are more easily stressed by temperature extremes than are young animals. The gerbils given enrichment experience were compared to control gerbils that were
held indoors in a small cage for an equivalent period of time.

SPECIFIC QUESTIONS OF THE LIFESPAN STUDIES

The lifespan studies were aimed at answering several specific questions and at examining the effects of environmental
influences on each of the following questions:

1. How long will gerbils live? The two small studies on
gerbil lifespan in the literature (Arrington et al., 1973;
Troup et al., 1969) are not consistent in that they report
median lifespan variously from 25 to 36 months of age. Therefore, more data on longevity of gerbils are needed.

2. When does growth stop? It is thought that rats continue to grow for much of their lifespan, and cessation of
growth has been used as a marker for senescence (Rockstein et
al., 1977). There are no data in the literature concerning
this question in gerbils.

3. What sex differences are there in gerbils? Do male
and female gerbils differ in longevity as would be expected
from other species? Both of the earlier studies of gerbil
longevity reported longer median lifespans for female gerbils
than for male gerbils. In one of the studies, however, the
authors felt that there were artifacts due to illness in the
male group (Troup et al., 1969).

It is well known that male gerbils are larger than female
gerbils, but differences have not been reported for specific
ages. Finally, few studies have examined sex differences in
gerbil behavior. In many of my studies with a model of attention, no sex differences were found, but gerbils used for those
studies were typically about fifteen weeks of age. There is
little information on older gerbils.

4. How do attributes of growth and behavior develop? To
understand changes associated with aging, it is first necessary
to know what changes occur in the same measures in development.

Therefore, these studies were designed to begin observations on the day of birth. The developmental data have been published (Cheal & Foley, 1985) and will not be discussed here.

5. <u>What changes are related to aging?</u> By comparing data from longitudinal and cross-sectional studies, it is possible to identify changes between different ages that are due to repeated experimental manipulations.

6. <u>Is there behavioral stability over the lifespan?</u> Recent research has shown stability of particular animal behaviors over fairly long periods (Cheal and Foley, 1985; MacDonald, 1983; Stevenson-Hinde et al., 1980), but no one has looked at stability throughout the lifespan.

7. <u>Are there predictors (or biomarkers) of aging?</u> Specifically, will some changes occur at predictable times prior to death rather than in relationship to chronological age?

Our data over the past three years have provided answers to some of these questions, partial answers to others, but have given no insight on other questions as yet. In the remainder of this paper a brief description of answers and partial answers to questions that could be answered to date are given, and some of the questions that require further data from these animals are suggested.

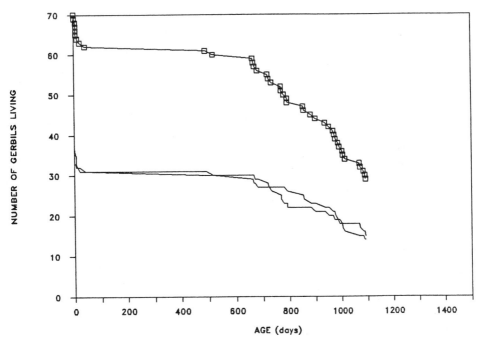

Fig. 1. Number of gerbils that were living at each day of age from birth to 36 months of age. Symbols indicate all gerbils. Separate lines indicate male and female gerbils. Sex differences were small with a few more male gerbils living at some ages than female gerbils.

Testing of 70 gerbils was begun on the day of birth. A total of 17 behavioral and allometric measurements were repeated at 1, 2, 3, and 4 weeks of age, and then each month thereafter as long as the gerbils lived. The loss of eight of the gerbil pups in infancy was not unusual. At weaning, there were 62 gerbils, 31 male and 31 female gerbils (Figure 1). There was no further loss until 16 months of age when two gerbils died. Further deaths occurred after the gerbils reached 22 months of age.

Median lifespan was 1092 days of age for male gerbils and 1078 days of age for female gerbils. The absolute number of male and female gerbils alive at any age has differed little up to 36 months of age at which time there were 14 female and 15 male gerbils. Median lifespan for enriched gerbils was 1090 days of age and was 1083 days of age for control gerbils. Thus, median lifespan was approximately 36 months of age for these gerbils. The oldest living gerbil reported in the literature was 48 months of age, and one female gerbil lived to more than 51 months of age in my laboratory.

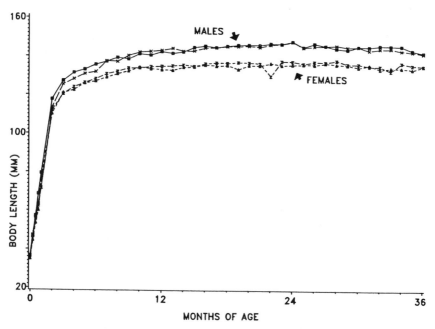

Fig. 2. Body length (mm) as a function of months of age for gerbils in the longitudinal study. Two lines for each sex represent Enriched and Control gerbils (no significant differences). The decrease in mean length at 23 months of age for Control females was due to one gerbil that died a few days later.

WHEN DOES GROWTH STOP?

As shown in Figure 2, these gerbils grew rapidly during
the first two months of age and then more slowly over the next
few months. There was no appreciable growth after twelve
months of age. Thus, gerbils do not continue to grow throughout life as do rats. At twelve months of age, only a third of
their median lifespan, the gerbils had reached the peak of
reproductive activity. Reproduction in female gerbils can
continue beyond two years of age, and a 36 month old male
gerbil sired a litter in my laboratory. Enrichment experience
had no effect on body length.

Data on body weight support the same conclusions on cessation of growth (Figure 3). Rapid growth from birth to two
months of age was followed by a slow increase over the first
year. There was no appreciable gain after twelve months of
age, although male gerbils were slightly heavier at about two
years of age.

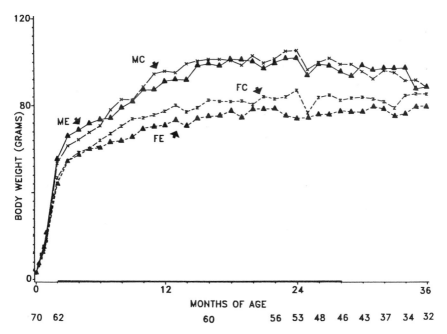

Fig. 3. Body weight as a function of months of
age for gerbils in the longitudinal study.
The number of gerbils living at different
ages are indicated by numbers along the
bottom of figure. Heavy line along abscissa
indicates months when enrichment (or control)
followed measurements. Male enriched, ME;
male control, MC; female enriched, FE;
female control, FC.

Enrichment experience affected body weight. In typical
enrichment experiments, rodents raised in large environments
weigh less than controls. To our surprise, in adolescence,
male gerbils given enrichment gained weight more rapidly than
male gerbils in the control condition. By seven months of age,
the controls had caught up with the enriched male gerbils.

Statistical analyses on these data have only been computed
to seven months of age. However, it appears that enrichment
had the typical effect on female gerbils in adulthood; that is,
enriched female gerbils weighed less than control female gerbils (Figure 3).

There was an apparent decrease in body weight of male
gerbils from two to three years of age (Figure 3). This decrease in weight could be due to weight loss late in life, or
it could be due to selective dying of heavier gerbils. Individual animal analysis suggested that both factors may be
involved. Nine of the fifteen male gerbils still living at 36
months of age weighed less at 36 months than they did at 24
months of age. The mean weight loss for these nine gerbils was
19.5 grams. The other six male gerbils gained a mean of 2.1
grams. In contrast, approximately equal numbers of female
gerbils increased weight, decreased weight, or stayed the same.

Additionally, a comparison was made between mean weights
at 24 months of age of the male gerbils that lived to 36 months
and those that did not live to 36 months. Those that lived
weighed a mean of 9.4 grams less at 24 months than did those
that died prior to 36 months of age ($t(24) = 1.88$, $p < .05$,
one-tailed). Thus, survival of male gerbils was related to
both weight loss and to lower body weight at younger ages.

This brief analysis will not suffice to determine either
the importance of early body weight to longevity or the pattern
of weight loss over the lifespan. It will be necessary to use
at least two additional analyses. One will be to examine longevity as a function of body weight at several early ages.
Another analysis will be to determine changes in body weight
for several months prior to death. These analyses will be made
after all the data have been collected.

WHAT SEX DIFFERENCES ARE THERE?

The data already show that there were no large sex differences in median lifespan for these gerbils (Figure 1).
Large sex differences in body weight first appeared at two
months of age (Figure 3). There were small significant differences at birth, one, two, and four weeks of age (Cheal &
Foley, 1985). Significant differences in body length were
found at birth, two, and three weeks of age, and at two months
of age, although large differences were only apparent from
three months of age (Figure 2).

These sex differences in body size were not unexpected.
However, sex differences in motor activity were not anticipated. I had never seen sex differences in attentional and
motor behaviors in gerbils, although I had tested thousands of

young gerbils. In accordance with these earlier studies, there were no differences between young male and female gerbils in number of lines crossed in a small arena, in number of rearings on the hind legs, or in latency to jump down from a small platform (Cheal & Foley, 1985).

On the other hand, the data in Figures 4, 5, and 6 suggest that female gerbils were more active than were male gerbils during the period when they would be most fertile even though these gerbils were sexually naive. Between six and eighteen months of age, females gerbils crossed more lines (Figure 4), reared on the hind legs more (Figure 5), and had shorter latencies to jump down from a platform than did male gerbils (Figure 6). Details of methods and statistical analyses were reported in Cheal (1987a).

No differences due to environmental effects were found at these ages. Statistical analyses have only been made on these behavioral data up to 18 months of age because of the confounding due to death of gerbils at later ages. Further analyses on these data must wait until the research is complete. However, it is apparent from the figures that these sex differences do not continue to late life.

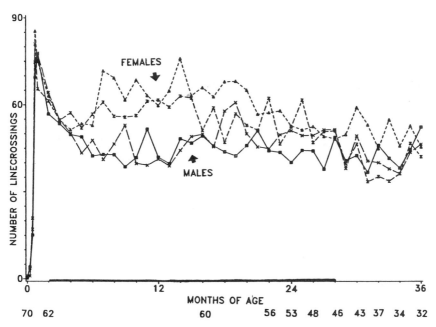

Fig. 4.   Number of linecrossings in a one minute test as a function of months of age for gerbils in the longitudinal study. The number of gerbils living at different ages are indicated by numbers along the bottom of the figure. Heavy line along abscissa indicates months when enrichment (or control) followed measurements.

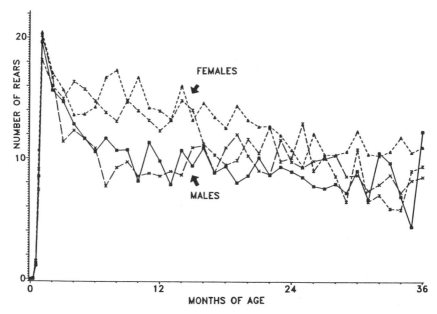

Fig. 5.   Number of rearings on hind legs in a one
          minute test as a function of months of age
          for gerbils in the longitudinal study.

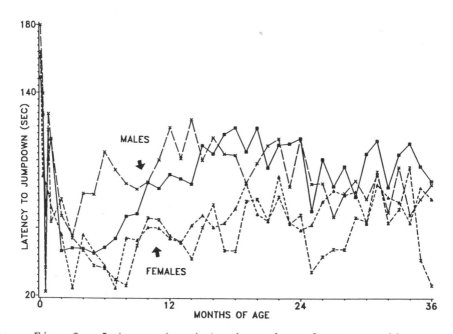

Fig. 6.   Latency (sec) to jump down from a small
          platform as a function of months of age for
          gerbils in longitudinal study.

WHAT EFFECTS ARE THERE OF REPEATED TESTING?

An effect of environmental treatment was found in separate
analyses of the repeated behavioral data in comparison with
data from the cross-sectional study. At each month from six to
18 months of age, gerbils given repeated testing crossed fewer
lines and reared on the hindlegs less than gerbils being tested
for the first time (Cheal, 1987a). These results point to an
important species difference between gerbils and rats. Unlike
a rat, a gerbil placed into a novel environment is very active,
and activity decreases with familiarity with the environment.

WHAT EFFECTS ARE DUE TO BRIEF EPISODES OF ENRICHED ENVIRONMENT?

The gerbil has a distinct ventral gland that is used to
mark objects in the environment. The gerbil lowers the abdomen
onto objects on the substrate, such as a stone or a peg in a
laboratory test, and deposits a sticky chemical called sebum.
Although both male and female gerbils mark with their ventral
gland, the male has a larger gland and marks more frequently
than does the female. Marking is thought to be a method of
identifying territory and of communication (Thiessen, 1973).

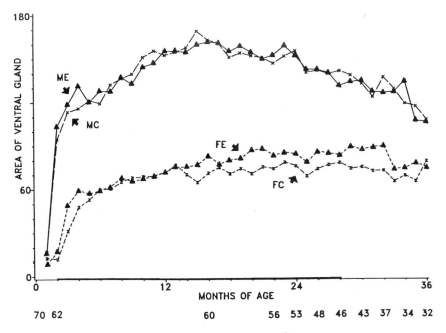

Fig. 7. Area of ventral gland (mm^2) as a function
          of months of age for gerbils in the
          longitudinal study. The number of gerbils
          living at different ages are indicated by
          numbers along the bottom of figure. Heavy
          line along abscissa indicates months when
          enrichment (or control) followed measure-
          ments. Male enriched, ME; male control, MC;
          female enriched, FE; female control, FC.

During adolescence, male gerbils that received enrichment had ventral glands that were approximately 13% larger than ventral glands of controls, and enriched females had glands that were more than 50% larger than those of control females (Figure 7). These differences due to environmental enrichment disappeared by five months of age.

Even though the ventral gland of enriched gerbils grew more rapidly in adolescence, at these early ages there was a lot of variability in the amount of marking, and differences between enriched and control gerbils were not significant (Cheal et al., 1986). Male gerbils marked much more than females at all ages, but significant differences due to environmental enrichment only occurred at later ages (Figure 8). Between six and eighteen months of age, male and female gerbils given enrichment marked significantly more than control gerbils (Cheal, 1987a). From Figure 8 it appears that the effects of an hour of enrichment monthly from two to 28 months of age continued to facilitate marking in male gerbils throughout the third year of life.

Another interesting point is that there was a significant correlation between the amount of marking behavior in male

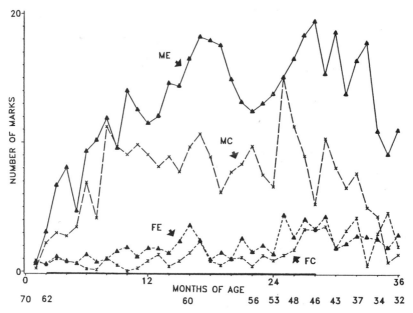

Fig. 8.   Number of marks with the ventral gland in a three minute test as a function of months of age by gerbils in the longitudinal study. The number of gerbils living at different ages are indicated by numbers along the bottom of figure. Heavy line along abscissa indicates months when enrichment (or control) followed measurements. Male enriched, ME; male control, MC; female enriched, FE; female control, FC.

gerbils at 18 months of age and the size of the ventral gland at four months of age. The biggest difference in size of the ventral gland between enriched and control male gerbils was observed at four months of age (Cheal et al., 1986). Both the ventral gland and marking behavior are known to be dependent on gonadal hormones (Cheal et al., 1984; Thiessen, 1973). The development of marking is also dependent on hormones during the perinatal period (Turner, 1975). The present data suggest that the amount of marking in adulthood may be partially dependent on the amount of hormone present during adolescence in male gerbils.

It should be noted that the sharp rise in the amount of marking behavior for male control and female enriched gerbils at 25 months of age (Figure 8) may be due to the two-week battery of tests that were conducted when these animals were 24 months of age. The drop in body weight of three groups of the gerbils at 25 months of age (Figure 3) may also be related to this testing. One of the tests necessitated single daily feedings for three consecutive days.

ADVANTAGES OF ENRICHMENT EFFECTS

It was suggested above that adolescent hormone levels might influence levels of marking behavior in adult male gerbils. Another possibility is that animals that grow more rapidly in the adolescent period may be more capable in competitions. This adolescent competence may in turn produce more dominant animals that mark more as adults. Earlier adolescence would increase the reproductive period and could increase the total number of offspring. Thus, there would be considerable selective advantage. The two possibilities, adolescent hormonal influences and developmental advantages, are not necessarily exclusive.

Effects of enrichment experience have been manifested in two other ways: in reducing seizures in male gerbils (Cheal, 1987a), and in reducing the time needed by male and female gerbils to find food (Cheal, 1987b). After nine months of age, fewer enriched male gerbils had seizures than in the other three groups (Figure 9). Control male, enriched female, and control female gerbils did not differ significantly in this measure between six and 18 months of age (Cheal, 1987a). The effect on enriched male gerbils was particularly apparent during "midlife" of the gerbils and is less evident at older ages. Of course, proportions are poor measures when group size is small as in the older ages.

Another large behavioral difference between the enriched and control conditions was found in a "search" test conducted when the gerbils were 24 months of age. When hungry, the gerbils were allowed to explore a small apparatus and search for food (Cheal, 1987b). The enriched gerbils found food much more quickly than did the control gerbils or than did a group of 8-month-old naive gerbils. The results were not due to differences in locomotor activity as there were no differences in activity scores or in amount of rearing on the hind legs from the same gerbils a few days earlier. These data were interpreted as reflecting more efficient foraging in gerbils that had received enrichment. Such efficiency could be due to improved ability to make use of environmental cues or to form a cognitive map. It is doubtful that they had more efficient olfactory systems because there were no differences in duration and frequency of investigation of conspecific odors in previous odor-elicited investigation studies (Cheal et al., 1982).

IS THERE BEHAVIORAL STABILITY?

Gerbil behavior is very stable within an animal over 13 months of adult life (Table 1; Cheal, 1987a). Two types of statistical analyses were calculated. Kendall's coefficient of concordance tested for stability of intraindividual behavior over the 13 months. Each gerbil's score was ranked at each age for each behavior, and the ranks were summed over ages (Riege, 1971). For additional support of stability, split half correlation coefficients tested for correlation between even and odd months. Four of the behavioral measures (marking, jumpdown, rearing, and activity) were used to calculate an individual profile score. This score was extremely stable over more than a third of the gerbils' median lifespan. Thus, it will be interesting to see if that stability continues into late life.

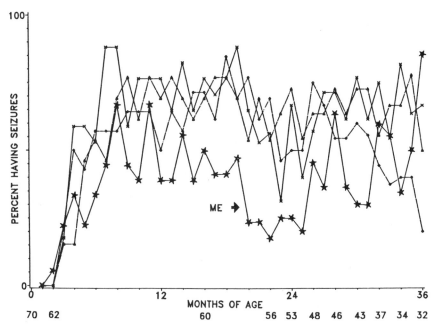

Fig. 9. Percent of gerbils that had seizures as a function of age in the longitudinal study. The number of gerbils living at different ages are indicated by numbers along the bottom of figure. Male enriched, ME.

Table 1.
Stability of individual gerbil behavior

Behavior	n	Tau	r	
			Males (n = 31)	Females (n = 31)
Marking	58	.65****	.94****	.88****
Jump Down	58	.53****	.93****	.78****
Rearing	60	.49****	.91****	.88****
Line Crossings	60	.43****	.81****	.89****
Climb Down	60	.28****	.19	.69****
Clinging	60	.17****	.17	.41*
Profile Score	60	.52****	.91****	.90****

Tau was based on rank order of each gerbil for each monthly measure from 6 to 18 months of age. Split-half correlation (r) compares each gerbil's even month measures with its own odd month measures. Profile scores were calculated from the sum of the z-scores for Rearing and Line Crossings divided by the sum of the z-scores for Marking and Jump Down. Taken from Cheal (1987a). $*p < .05$, $****p < .00001$.

FUTURE ANALYSES

As stated earlier, it will not be possible to interpret these data and those yet to be collected without considerable additional analyses. In order to determine the effects of enrichment experience on aging, it will be necessary to look at individual changes in the longitudinal animals. Changes that occur within long-lived animals will suggest different conclusions than changes that occur due to selective death of short-lived animals.

It will also be important to compare the data from the longitudinal gerbils with comparable data from cross-sectional gerbils. These data will be collected in the next months. We have already learned that adolescent and young adult gerbils given repeated testing differ remarkably in some measures (locomotor activity, rearing, jumpdown) from gerbils that are experimentally naive (Cheal and Foley, 1985; Cheal, 1987a). Thus, it is possible that decreases in activity are not due to motor impairment of the older gerbils but to adaptation to the testing situation. Many old gerbils may be capable of activity when placed into a new situation.

ARE THERE BIOMARKERS OF AGING?

In addition to examining changes over age, it will also be important to look at the relationship between levels of behavior and longevity. Are there changes predictive of death? To answer this question, data will be analyzed backwards from age at death. Correlations between measures in early life and longevity may suggest useful biomarkers of aging.

To make full use of these animals, all tissue has been saved for histopathology. Ideally, histopathology will be done on all the longitudinal animals and on the tissue from the cross-sectional gerbils. In this way it will be possible to separate pathologies that are compatible with life from those that are not. It will then also be possible to look at correlations between the behavioral and allometric measures that we have recorded and the pathologies suggested by the histological assessments.

CONCLUSION

In summary, this research has already provided some new and interesting effects of enrichment on the life of gerbils from early development to the median lifespan. The data support much research that has been published previously in which advantageous effects of environmental enrichment have been demonstrated. The most exciting part of the present study is that a very small amount of enrichment can have far reaching effects, and that the effects were apparent months after the enrichment was ended. A 36 month median lifespan for gerbils may be roughly analogous to 75 years as median lifespan in humans. One might ask if one hour a month for 27 months can affect the life of a gerbil, what affect would 12 hours of enrichment each year for 56 years have on the life of a human being? At this stage of the research, such a question can only lead to conjecture. Much additional research, including replication of these results, is needed before such a question is meaningful.

REFERENCES

Arrington, L. R., Beaty, T. C., and Kelley, K. C., 1973, Growth, longevity, and reproductive life of the Mongolian gerbil, Laboratory Animal Care, 10:262-265.
Cheal, M. L., 1986, The gerbil: A unique model for research on aging, Experimental Aging Research, 12:3-21.
Cheal, M. L., 1987a, Adult development: Plasticity of stable behavior, Experimental Aging Research, 13:in press.
Cheal, M. L., 1987b, Environmental enrichment facilitates foraging behavior, Physiology & Behavior, 39:in press.
Cheal, M. L., and Foley, K., 1985, Developmental and experiential influences on ontogeny: The gerbil (Meriones unguiculatus) as a model, Journal of Comparative Psychology, 99:289-305.
Cheal, M. L., Foley, K., and Kastenbaum, R., 1986, Brief periods of environmental enrichment facilitate adolescent growth of gerbils, Physiology & Behavior, 36:1047-1051.
Cheal, M. L., Johnson, M. O., Ellingboe, J., and Skupny, A. S. T., 1984, Perseveration of attention to conspecific odors and novel objects in castrated gerbils, Physiology and Behavior, 33:563-570.

Cheal, M. L., Klestzick, J., and Domesick, V. B., 1982, Attention and habituation: Odor preferences, long-term memory, and multiple sensory cues of novel stimuli, _Journal of Comparative and Physiological Psychology_, 96:47-60.

Diamond, M. C., Livesey, P. J., and Bell, J. A., 1985, Plasticity in the 904 day old male rat cerebral cortex, _Experimental Neurology_, 15:187-195.

Diamond, M. C., Rosenzweig, M. R., and Krech, D., 1965, Relationships between body weight and skull development in rats raised in enriched and impoverished conditions, _Journal of Experimental Zoology_, 160:29-36.

Levine, S., Haltmeyer, G. C., Karas, G. G., and Denenberg, V. H., 1967, Physiological and behavioral effects of infantile stimulation, _Physiology & Behavior_, 2:55-59.

MacDonald, K., 1983, Stability of individual differences in behavior in a litter of wolf cubs (_Canis lupis_), _Journal of Comparative Psychology_, 97:99-106.

McManus, J. J., 1971, Early postnatal growth and the development of temperature regulation in the Mongolian gerbil (_Meriones unguiculatlus_), _Journal of Mammalogy_, 52:782-792.

Riege, W. H., 1971, Environmental influences on brain and behavior of year-old rats, _Developmental Psychobiology_, 4:157-167.

Rockstein, M., Chesky, J. A., and Sussman, M. L., 1977, Comparative biology and evolution of aging, _in_: "Handbook of the Biology of Aging," C. E. Finch and L. Hayflick, eds., Van Nostrand Reinhold, New York.

Stevenson-Hinde, J., Stillwell-Barnes, R., and Zunz, M., 1980, Subjective assessment of rhesus monkeys over four successive years, _Primates_, 21:66-82.

Thiessen, D. D., 1973, Footholds for survival, _American Scientist_, 61:346-351.

Troup, G. M., Smith, G. S., and Walford, R. L., 1969, Life span, chronologic disease patterns, and age-related changes in relative spleen weight for the Mongolian gerbil (_Meriones unguiculatus_), _Experimental Gerontology_, 4:139-143.

Turner, J. W., 1975, Influence of neonatal androgen on the display of territorial marking behavior in the gerbil, _Physiology & Behavior_, 15:265-270.

LONGEVITY IN FISH: SOME ECOLOGICAL AND

EVOLUTIONARY CONSIDERATIONS

Raymond J. H. Beverton

Department of Applied Biology
UWIST, P.O. Box 13
Cardiff, U.K.

INTRODUCTION

My interest in longevity in fish arose originally from its significance in fish resource dynamics and its relationships to growth, maturation and fecundity. My first opportunity to perceive the wider implications of the phenomenon of longevity came at the 1959 Conference on Lifespan in Man and Animals sponsored by the CIBA Foundation. Holt and I (Beverton and Holt, 1959) gave a paper on life-spans of fish in relation to growth, and the contributors included the late George Sacher whose paper on mammalian size and life-span has been referred to at this conference. The present symposium in its aims and multi-disciplinary character has much in common with the 1959 CIBA Conference. I shall again approach my subject primarily from the demographic standpoint, but this time exploring certain evolutionary implications.

MEASUREMENT OF LONGEVITY IN FISH

The rigor with which the demographic evidence of longevity in fish can be documented and interpreted depends on the reliability with which the age of individuals can be determined. The seasonality in metabolic activity of fish and hence in their growth, in middle and high latitudes often leaves its mark (literally) as annual or quasi-annual regularities in the structure of their hard parts - scales, bones and, especially, the otolith of the middle ear.

Age determination of fish such as the herring with well-developed scales was established at the turn of the century by the pioneer Norwegian fisheries scientist Einear Lea (1913), and significant advances have been made in the last two decades. Christensen (1964) developed the technique of carbonizing (charring) the organic membrane laid down annually in the otolith of some species of fish by exposing to gentle heat the broken surface of the otolith. This approach was later refined by sectioning the otolith with a diamond saw after embedding in resin. The techniques are summarized by Blacker (1974) and Williams and Bedford (1974).

More attention was given in recent years to the validation of age determination from annular structures, which are not always laid down on a strict yearly basis, even in temperate regions. Chilton and Beamish (1982)

give an up-to-date critique of validation methodology. Of particular interest is the use of ratios of radioisotopes of lead (^{210}Pb) and radium (^{226}Ra)
found in trace quantities in fish otoliths (Bennett et al., 1982).

The effect of these various advances in the techniques of age-determination has extended the recorded ages of older fish, sometimes dramatically
so. For example, it was rare to record an age greater than 10 years for the
common sole (Solea solea) from the North Sea by counting such rings as are
visible in the whole (uncut) otolith; after sectioning and charring the otolith, ages of up to 20 years were not uncommon. Leaman and Beamish (1984)
give a particular dramatic example of the difference in age-composition of
ocean perch (Sebastes spp) from the North Pacific, using first whole otoliths and then sectioning the same otoliths and reading them again. In this
exceptionally long-lived genus, age determination from sectioned compared
with whole otoliths resulted in the maximum recorded age of fish in the
sample increasing from 40 to over 80 years.

Such extension of maximum recorded age has had the effect of reducing
the perceived annual mortality rate. In an ocean perch sample, for example,
the mortality rate was 12% per year from the age-composition based on whole
otoliths, but only 3% when sectioned otoliths were used. Since the increase
in recorded age is progressively more marked in older fish, the effect also
tends to straighten out what previously appeared to be a Gompertz-like life-
table, with the annual mortality rate apparently increasing with age. Thus,
Bidder's (1932) original proposition, that some species of fish are
"immortal" because there is no increase of their mortality rate with age, is
given a new lease of life! The difficulty is that a combination of the
limitations of sampling and accurate age determination at the top end of the
age spectrum of long-lived species makes it difficult to establish convincingly whether or not the trend of mortality rate with age departs significantly from linearity.

LONGEVITY AND THE EVOLUTIONARY RECORD

Although, in certain instances, scales are preserved from which age may
be inferred, it is scarcely feasible to attempt to trace the evolution of
longevity of fish direct from the fossil record - which is itself imperfect. Some inferences can be drawn by combining modern evidence of longevity and the evolutionary history of fish as documented in the standard ich-
thyological textbooks such as those of Norman (1975), Nelson (1984) and
Moyle and Cech (1982).

The earliest known fish, from Cambrian deposits some 450-500 m years
ago, were typically small, bottom-living, jawless (Agnatha) forms distantly
related to the modern cyclostomes (hagfish and lampreys). The probability
is that they were short-lived, but confirmation is lacking.

Some interesting clues however can be gained from the distribution of
life-span among living representatives of the main evolutionary lines. In
exploring this I admit to being unaware of any published evidence on longevity in some of the rarer groups. Fig. 1 is a highly simplified picture of
the evolutionary tree for fish, with the living groups in the right-hand
column (with the exception of the lungfish and coelocanths) arranged roughly
in the order of decreasing "primitiveness", reading downwards.

The most primitive groups, the hagfish and lampreys, are scaleless and
cartilaginous, making age-determination from structures problematic, if not
impossible. The importance of some species (e.g., the sea lamprey, Petromyzon marinus) as predators on fish however, has caused their life-cycle to
be well understood (Applegate, 1950). It is unlike that of true fish in

162

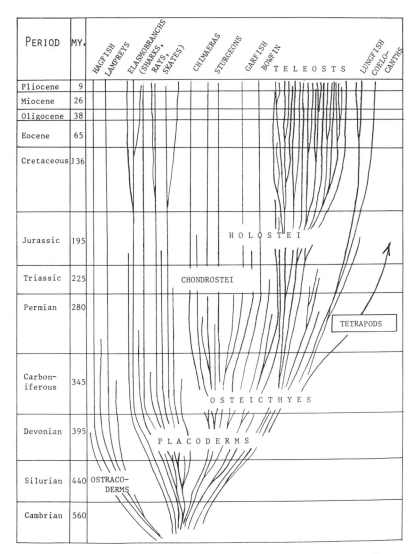

Period	MY.															
Pliocene	9															
Miocene	26															
Oligocene	38															
Eocene	65															
Cretaceous	136															
Jurassic	195															
Triassic	225															
Permian	280															
Carboniferous	345															
Devonian	395															
Silurian	440															
Cambrian	560															

Fig. 1. Simplified representation of the "evolutionary tree" of fish.

that the ammocoete larval stage is greatly prolonged, lasting from 3 to 5 years, but the adult phase is brief, lasting from 6 months to 2 years, with death following the first and only spawning act.

Sharks and rays (Elasmobranchs), generally accepted as the most primitive of the true fishes, also have a cartilaginous skeleton, but the vertebrae of sharks and the dorsal spines possessed by some species, e.g., the spur dogfish Squalus acanthias, have annual structures from which age can be determined (Ketchen, 1974). This species, on the small side for sharks, was shown to be very long-lived and slow-growing, with ages of up to 60 years recorded for specimens of 1 m in length. It is reasonable to suppose that the largest of all fish, the whale shark (Rhincodon typus) which grows to 18 m in the tropics, and the Greenland shark (Simniosus microcephalus) which reaches 6 m in the sub-Arctic, have life-spans as long or longer. Despite their "primitive" character, elasmobranchs are highly successful top predators which have colonised all the world's oceans. They are typically large

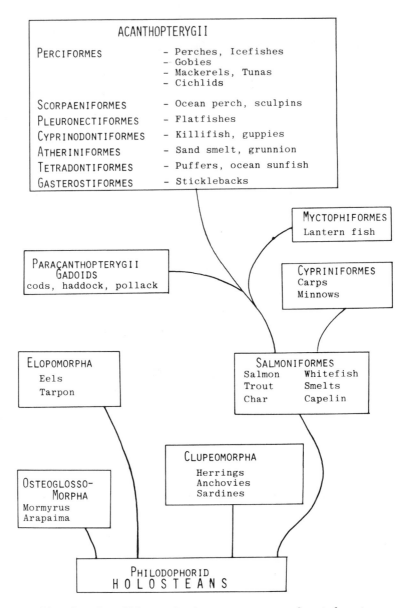

Fig. 2. Possible evolutionary sequence for teleosts.

- even the smallest (<u>Squaliolus laticaudus</u>) reaches 24 cm fully grown - and, so far as the limited evidence goes, long-lived, with no suggestion of increased post-spawning or senescent mortality.

The sturgeons (<u>Acipenseriformes</u>) are unrelated to the Elasmobranchs, having evolved from a primitive stock of bony fish (Teleosts) some 200 m years ago, but in size and longevity they have much in common. They are also cartilaginous, having lost calcium from their bones secondarily, but this may be why age determination, e.g., from their vertebrae, is relatively reliable. The largest species of sturgeon (and the largest freshwater fish)

the beluga (Husa husa) from the Black, Azov and Caspian Seas, has been
reported up to 118 years and over 5 m in length (Tspekin and Zokolou,
1971). Ages in the region of 100 years were also reported for the largest
of the North American species, the white sturgeon (Acipenser transmon-
tanus). Life-spans in the range of 40-80 years are not uncommon in other
species of sturgeon, while even the smallest (the sterlet, A. ruthenus)
lives up to 20 years and grows to some 50 cm in length (Doroshov, 1985).
Although their reproduction is quite different from that of the elasmobranchs, being highly fecund egg producers, they are like elasmobranchs in
being repeated spawners (iteroparous) with no significant evidence of post-
spawning mortality.

The remaining group other than the teleosts - the garfish (Lepidosteus
spp), bowfin (Amia calva), lungfish (African, Prototerus spp, and
S. American, Lepidosiren paradona) birchirs (Polypterus spp) and the coelo-
canth (Latimaeria chalumnae) are typically large predators, mostly freshwater. Each is represented by a small number of species (some by only one)
covering a limited size range. I have been unable to find longevity data
for these fishes but it could be anticipated that their life-spans extend to
tens of years.

Something in the region of 95% of all the 21,000 recorded species of
fish are teleosts, within which a gradation from the more primitive or generalised to the "advanced" and specialised can be traced, albeit in only a
very rough (and by no means generally accepted) way. Fig. 2 represents a
possible order, starting with the most generalised at the top, as in Fig. 1.

Reliable records of longevity are much commoner in the teleosts than in
the groups discussed above, partly because many species are of high economic
importance justifying research on them. Even so, the evidence is patchy,
since neither scales (if present) nor otoliths can be relied on in every
species to carry reliably annual and easily interpreted structures, especially in the tropics.

Of the three more generalised groups, lying to one side of the main
teleostean evolution, the Osteoglossomorpha includes one of the largest
truly freshwater scaly fish, the S. American Arapaima gigas, but I have been
unable to find records of its age. The Elopomorpha include the eels
(Anguilla spp) whose age is difficult to determine but is certainly long-
lived, with a potential life-span up to 20 years and probably more. The
Clupeomorpha include the herring, sardines and anchovies whose scales (in
temperate regions) are among the most easily read. Unlike the previously
mentioned groups, the Clupeomorpha include nearly 400 species the majority
of which are fairly (though not extremely) small and planktivorous, with
lengths in the range 10-30 cm. A few of the largest species (about 50 cm
maximum) are piscivorous but only one, the wolf herring (Chirocentrus dorab)
is a large, voracious carnivore, growing to over 3 m. As a group, for their
size the true herring (Clupea harengus) are relatively long-lived, the
Atlanto-Scandian (Icelandic-Norwegian) herring living to approaching 30
years although rarely exceeding 35 cm in length. On the other hand, the
life-span of the small tropical clupeids and anchovies is short, in the
region of 3-5 years.

The salmoniformes, on the main teleostean evolutionary line, are typically inhabitants of northerly regions and the sub-Arctic. Perhaps partly
for this reason, some species such as the char (Salvelinus spp) and whitefish (Coregonus spp), like the northern herrings are unusually long-lived
for their size, reaching ages well into the 30's. Others, such as smelts
(Osmeridae) and capelin (Mallotus villosus) although also northerly, have
life-spans in the range of 5-10 years. The salmonidae are especially
remarkable for the wide variation in their longevity within closely related

genera. Thus, in contrast to the long-lived chars, Pacific salmon (Oncorhynchus spp) grow larger but are much shorter-lived and strictly semelparous, all dying very soon after the first spawning. The extreme case is the pink salmon (O. gorbuscha) which has a strict 2-year life-span. Both the salmonids (Thorpe et al., 1982) and the salvelinids (Nordeng, 1983) are remarkable for the plasticity of their growth, maturation and longevity within the same gene pool.

The orders of higher teleosts shown in Fig. 2 (except for the Myctophiformes which are small) include species covering a range of size and life-spans. This characteristic reaches its ultimate expression in the sub-order Acanthopterygii, which includes the most prolific (in terms of species) of all orders, the Perciformes, which has over 7000 species. Several of the orders comprising the Acanthopterygii include the shortest-lived of all fish, with a life-span of a year or, possibly a little less. Among these are Cynolebias spp and Notobranchius spp of the Cyprinodontiformes, the grunion (Leuresthes tenuis) of the Atheriniformes, some of the tropical gobies in the Perciformes (e.g., the world's smallest fish, Triminatom nanus, which is fully grown and mature at 8 mm) and some sticklebacks (Gasterostiformes).

The Acanthopterygii also include very long-lived species. Among the Pleuronectiformes are fish such as halibut, (Hippoglossus spp), plaice (Pleuronectes platessa) and sole (Microstomus pacificus), which have been reliably recorded up to 35-45 years of age, while the large tunnies (Perciformes) have a similar life-span. But the record goes to a species of rockfish (Sebastes aleutianus) of the Scorpaeniformes, with a maximum recorded age of 140 years (Chilton and Beamish, 1982). Ages between 60 and 120 years were recorded by these authors for several other Sebastes species from the north Pacific. The extreme longevity of some species of the genus Sebastes is even more remarkable in that they do not grow to particularly large sizes; thus Sandeman (1969) records 50 year old S. mentella from Labrador of no more than 40 cm in length. There is no doubt that the genus Sebastes comes nearest to Bidder's concept of immortality!

Patchy though the evolutionary record is, some conclusions can be drawn from this necessarily brief review of the evidence:

(a) Apart from the cyclostomes, long life and (usually) large size, are characteristic of the living representatives of the primitive fish groups. Conversely, short life and small size are rare outside the teleosts; this is true even for the elasmobranchs which are highly successful colonisers of all parts of the marine environment (though surprisingly, not of freshwaters, except for a few species in Central and South America).

(b) Some limitation of range of longevity also occurs among the most primitive teleost groups, but in some, this feature tends to be offset by plasticity of longevity and other life-history characteristics within the genetic repertoire of the species. The greatly increased speciation that accompanied later teleost evolution has seen a widening of the range of interspecific longevity, the extremes of both short-and long life-spans being found in the most advanced acanthopterygian groups. On the other hand, the high degree of intraspecific plasticity of the salmonoids seem to have been lost.

(c) There is a tendency for longevity, and to a lesser extent large size, to be associated with cold environments, and vice-versa. This is seen most clearly within the environmental range of one species, or between closely related species of one genus. The association becomes weaker between less closely related groups. The most extreme

examples of short and long life are indeed found in fishes living in
warm and cold (or, at least, temperate) environments, respectively;
but the next longest and shortest life spans are widely distributed.

(d) Perhaps surprisingly, the mode of reproduction seems weakly, if
at all, related to longevity. Among the very long-lived species are
both highly fecund oviparous fishes (e.g., sturgeons) and viviparous
or ovo-viviparous fishes (e.g., sharks and Sebastes spp.) oviparity
and viviparity is also found among the extremely short-lived species,
e.g., Cyprinidontidae (killifish) and Poecillidae (mollies)
respectively. Apart from these very small annual fishes, the
incidence of semelparity, with an abrupt end of the life-span after a
single spawning, is infrequent and found mainly in more primitive
groups (cyclostomes, eels, salmonids and some clupeids).

(e) It could therefore be conjectured that semelparity and short
life (despite, perhaps, a fairly large size) was the primordial
reproductive strategy of the early vertebrates, and its replacement
by iteroparity and increased longevity presumably conveying greater
ecological versatility and evolutionary fitness. To take full
advantage of iteroparity, it would be necessary for an adequate food
supply to be available to support the continued growth as adults,
which characterizes fish. Nellen (1985) argues in this connection
that for larger individuals, consumption of smaller members of their
own species might well have been the only feasible source of food,
and that the high fecundity typical of bony fish evolved to meet this
requirement. Cannibalism is still, of course, very common in such
fish and a major source of food.

LONGEVITY AND NATURAL SELECTION - THE DEMOGRAPHIC EVIDENCE

The evolutionary evidence I summarised points to the conclusion that,
in general, it has been of evolutionary value to live longer. If this is
indeed the case, it is presumably because greater longevity conveys a selective advantage by increasing the cumulative life-time fecundity (egg production) of the longer-lived female parent. For this to happen two sets of
demographic criteria have to be satisfied:

(a) There has to be a favourable trade-off between growth, the onset
of maturation, and subsequent reproduction and survival within the
adult (mature) phase of the life cycle.

(b) Any such changes tending to increase life-time egg-production
must be at least neutral, if not favourable, to the many events which
must also be successfully completed during reproduction itself and
the pre-mature phase of the life-cycle.

This second criterion is particularly significant in all highly fecund
fish where mortality is very high in early life. However, practical difficulties of sampling, have meant that much less quantitative data exist for
the pre-mature stage of the life-cycle in fish than for the mature phase,
and almost nothing is known about a possible causal connection between these
two criteria. In confining attention to the mature phase of the life-cycle,
as in what follows and in the vast majority of papers on reproductive strategies in fish, it must be remembered therefore that conclusions about
"evolutionary fitness" deriving therefrom may not necessarily be decisive
until their possible connections (if any) with pre-mature survival can be
established.

It is clearly impossible to test from the fossil record whether the trade-offs embodied in criteria (a) have been instrumental in the evolution of species. Furthermore, the contemporary "rate of evolution" in fish is too slow to expect to see and assess their significance except in very favourable circumstances. It seems to me, however, that an ecological approach offers another line of attack which may throw further light on the problem. Two starting postulates are needed:

(a) That evolution has been moulded (often brutally) by major climatic events (e.g., glacial periods).

(b) That the problems facing a species attempting to maintain self-reproducing populations at the extremes of its environmental range are similar in kind, if not in magnitude, to those of the whole species if confronted with a major climatic change.

Life-time Cohort Egg-production (LCE)

To the extent that the above postulates are valid, it is reasonable to suppose that a species adapts its reproductive strategy at the extremes of the range in accordance with criteria (a) above, within the limits of its contemporary genetic repertoire. To test this hypothesis it is first necessary to express these criteria in quantitative form which permits comparisons to be made. The formations are well established and already have been used to explore theoretically the concepts of reproductive strategy in fish, notably by Stearns and Crandall (1984).

If the number of female fish surviving to age t from a total of $R_m^{\female}$ of a cohort (e.g., year-class) reaching maturity at age t_m is N_t, and the fecundity of an individual at age t is F_t, then the Life-time Cohort Egg-production (LCE) is:

$$LCE = \int_{t_m}^{\infty} N_t E_t \cdot dt \qquad \ldots\ldots(1)$$

$$t \geq t_m$$

This will be recognised as the Euler-Lotka equation but without (as intended) the rate of increase term e^{-rt} and the condition for equilibrium that the integral should equal unity.

The development of equation (1) in a form appropriate to fish population dynamics derives from the methodology of Beverton and Holt (1957, 1964). It was subsequently extended and applied to the analysis of population biomass and fecundity by Iles (1973), Schopka and Hempel (1973) and Jensen (1981). Some further definitions and adaptations presently required are:

(a) The natural mortality rate in mature fish populations probably increases with age (i.e., is Gompertzian) even when there is no abrupt end to the life-span, but the evidence is problematic. It is sufficient for the present purposes to postulate a constant average mortality coefficient M over the mature phase (Beverton, 1963). The quantity N_t of (1) can then be expressed as:

$$N_t = R_m^{\female} e^{-M(t-t_m)} \qquad \ldots\ldots(2)$$

$$(t \geq t_m)$$

(b) In most fish, and especially in the highly fecund oviparous species, fecundity is fairly closely proportional to body weight (Bagenal, 1973), so that it is possible to write, as a reasonable approximation:

$$E_t = qwt \qquad \qquad ....(3)$$

where w_t is the weight of a female fish of age t.

(c) <u>Growth</u> is continuous in fish but the rate declines as the asymptotic size is approached. The average growth in length of fish is well described, neglecting seasonal and other possible transient irregularities, by the von Bertalanffy equation:

$$l_t = L_\infty (1-e^{-K(t-t_o)}) \qquad \qquad ....(4)$$

where L_{oo} is the asymptotic length, K a constant determining the rate at which that asymptotic length is approached, i.e., the "curvature" of the growth curve, and t_o is an arbitrary constant defining the age at which length is theoretically zero. Since weight is closely proportional to the cube of length in most fish, the equation for growth in weight corresponding to (4) is:

$$w_t = p\, L_\infty \,(1-e^{-K(t-t_o)})^3 \qquad \qquad ....(5)$$

in which p = constant. Equation (5) can be more conveniently written in summation form as:

$$w_t = pL_\infty^3 \sum_{n=0}^{3} U_n e^{-nK(t-t_o)} \qquad \qquad ....(6)$$

in which $U_o = 1$, $U_1 = -3$, $U_2 = +3$, and $U_3 = -1$.

The conventional form of the equation for LCE of a cohort R_m^o of female fish maturing at age T_m can now be obtained by substituting for N_t from (2), E_t from (3) and w_t from (6), in (1) and integrating over the mature life-span, giving:

$$LCE = R_m q p L_\infty^3 \sum_{n=0}^{3} \frac{U_n e^{nK(T_m-t_o)}}{M + nK} \qquad \qquad ....(7)$$

I shall now make four modifications to this equation so that it is more convenient for the analysis of the reproductive strategy "trade-off." Two are purely algebraic, viz:

(i)   to take $1/M$ out of the summation term, and

(ii)   to substitute, from (3),

$$e^{-nK(T_m-t_o)} = (1-L_m/L_\infty)^n \qquad \qquad ....(8)$$

where L_m is the length at which 50% of the female cohort attains maturity.

(iii) The third is to replace the mortality coefficient M by the inverse of the characteristic maximum observed age T_{max}, to which is dimensionally equivalent (Beverton, 1963). Hoenig (1983) showed that data of M and T_{max} in fish are adequately graduated by simple inverse proportionality, i.e., it is possible to write:

$$M = g/T_{max} \qquad \qquad ....(9)$$

where g is a constant having a value of about 4.

(iv)   The last modification to (6) is conceptual, and is to define by T^*_m the lowest mean age at which the species is physiologically capable of maturing and by R^*_m the cohort numbers at that age. The natural mortality rate operative in the age span between T^*_m and the actual mean age at maturity T_m will be assumed to be the same as the mortality rate after maturity. The life-span thus formulated is shown in schematic form in Fig. 3.

With these substitutions and modifications, the Life-time Cohort Egg-production per female reaching maturity, referred back to the number at the minimum possible maturation age T^*_m, becomes:-

$$\frac{LCE}{R^*_m} = qpL_\infty^3 \cdot \frac{T_{max}}{4} \exp\left[-4\left(\frac{T_m - T^*_m}{T_{max}}\right)\right] \times \sum_{n=0}^{3} \frac{U_n\left(1 - \frac{L_m}{L_\infty}\right)^n}{1 + \frac{nKT_{max}}{4}} \qquad ....(10)$$

Inspection of this equation shows that, dimensionally, the life-time egg-production is proportional to the product of weight and age (pL_∞^3 and T_{max}), as it should be. All other terms:

$$\frac{T_m - T^*_m}{T_{max}} \quad , \quad L_m/L_\infty \quad , \quad KT_{max} \qquad ....(11)$$

are dimensionless, but their respective numerical values for a given population moderates the otherwise direct relationship between life-time egg-production on the one hand and weight and longevity on the other. Thus equation (10) provides a quantitative basis for examining how well a species has adapted its life-time reproductive strategy, measured in terms of the trade-off between maturity, growth, fecundity and longevity, to the various conditions encountered across its environmental range.[*]

Application to Walleye (Stizostedion vitreum vitreum)

The idea that the life-history characteristics of species would be expected to change in a regular way across the latitudinal range of a species is not new. It was elegantly developed by the great Russian ichthyologist G. V. Nikolskii in his book on Fish Population Dynamics

---

[*] The lack of a Gompertzian representation of the age-specificity of mortality rate leads to the somewhat incongruous inclusion of an implicitly limited life-span (T_{max}) in an equation integrated to infinity. A check on whether any significant distortion is thereby introduced can be obtained by repeating calculations with integration terminated at an upper life-span limit of $T\lambda$, where $T\lambda$ is set at the observed characteristic maximum age T_{max} plus, say, 10%. In the following analysis the difference amounted to a few per cent at all except the lowest values of T_{max} (see Table 2), and did not affect significantly the conclusions.

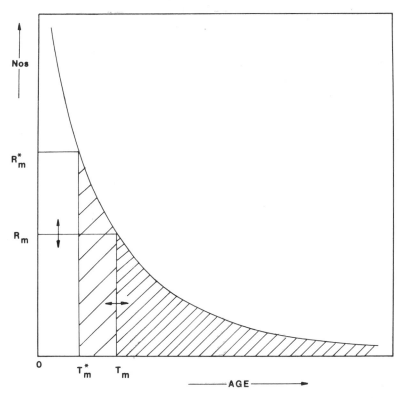

Fig. 3.   Schematic representation of the life-span, showing lowest possible age at maturity T_m^* and actual age at maturity T_m.

(1969). Since then a number of studies showed that one or more of the "reproductive strategy" parameters do indeed vary in this way (e.g., Leggett and Carscadden (1978), for the American shad, <u>Alosa sapidissima</u>). To my knowledge, however, estimation of the Life-time Cohort Egg-production across the range of a single species has not hitherto been attempted. No doubt the reason is that the instances in which the full suite of parameters needed to compute the LCE from equation (10) are few and far between.

There is one species for which such an analysis is possible. This is the north American pikeperch or walleye, <u>Stizostedion vitreum vitreum</u>. The walleye, a member of the perch family which can reach a length approaching a metre and a weight of 15 kg, has been extensively studied because of its importance for sport fishing. The comparative population biology of a number of self-contained populations, from the extreme southernmost limits of the species in California to the northerly limit of its range in Canada, is well-documented and analysed by Colby et al. (1979) and Colby and Nepszy (1981).

The full suite of parameters for female fish needed to calculate the Life-time Cohort Egg-production (as defined by equation (10)) can be estimated from the data given in these two sources for a number of locations across the environmental range, with two qualifications. One is that direct observations of the length at 50% maturity, L_m, are not quoted; however, the corresponding age at 50% maturity is given, which together with length-at-age data, allows L_m to be estimated sufficiently well for the present purpose. The other is that some of the populations in question support sport

Table 1. Ages of maturity and maximum ages of female walleye at various ambient temperatures (from Colby and Nepszy, 1981, Fig. 4 and Table 2).

Temp. (GDDx10^{-3})	T_{max}(yr)	Temp. (GDDx10^{-3})	T_m(yr)
1.15	19	0.97	8.5
1.4	15	1.01	9
1.65	14	1.02	9
1.9	11	1.04	6
2.15	15	1.16	6.5
2.4	12	1.18	7
2.65	7	1.28	7.5
2.9	11	1.29	5.5
3.15	9	1.42	7
3.4	8	1.90	4.5
3.65	11	2.19	3.5
3.9	8	2.60	2.5
4.15	8	3.69	2.5
4.4	-	4.08	(2.5)
4.65	6	4.15	(2.5)
4.9	3	4.44	(2)
5.15	4	5.68	(2)
5.4	3		
5.65	3		

fisheries, which may have lowered to some degree the observed maximum ages. On the other hand, of particular value is that a physiologically relevant index of the ambient temperature for each location has been derived by Colby and Nepszy (1981), namely the sum of the products of days x degrees above 5°C, this being the minimum temperature in the growing season which allows growth to take place.

The most extensive set of data with associated temperatures are of maximum age (T_{max}) and age at 50% maturity (T_m). These are given in Table I, being derived from Fig. 4 and Table II of Colby and Nepszy (1981).

Fig. 4 shows T_{max} and T_m plotted against the temperature index GDD x 10^{-3}. The lower bound to T_m (and presumably, to T_{max}) at the highest observed temperatures is particularly important, since it provides an estimate of T_m^* the lowest physiologically possible age at maturity, of 2 years. Interpolation from the curve of Fig. 4 also provides a better estimate of T_{max} and T_m than are available directly for the 13 locations for which growth and temperature are given in Appendix I of Colby et al. (1979). Table 2 gives the resultant suite of parameter values of growth, maturity and longevity, estimated for each location, together with the associated temperature indices as GDD x 10^{-3}.

The relationships between T_{max} and T_m (the curve being derived from Fig. 4) and between L_m and L_∞, are shown in Figs. 5(a) and 5(b) respectively. In Fig. 5(b) the points are labelled according to the serial number of the location listed in Table 2. T_m falls more or less linearly with T_{max} as the temperature increases, until the lower limit of $T_m^* = 2$ yr is reached. In contrast, L_m remains effectively constant, even though L_∞ at the high temperatures is only about half that at the lowest temperature (50 cm compared with 110 cm).

Table 2. Estimates of parameters of growth, maturity and longevity, of walleye and values of Life-time Cohort Egg-production, LCE/Rm$^{\circ}_{+}$ at 13 locations, with ambient temperatures (GDDx10^{-3}).

No.	Location	Temp. GDDx10^{-3}	T_{max}[a] yr	T_m[a] yr	K yr^{-1}	L_∞ cm	L_m cm	KT_{max}	LCE/R$_m$$^{\circ}_{+}$ (eggsx10^{-3})
1	Big Trout Lake, Ont	1.04	20	8.0	0.05	85	44	1.0	223
2	N.Caribou Lake, Ont	1.16	19	7.3	0.09	72	39	1.7	167
3	Lac La Ronge, Sask	1.18	18	7.1	0.06	108	46	1.1	296
4	Deer Lake, Ont	1.28	17.5	6.4	0.09	88	38	1.6	209
5	Escanaba Lake, Wis	1.90	14	4.3	0.21	62	41	2.9	194
6	Lake Winibago, Wis	2.19	13	3.6	0.21	64	39	2.7	210
7	Pike Lake, Wis	2.27	12.5	3.6	0.16	80	41	2.0	282
8	Current River, Miss	3.60	8	2.3	0.22	70	39	1.8	180
9	Lake Meredith, TX	3.69	8	2.2	0.40	60	46	3.2	225
10	Center Hill Res, TN	4.08	6.5	2.1	0.32	75	46	2.1	235
11	El Capitan Res, CA	4.44	6.0	2.1	0.69	62	50	4.1	214
12	Belton Res, TX	5.30	3.5	2.0	1.19	54	50	3.6	101
13	Canyon Res, TX	5.68	3.0	2.0	1.10	47	42	3.3	56

[a] Estimates of T_m and T_{max} are obtained by interpolation from Fig. 4.

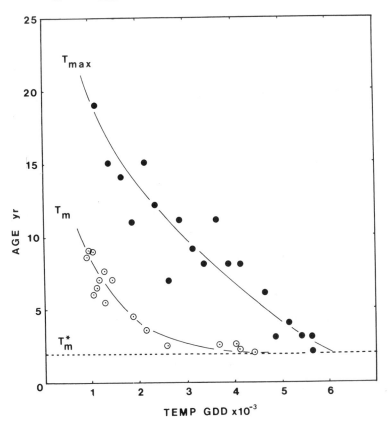

Fig. 4. Relationships beween T_{max}, T_m and ambient temperature (GDDx10^{-3}) in walleye (from Table 1).

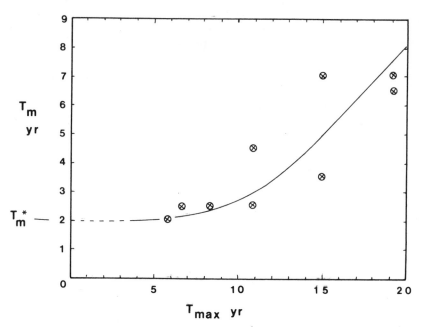

Fig. 5 (a). Relationship between T_m and T_{max} in walleye generated over a range of ambient temperature; from Table I and Fig. 4.

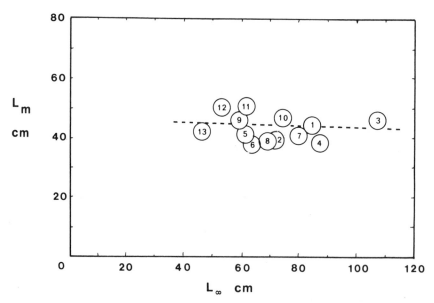

Fig. 5 (b). Relationship between L_m and L_∞ in walleye generated over the range of ambient temperature shown in Table II.

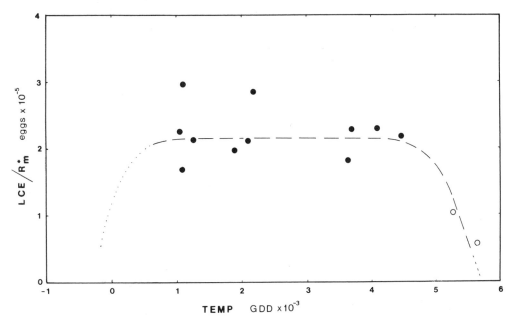

Fig. 6. Values of Life-time Cohort Egg-production per female recruit at age
T_m^*, i.e., LCE/R$_m^*$♀ from eq. (10) calculated from the parameter
values listed in Table 2 and plotted against ambient temperature.

Growth data for walleye taken from Appendix I of Colby et al., provide
the estimates of K and L_∞ listed in Table 2. Estimates of both parameters
become rather uncertain at the highest temperatures because of the extreme
shortening of the life-span, but the general tendency for K to increase
sharply with temperature, and L_∞ much less so, is clear.

Colby et al., (1979) report that the fecundity of walleye is closely
proportional to body weight, so that equation (3) is applicable. Also there
seems to be no significant trend in specific fecundity (i.e., in value of q
in equation (3)) with location nor hence with temperature. The mean value
of q from Table III of Colby et al., is 57,000 (eggs per gm female), which
is used for computing the LCE in Table 2. Calculations of the Life-time
Cohort Egg-production of mature females per recruit reaching the threshold
maturation age T_m^*, i.e., LCE/R$_m^*$♀ as defined by equation (10), are shown for
each location in the last column of Table 2 and plotted against temperature
in Fig. 6. Despite the fluctuations (due in part to variations in L_∞ which
are magnified in the cubic form qL_∞^3), the life-time fecundity per recruit
remains roughly at the same level at all temperatures except the two highest, where it falls dramatically.

It can be concluded that the walleye has a well-adapted reproductive
strategy, in that the mutual adjustment of growth, maturation, fecundity and
longevity across most of the enviromental range of the species is such as to
maintain a nearly constant life-time egg-production per recruit. This is so
despite a six-fold change in longevity. Indeed, the strong impression is of
a temperature-driven "rate of living," an old concept but one which nevertheless provides a simple description of the observed phenomena as Woodhead
(1978) pointed out with reference to temperature and longevity in other fish
species.

A further illustration of this concept is provided by the way in which the other "rate" variable, the growth coefficient K, which measures the rate at which the asymptotic length L_∞ is approached, changes with temperature. This is shown in Fig. 7(a), together with the reciprocal of longevity ($1/T_{max}$) from Fig. 4 for comparison. The close correspondence between the two temperature-driven relationships is noteworthy, and adds further confirmation to the association between temperature, mortality and growth derived by Pauly (1980) from analysis of 175 fish stocks covering a wide range of species.

In view of the fact that the quantity $4/KT_{max}$ ($\simeq M/K$) appears in the Life-time Cohort Egg-production equation (10), it is of particular interest that the relative change in K over the temperature range is greater than that of $1/T_{max}$ (i.e., 0.05 to 1.2, or about x 25 compared with 0.05 to 0.33, or about x 7). Thus the product KT_{max} itself tends to increase with temperature and its reciprocal to decrease, as shown in Fig. 7(b).

Temperature or food?

An important qualification now must be considered, namely that other environmental conditions - notably food supply - may have been correlated with temperature and had a direct effect on at least some of these parameters. Level of feeding has a powerful influence on the ultimate size (L_∞) but much less on K - unless the shape of the growth curve is distorted by marked changes in the availability of food during life. The classic experiments of Comfort (1963) on the effect of feeding on the growth and longevity of guppies (Lebistes reticulatus) shows that feeding at less than satiation increased the mean life-span by about 10% - a highly significant change but a trivial one compared with the 7-fold change in T_{max} recorded in Table 1 for walleye. Again, Edwards et al. (1979) applied experimental data of Elliott (1976) to show that ambient temperature, not availability of food was mainly responsible for observed geographical variations in the growth rate of brown trout (Salmo trutta) in contrasting rivers and streams in Britain.

From this limited evidence it would seem reasonable to surmise that although the food supply in the more northerly locations was more limited than in the highly productive southern habitats, food supply alone is unlikely to explain the much greater longevity of walleye in the northern localities or the remarkably regular increase of longevity with decreasing temperature (Fig. 4).

Another way to resolve this question would be to observe the effect of temperature on growth and longevity under conditions in which other factors are kept constant. There are numerous references in the literature to temperature-induced changes in growth and/or longevity of fish, but I cannot find any comprehensive study covering the life-time growth, maturation and survival history of even short-lived species under a range of controlled conditions of temperature and feeding. For example, Comfort (1963) made only passing reference to maturation in his guppies, and did not treat temperature as an experimental variable. Elliott's (1976) studies on growth and feeding of trout (S. trutta) in relation to temperature covered only the first two years of life in a fairly long-lived species. The nearest experimental evidence which can be compared directly with the above analysis for walleye is that of Kinne (1960) on growth and temperature in the desert pupfish (Cyprinodon macularias).

Kinne maintained populations of C. macularias at five different temperatures for 26 weeks, by which time enough of the growth span was completed to enable accurate estimates of K and L_∞ to be obtained from his published

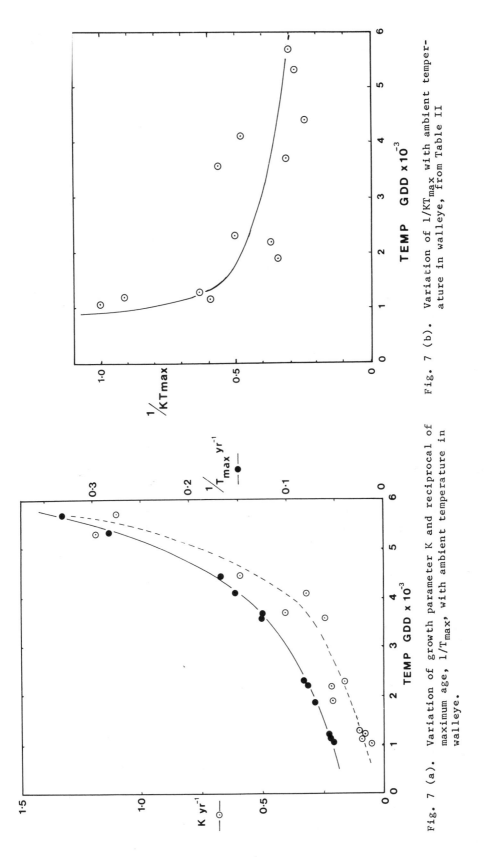

Fig. 7 (a). Variation of growth parameter K and reciprocal of maximum age, $1/T_{max}$, with ambient temperature in walleye.

Fig. 7 (b). Variation of $1/KT_{max}$ with ambient temperature in walleye, from Table II

Table 3. Estimates of K and L_∞ for desert pupfish (<u>Cyprinodon macularias</u>) reared at various temperatures (from Kinne, 1960)

Temp. $^\circ$C	L_∞ mm	K yr^{-1}
15	24.0	1.6
20	29.0	1.6
25	31.0	3.7
30	31.7	3.9
35	24.0	6.2

data. The growth curves are shown in Fig. 8 and the estimates of K and L_∞ derived from them in Table 3.

Fig. 9(a) shows those estiamtes of K and L_∞ for <u>C. macularias</u> plotted against temperature, while Fig. 9(b) shows the same plot for walleye (taken from Table 2). Fig. 9(c) shows estimates of K and L_∞ for North Atlantic cod (<u>Gadus morhua</u>) modified from Taylor (1958). When it is remembered that these results refer to three quite unrelated species, and we compare marine and freshwater field data obtained by many observers with precisely controlled experimental data, the similarity in the way that the two parameters change with temperature is rather striking.

The first function to fail at both the cold and warm extremes of the environmental range of walleye appear to be maturation - or, at least, the regular production of viable eggs. Thus the walleye in the warmest location (Canyon Reservoir, Texas) and perhaps those in the next warmest (Belton Reservoir, Texas) fail to produce viable offspring, the population having to be maintained by stocking. At temperatures much lower than in the most northerly locations listed in Table 2 growth is evidently so slow that the threshold size for maturation either is never reached or, if it is, there are insufficient metabolic resources available for oocyte development. In some other species, of which the European sculpin (<u>Cottus gobio</u>) and loach (<u>Noemacheilus barbatulus</u>) are examples, egg production at the "cold" extreme of their range is maintained - albeit at reduced level - by reducing the number of "batches" of eggs spawned per season (Mann et al., 1984); but walleye are not "batch spawners" and cannot use this tactic.

Heritability of reproductive strategies

If there were any genetic basis to the mutual adjustment between growth, maturation and longevity - and perhaps fecundity as well - which exists across the environmental range of the walleye, it would be tempting to interpret this as incipient speciation. Despite the fact that the walleye occupies lakes and streams of which many are geographically isolated and widely separated, attempts to identify races or strains having some degree of genetic differentiation have met with relatively little success. As Colby and Nepszy (1981) put it ... "Although there is some genotypic evidence for stock discreteness, most evidence points to differences (age, growth, fecundity, maturity) which are believed to be phenotypic expressions induced by the environment."

Surprising though this conclusion may seem, it is in keeping with the growing body of evidence for the plasticity of the parameters governing reproductive strategy. This acid test, which is whether individuals and their offspring which are either transplanted from one part of their range

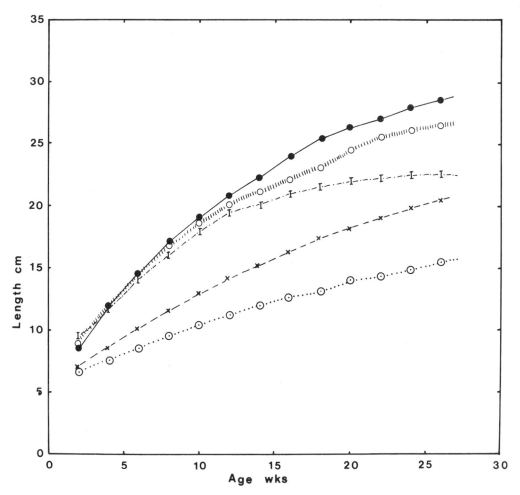

Fig. 8. Growth in length of <u>Cyprinodon macularias</u> at various temperatures
(from Kinne, 1960).

to another or are reared in controlled conditions, retain their reproductive
characteristics, does not appear to have been carried out in walleye.

There is, however, abundant evidence in other species to show that much
of the observed intraspecific variation in reproductive characteristics,
even between geographically isolated species, is mainly or wholly phenotypic. The plasticity of salmonids and salvelinids has been referred to.
Mann et al. (1984) report that when sculpins (<u>Cottus gobio</u>) were transferred from streams in the south of England to the north and vice-versa, the
transferred fish tended to take on the reproductive strategies of the local
fish; so these authors concluded that the differences were essentially
phenotypic. Again, Godø and Moksness (1985) showed that by rearing cod
(<u>Gadus morhua</u>) from the Arcto-Norwegian and coastal populations in aquaria
in optimal conditions of feeding and temperature, the large differences in
growth and age at maturation between the two populations in the wild could
be eliminated. Of particular significance was that the two cod populations
in the wild can be separated by haemoglobin polymorphism, a fact which
throws doubt on the use of this character as a true diagnostic of genetic
differentiation.

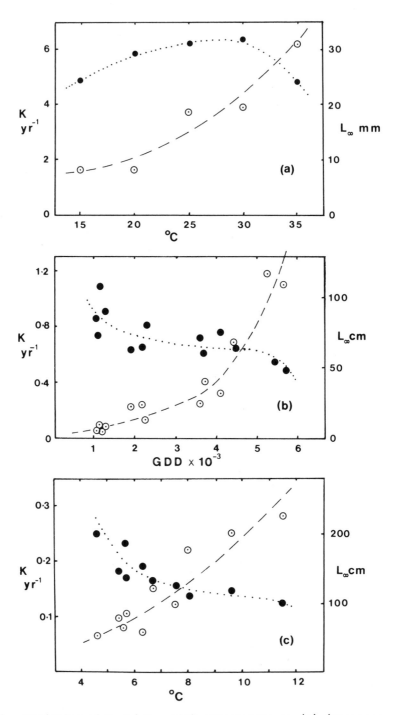

Fig. 9. Variation of K and L_∞ with temperature in (a) (Cyprinodon macularias) from Table III, (b) Walleye, from Table II, (c) cod (G. morhua), modified from Taylor (1958).

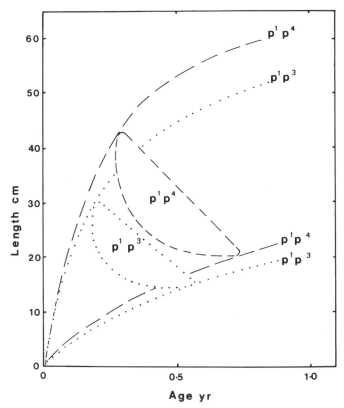

Fig. 10.   Envelopes bounding range of age and length at first maturity in
two genotypes of platyfish (<u>X. maculatus</u>) under different feeding
conditions, with presumed curves of growth in length. (Adapted
from McKenzie et al., 1983).

There are, however, a few instances in which genetically based differences of reproductive strategy parameters within a single species have been
demonstrated. One is of populations of mosquito fish (<u>Gambusia affinis</u>)
which have survived through some 140 generations in reservoirs in Hawaii
from an initial stock of 150 fish introduced in 1905 for mosquito control.
Stearns (1983) showed that female fish from reservoirs with fluctuating
water levels mature at a later age (8% greater) and at a little smaller size
(3% smaller) than those from stable reservoirs, when both are reared under
controlled conditions. In males, both the age and length at maturity of
fish from the fluctuating reservoirs was greater than from the stable ones
(16% and 6%, respectively).

Other evidence of intraspecific genotypic differentiation of maturation
comes from the work of McKenzie et al. (1983) on the platyfish (<u>Xiphophorus
maculatus</u>). By rearing them under a wide range of feeding conditions, they
showed that the weight-age relationship at maturation was almost completely
distinguishable in two genotypes which differed at a sex-linked P locus.
For comparison with other data in this paper I converted their weight data
to length, the resulting length-age envelopes being shown in Fig. 10.
McKenzie et al. (1983) do not give the full growth curves, but it may be
surmised that they are something like those shown by the broken lines.
These results show that size at maturity can be influenced by large differences in food supply, and that under these conditions it is the size-age
relationship rather than size (or age) as such which is the distinguishing
characteristic of the two genotypes. I hope that the full life-time growth

and longevity data for these populations soon will be published, since they promise to be of exceptional interest.

While a high degree of phenotypic plasticity of the parameters governing reproductive strategy in fish is established, the above analysis suggests that not all parameters are equally plastic, nor is the influence of the two main environmental factors, temperature and food, the same. Thus because temperature determines the "rate of living" (and of dying), longevity (T_{max}), age at maturity (T_m) and the rate of completion of the growth pattern (K) are all directly temperature-dependent, whereas the two size "markers," length at maturity (L_m) and asymptotic length (L_∞), are relatively insensitive. In contrast, food supply has the most marked effect on those size markers, particularly on L_∞, and a relatively minor effect on longevity.

The "robustness" of L_m with respect to ambient temperature across the environmental range of a species is in harmony with the results obtained by Stearns (1983) in further experiments with the mosquito fish from Hawaii raised at temperatures between 24°C and 28°C. Whereas age at maturity decreased by some 30% over this temperature range, the length at first maturity hardly changed. This robustness of length at maturity is also consistent with the conclusion reached by Alm (1959, Fig. 58) in his classic study of growth and maturation of various species of fish (particularly trout, S. trutta) in Swedish lakes when making intraspecific comparisons, i.e., beween cohorts of the same population or between populations. Where there are known genetic differences however, Alm found that length at maturity was more variable. Similarly Beverton and Holt (1959) in their review of widely differing species of fish, found that both L_m and L_∞ tended to vary together. Again, Beverton (1963) found a rather closely proportional relationship between L_m and L_∞ among different species and genera of clupeids (herrings) and engraulids (anchovies).

It is impossible to reconstruct with any confidence the precise kind of environmental influences that have shaped evolution, but the general conclusion seems to be that climatic trends have predominated (Clemens, 1986). Again, temperature is not the only manifestation of climatic change but it is likely to be the most consistent. In contrast, the connection between food supply and environmental extremes or climatic change is much less regular or predictable. Therefore, if true genetic speciation is now occurring at the extremes of the contemporary range of a species, or has done so in the past, it may be that the crucial step is the physiological release of the incipient "new" species from the straightjacket (in reproductive strategy terms) of a tightly confined size at maturity.

CONCLUDING REMARKS

While this analysis shows that a trade-off between growth, maturity and longevity can be conceived which, in given conditions, maximises the potential Life-time Cohort Egg-production it is not a sufficient explanation of the precise mechanism of speciation. This must work through the enhanced evolutionary fitness imparted to the individual. It requires that not only that fitness is sufficiently heritable, but also that heritability is transmitted preferentially to a limited progeny and not dissipated among the population at large.

The key presumably lies in the variaton of reproductive strategy that exists between the individuals of one and the same cohort. Wide variation in size and maturation among individuals of the same age is characteristic of fish populations, but little is known about the corresponding variation of growth pattern, mortality and longevity within cohorts.

The ultimate test of the capacity of a fish species to survive at environmental extremes, or to adapt to an environmental change, may not lie in
the adult reproductive strategy at all but in the earlier stages of the
life-history, wherein lie the main determinants of the size of the cohort
when it eventually reaches maturity in the next generation. Apart from a
few intriguing clues (e.g., Thorpe et al., 1984, on egg size and larval
growth in salmon) the association in fish between the criteria for evolutionary fitness in the pre-mature phase and adult reproductive strategy in
terms of egg production is largely uncharted territory.

REFERENCES

Alm, G., 1959, Connection between maturity, size and age in fishes, Rep.
    Inst. Freshwater Res. Drottningholm, 40:5.
Applegate, V. C., 1950, Natural history of the sea lamprey (Petromyzon
    marinus) in Michigan, U.S. Fish Wildl. Serv. Spec. Sci. Rep. Fish,
    555:1.
Bagenal, T. B., 1973, Fish fecundity and its relations with stock and
    recruitment, Rapp. P-V. Reun. Cons. Int. Explor. Mer., 164:247.
Bennett, J. T., Boehlert, G. W., and Turekian, K. K., 1982, Confirmation of
    longevity in Sebastes diploproa (Pisces: Scorpaenidae) from
    $^{210}Pb/^{226}Ra$ measurements in otoliths, Mar. Biol., 71:209.
Beverton, R. J. H., 1963, Maturation, growth and mortality of Clupeid and
    Engraulid stocks in relation to fishing, J. Cons. Cons. Int. Explor.
    Mer, 154:44.
Beverton, R. J. H., and Holt, S. J., 1957, On the dynamics of exploited
    fish populations, Fish. Invest. Ser. II, Vol. XIX, HMSO, 553.
Beverton, R. J. H., and Holt, S. J., 1959, A review of the lifespans and
    mortality rates of fish in nature, and their relationship to growth
    and other physiological characteristics, Ciba Found. Colloq. Ageing,
    5:142.
Beverton, R. J. H., and Holt, S. J., 1964, Tables of yield functions for
    fishery assessment, FAO Fish. Tech. Pap., No. 38.
Bidder, G. P., 1932, Senescence, Brit. Med. J., ii: 583.
Blacker, R. W., 1974, Recent advances in otolith studies, in: "Sea Fisheries
    Research," F. R. Harden Jones, ed., Elek Science, London.
Chilton, D. E., and Beamish, R. J., 1982, Age determination methods for
    fishes studied by the groundfish program at the Pacific Biological
    Station, Can. Spec. Publ. Fish. Aquat. Sci., 60.
Christensen, J. M., 1964, Burning of otoliths, a technique for age determin-
    ation of soles and other fish. J. Cons. Cons. Int. Explor. Mer., 29:
    73.
Clemens, W. A., 1986, Evolution of the terrestrial vertebrate fauna during
    the Cretaceous-Tertiary Transition in:"Dynamics of Extinction," D. K.
    Elliott, ed., John Wiley, New York.
Colby, P. J., McNicol, R. E., and Ryder, R. A., 1979, Synopsis of biological
    data on the walleye Stizostedion v. vitreum (Mitchell 1818), FAO
    Fish. Syn. No., 119:139.
Colby, P. J., and Nepszy, S. J., 1981, Variation among stocks of Walleye
    (Stizostedion vitreum vitreum), Management implications, Can. J.
    Fish. Aquat. Sci., 38:1814.
Comfort, A., 1963, Effect of delayed and resumed growth on the longevity of
    a fish (Lebistes reticulatus, Peters) in captivity, Gerontologia,
    8:150.
Doroshov, S. I., 1985, Biology and culture of sturgeon Acipenseriformes,
    in: "Recent Advances in Aquaculture 2," J. F. Muir and R. J. Roberts,
    eds., Croom Helm, London.
Edwards, R. W., Densem, J. W., and Russell, P. A., 1979, An assessment of
    the importance of temperature as a factor controlling the growth rate
    of brown trout in streams, J. Anim. Ecol., 48:501.

Elliott, J. M., 1976, The energetics of feeding metabolism and growth of
brown trout (Salmo trutta L.) in relation to body weight, water
temperature and ration size, J. Anim. Ecol., 45:923.

Godø, O. R., and Moksness, E., 1985, Growth and maturation of Norwegian
coastal cod and Arctic-Norwegian cod under different conditions, in:
"Proc. Workshop on Comp. Biol. Assess Manag. of Gadoids from N. Pac.
and Atl. Oceans, Part II," Seattle, Washington.

Hoenig, J. M., 1983, Empirical use of longevity data to estimate mortality
rates, Fish. Bull., 82: No. 1.

Iles, T. D., 1973, Dwarfing or stunting in the Genus Tilapia (Cichlidae):
a possibly unique recruitment mechanism, Rapp. p-V. Reun. Cons. Int.
Explor. Mer., 164:247.

Jensen, A. L., 1981, Population regulation in lake whitefish, Coregonus
clupeaformis (Mitchill), J. Fish. Biol., 19:557.

Ketchen, K. S. 1974, Age and growth of dogfish Squalus acanthias in British
Columbia Waters, J. Fish. Res. Board Can., 32:43.

Kinne, O., 1960, Growth, food intake, and food conversion in a euryplastic
fish exposed to different temperatures and salinities, Physiol.
Zool., 33:288.

Kristinsson, J. B. Saunders, R. L., and Wiggs, A. J., 1985, Growth dynamics
during the development of bimodal length-frequency distribution in
juvenile Atlantic Salmon (Salmo salar L.), Aquaculture, 45:1.

Lea, E., 1913, Further studies concerning the methods of calculating the
growth of herring, Publs. Circonst. Cons. Int. Explor. Mer., 66:1.

Leaman, B. M., and Beamish, R. J., 1984, Ecological and management
implications of longevity in some northeast Pacific ground fishes,
Bull. Int. North Pacific Fish. Commission, 42:85.

Leggett, W. C., and Carscadden, J. E., 1978, Latitudinal variation in
reproductive characteristics of American Shad (Alosa sapidissima):
Evidence for population specific life history strategies in fish,
J. Fish. Res. Board. Can., 35:1469.

Mann, R. H. K., Mills, C. A., and Crisp, D. T., 1984, Geographical variation
in the life-history tactics of some species of freshwater fish, in:
"Fish Reproduction: Strategies and Tactics," G. W. Potts, and R. J.
Wooton, eds., Academic Press, London.

McKenzie, W. Jr., Crews, D., and Kallman, K. D., 1983, Age, weight and
genetics of sexual maturation in the platyfish, Amer. Soc. Ichthy.
Herp., 770.

Moyle, P. B., and Cech, J. J., 1982, "Fishes: An Introduction to Ichthy-
ology," Prentice-Hall Inc., New Jersey.

Nellen, W., 1986, A hypothesis on the fecundity of bony fish,
Meeresforch., 31:75.

Nelson, J. S., 1984, "Fishes of the World," John Wiley, Interscience Pub.,
New York.

Nikolskii, G. V., 1969, "The Theory of Fish Population Dynamics," R. Jones,
ed., Oliver and Boyd, Edinburgh.

Nordeng, H., 1983, Solution to the "char problem" based on Arctic Char
(Salvelinus alpinus) in Norway, Can. J. Fish. Aquat. Sci., 40:1372.

Norman, J. R., 1975, "A History of Fishes," 3rd Ed., P. H. Greenwood, ed.,
Ernest Benn, London.

Pauly, D., 1980, On the interrelationships between natural mortality, growth
parameters and mean environmental temperature in 175 fish stocks,
J. Cons. Cons. Int. Explor. Mer., 39:175.

Sandeman, E. J., 1969, Age determination and growth rate of redfish,
Sebastes spp., from selected areas around Newfoundland, Int. Comm.
N. W. Atl. Fish Res. Bull., 6:79.

Schopka, S. A., and Hempel, G., 1973, The spawning potential of populations
of herring (Clupea harengus L.) and cod (Gadus morhua L.) in relation
to the rate of exploitation, Rapp p-v. Reun. Cons. Int. Explor. Mer.,
164:236.

Stearns, S. C., 1983, The evolution of life-history traits in mosquitofish since their introduction to Hawaii in 1905: Rates of evolution, heritabilities, and developmental plasticity, Amer. Zool., 23:65.

Stearns, S. C., and Crandall, R. E., 1984, Plasticity for age and size at sexual maturity: A life-history response to unavoidable stress, in: "Fish Reproduction: Strategies and Tactics," G. W. Potts and R. J. Wooton, eds., Academic Press, London.

Taylor, C. C., 1958, Cod growth and temperature, J. Cons. Cons. Int. Explor. Mer., 23:366.

Thorpe, J. E., Miles, M. S., and Keay, D. S., 1984, Developmental rate, fecundity and egg size in Atlantic Salmon, Salmo salar L., Aquaculture, 43:289.

Thorpe, J. E., Talbot, C., and Villarreal, C., 1982, Bimodality of growth and smolting in Atlantic Salmon, Salmo salar L., Aquaculture 28:123.

Tsepkin, E. A., and Sokolov., L. I., 1971, The maximum size and age of some sturgeon, Vopr. Ikhthiol., 11:444.

Williams, R., and Bedford, B. C., 1974, The use of otoliths for age determination, in: "The Ageing of Fish," T. Bagenal, ed., Unwin Brothers Ltd., London.

Woodhead, A. D., 1978, Fish in studies of aging, Exp. Geront., 13:125.

EVOLUTIONARY RELIABILITY THEORY

Arnold R. Miller

Department of Biological Sciences
University of Denver
Denver, CO   80208

INTRODUCTION

I am developing a new branch of reliability theory called evolutionary reliability theory that concerns the evolution of reliability in
populations of systems, such as organisms, that evolve. It subsumes the
standard reliability theory but has a higher dimension of time, namely,
evolutionary time. In reliability theory, failure phenomena are usually
classified according to the monotone properties of the hazard rate
$h(x) = g(x)/R(x)$, where h is the hazard rate, x is the age at failure, g
is the failure density function, and R is the reliability, where $R(x) =$
$P(X > x)$. Following this method of classification, we have three kinds of
evolutionary reliability phenomena: failure events that exhibit (1) a
decreasing hazard rate, (2) a constant hazard rate, and (3) an increasing
hazard rate. An example of (1) is the reliability of biological
development--the selection forces that have evolved safeguards, such as
redundancy, so that developmental errors are maintained at a tolerable
level. An example of (2) is the reliability of the fully developed system
as it faces random failure processes, e.g., accidents, disease, and
competition, and it thus concerns the evolution of structural and
functional redundancy (e.g., two kidneys and two lungs). Category (3)
concerns the reliability of the system with respect to wearout (aging) and
this is the main subject of this paper.

Wearout is a mathematical concept--it means simply that the system
experiences an increasing hazard rate--and does not necessarily imply
mechanical wearout (Birnbaum, et al., 1966). There can be chemical and
electrical wearout. Aging is a synonymous term. The main questions of
interest in regard to aging are the following: Why have organisms evolved
aging, why do they have life tables of given forms, and how extensible (in
terms of cost) are their lifespans once they have evolved? To answer
these questions, we need the concept of the heterogeneous wearout
distribution, a new reliability-theoretic concept in the evolution of
aging.

The wearout failure-time distribution of an infinite population of
genetically homogeneous components i (i = 1, 2,..., n from an n-component
system) in a constant environment is known (Barlow and Proschan, 1981;
Smith, 1983), at least for nonbiological components, to be approximately
normal with mean lifetime w_i and standard deviation s_i. The standard

deviation s_i is nonzero only because the components are not completely homogeneous due to manufacturing errors (or analogous developmental errors in the biological case) or because the environment is not perfectly homogeneous. Since for evolutionary systems these sources of variation are of minor importance compared to a much greater source, genetic heterogeneity, we assume in this work that $s_i = 0$. Consider the wearout failure distribution of genetically heterogeneous components i for an evolutionary system. This distribution is a function of the population's distribution of genotypes affecting the reliability of component i and is determined by natural selection. Let continuous random variable W_i be the wearout failure-time of genetically heterogeneous components i; each value $W_i = w_i$ corresponds to the above mean wearout lifetime w_i of a genetically homogeneous component subpopulation with $s_i = 0$. The heterogeneous wearout distribution of the system, describing the distribution of wearout over the reliability structure, is the probability density f of the random vector $\underset{\sim}{W} = (W_1, W_2, \ldots, W_n)$, where $\underset{\sim}{w}$ belongs to the Euclidean n-space $\mathcal{W} = \{\underset{\sim}{w}: w_1 > 0, w_2 > 0, \ldots, w_n > 0\}$. Any particular system or homogeneous subpopulation of systems is represented as a point $\underset{\sim}{w} = (w_1, w_2, \ldots, w_n)$ in wearout space $\mathcal{W}$.

Fundamental reliability and maintainability properties of a species depend on its heterogeneous wearout distribution. Multidimensional density f, by statistically governing all component wearout of the system, governs virtually all aging properties of the evolved system. In this model, the seemingly enigmatic fact of the evolution of biological components that self-repair yet nonetheless age--i.e., the evolution of finite-valued random variables W_i--is explicable in terms of the stationarity conditions of density f. The shape of the survival curve, or the reliability function, and the expected lifespan for the species are determined by the shape and location of f. The maintainability of the system once it has evolved aging depends on dispersion properties of the distribution: Intuitively, the number of component repairs necessary to extend the system life by a given increment depends on the correlation of random variables W_i (i = 1, 2, ..., n). Thus if we understood how f evolves under natural selection, we would gain deep insight into the most fundamental characteristics of aging in evolutionary systems.

MULTIPLE-INTEGRAL EQUATION

Our objective is to derive a mathematical expression for multidimensional density function f. I have accomplished this result, and details can be found in another paper that is submitted for publication elsewhere. The theory is developed from the following ten assumptions regarding the reliability and self-reproduction of evolutionary systems:

(1) The population consists of binary, coherent, order-n, isomorphic systems (Barlow and Proschan, 1981). Being coherent implies that a system fails only because one or more of its components fails. Isomorphic systems have the same reliability structure (e.g., whether the system is a series structure, parallel structure, etc.).

(2) There are two independent, superimposed modes of component failure: (a) random failure having a constant failure rate and (b) wearout failure having an increasing failure rate. Random failure of components arises from accidents, competition, predation, disease, and other random events.

(3) The failure of components is statistically independent.

(4) All components have the same random (exponential) failure rate
      λ, assumed given.

(5) The standard deviation s_i ($i = 1, 2,\ldots, n$) for the wearout failure-time of homogeneous components is zero. This is equivalent to a degenerate distribution with mean w_i. As is characteristic of wearout, the component failure rate is increasing since it has the value zero before age w_i and infinity at w_i.

(6) Probability density function f, the heterogeneous wearout distribution, is stationary in evolutionary time t. Since this requires that the probability of birth always equals the probability of death at each $\underset{\sim}{w} \in \mathcal{W}$, it implies that reproduction is a continuous process.

(7) The population size is infinite.

(8) At any time t, the systems that self-reproduce, called parents, are a random sample, with replacement, from the subpopulation for which age $Y \geqslant r$, where Y is a continuous random variable and r is a real parameter. Because the sampling is with replacement, a given parent can reproduce repeatedly; since sampling is random, fecundity is independent of age. Parameter r is the earliest age of reproduction for all individuals of the population.

(9) Reproduction occurs component-wise as follows. Let random variable W_i' be the wearout life of component i ($i = 1, 2,\ldots, n$) of an offspring and v_i be that of the parent. Then there exists a probability density function τ_W, assumed given, such that

$$P(a \leqslant W_i' \leqslant b) = \int_a^b \tau_W(w_i, v_i) dw_i \qquad (1)$$

where a and b are real numbers.

(10) Random variables W_i' ($i = 1, 2,\ldots, n$) are statistically independent.

From these ten assumptions, I have solved the problem by deriving (in many steps) the following multiple-integral equation whose solution is density f:

$$f(\underset{\sim}{w}) = \frac{\int_W \phi(\underset{\sim}{w}) f(\underset{\sim}{w}) d\underset{\sim}{w} \int_\gamma \tau_W(\underset{\sim}{w}, \underset{\sim}{y}) \Gamma(\underset{\sim}{y}) f(\underset{\sim}{y}) d\underset{\sim}{y}}{\phi(\underset{\sim}{w}) \int_\gamma \Gamma(\underset{\sim}{y}) f(\underset{\sim}{y}) d\underset{\sim}{y}} \qquad (2)$$

where ϕ, τ_W, and Γ are known, computable functions, $d\underset{\sim}{w} = dw_1 dw_2 \ldots dw_n$, $\mathcal{W}$ is the n-dimensional wearout space for the population, and γ is an n-dimensional subspace of $\mathcal{W}$. The only unknown quantity is the desired function f. Integral equations are analogous to differential equations (an integral equation is related to a differential equation as an integral is related to a derivative), and as for differential equations, the unknown is a function.

Equation (2), in the form of its discrete analog, is solved numerically by the method of successive approximations (Jerri, 1985). Although the theory includes broader classes of structures, the computations discussed here model organisms as series systems. Solution of equation (2) is computationally intensive, and generally a supercomputer is required. For this reason, the dimension of wearout space in these computations was limited to two or three; that is, the organisms were modeled as systems consisting of two or three modules (groups of components behaving as a single component) in series. Thus, we assume that we can partition an organism into two or three modules such that each has random failure rate λ (required by assumption 4). Besides λ, five additional parameters are required for each species (one of these is parameter r described in assumption 8). A wearout space of four dimensions is probably the practical limit for today's computer technology, if the species being modeled is relatively long-lived. The solution, density f, the heterogeneous wearout distribution, for series systems is a bell-shaped density function whose constant-probability contours are ellipse-shaped (but they are not true ellipses). The ellipse-like major axis lies along the line $w_1 = w_2$ (n = 2).

VALIDATION

From the computed density f, one can compute the life table for a species and thereby test the realism of equation (2). Life tables give the most available statistical information about the wearout of organisms. For a life table to be usable for a validation study of (2), it must satisfy the following criteria: (1) It must be statistically satisfactory. (2) Generally, the survival function should be concave, that is, not everywhere convex. The individuals of a species with a convex (exponential-like) survival function die principally from random events and thus the life table tells little about aging. (3) The observed table should be largely the product of natural selection. This would exclude, for example, species whose mortality is artificially high because of over-hunting or artificially low (in the case of humans) because of cultural changes that were instantaneous on the evolutionary time scale. Although there are at least one-hundred mammalian life tables in the literature, very few satisfy these criteria. We have found four that are suitable for the validation study. The species are all ungulates: domestic sheep, Dall sheep, African (or Cape) buffalo, and hippopotamus. A fifth, for the wild boar, being strongly convex, fails only criterion (2). Since the wild boar table is the best convex table I have found for ungulates, it is included as a limiting case. Thus, these five species represent a broad range of survival characteristics, ranging from convex to strongly concave.

The basic realism of multiple-integral equation (2) is demonstrated by its ability to predict the life tables of the ungulates wild boar, Dall sheep, African buffalo, and hippopotamus. (The fifth ungulate life table--for domestic sheep--was used to estimate empirically density function τ_W, which is then used for the other four.) The equation is satisfactorily able to predict the survival functions, both in shape and location, for the four test species. The agreement between the theoretical and empirical expected lifespans is excellent, the maximum relative error being less than 3%.

DISCUSSION

This problem, derivation of an equation describing the heterogeneous wearout distribution, leads to a multiple-integral equation, a generalization of the more common one-dimensional integral equation (Jerri, 1985), as the natural mathematical expression of the theory. Because systems are multicomponent, they are represented as points in a multidimensional Euclidean space, wearout space $\mathcal{W}$. Since the probabilities of birth and death at a point w involve integrals over subspaces of $\mathcal{W}$, density function f occurs behind multiple integral signs. The solution f of the multiple-integral equation, equation (2), is the desired heterogeneous wearout distribution at stationarity.

Since the equation has been derived exactly from the assumptions, its scope of applicability is determined by the scope of the assumptions. Thus, the equation does not apply to all organisms (for example, to species that are not fixed systems, such as bacteria, to the juvenile period of insect development, and to semelparous organisms). However, since the assumptions were developed so as to be satisfactory approximations for mammals, it does apply, in addition to others, to mammalian species.

The validation results show that a potential application of the equation is the computation of life tables *ab initio*, i.e., from the beginning, from the fundamental heterogeneous wearout distribution. However, probably a theoretically more important application concerns the question of how costly it is to extend the lifespan of an evolutionary system once it has evolved. Williams (1957) and Maynard Smith (1959) have qualitatively suggested that it would be very costly because of a proposed synchronism of the aging rates of the components of an organism: Natural selection, by acting only on the shortest-lived subsystem of an organism, should tend to bring all subsystem lifetimes to similar values. (Although the arguments were not in reliability-theoretic terms, series systems were implied.) It was even proposed that this phenomenon would make extension of the lifespan as impossible as creating a perpetual-motion machine. If such a phenomenon exists, then it should be observed in density f. And this is indeed what is observed: Random variables W_i are correlated, i.e., in any particular system, the wearout lifetimes of the components tend to be similar. Moreover, the effect increases as a function of the evolved expected lifespan of the species. Thus at least for long-lived order-2 series systems (the type studied), evolution of wearout lifetime appears to be conservative: The lifetime evolves in such a way as to make it difficult to change. I believe this is the first time such a phenomenon has been demonstrated. However, it should be noted that the results apply only to series systems, and biological organisms are only roughly series structures. Because they have substantial parallelism, they are more realistically modeled as mixed, or series-parallel, systems. Since I have also demonstrated that synchronism does not occur in parallel systems, it will be interesting to see the net effect of synchronism in series-parallel systems, as well as other types of structures not categorizable as such.

No other theory of the evolution of aging is able to predict life tables. The best developed, most plausible, and most experimentally tested hypothesis is a population-genetic theory, originally due to Medawar (1957), postulating the accumulation of deleterious pleiotropic genes or mutations due to a restriction of selection pressure on late-acting characters (aging) in organisms that have a finite probability of dying due to strictly random (non-aging) causes. In contrast, the theory of this paper is an abstract mathematical theory that assumes no physical, biological, or genetic mechanisms. It could apply to self-replicating machines that reproduce via means completely different from those of biological organisms. Nonetheless it probably subsumes the population-genetic theory as a special case or realization. The hypothesis of a restriction of natural selection is surely true, and a population obeying our assumptions presumably exhibits the phenomenon. However, instead of the hypothesis that selection fails to select against deleterious effects, a more direct and simpler hypothesis is that it fails to select for component reliability. This second viewpoint has been discussed, though not from a reliability-theoretic perspective, in the gerontological literature (Cutler, 1976; Sacher, 1978). The population-genetic theory treats organisms as systems without reliability structure, and it therefore cannot account for system details such as the shape of density f corresponding to synchronism. In contrast, the new theory is a reliability theory, an evolutionary reliability theory, and the important property of system structure is central.

I believe that multiple-integral equation (2), if it withstands further experimental testing, is the first theoretical advance in the evolution of aging at the level of detail—at the level of reliability structure—necessary to address the fundamental questions of the biology of aging asked above.

Acknowledgement. This work was supported by the National Institute on Aging through Grant AG03331 and was performed at the University of Illinois, Urbana. Computer time was provided in part by the Research Board and the National Center for Supercomputing Applications (funded by the National Science Foundation), both of the University of Illinois, Urbana.

REFERENCES

Barlow, R. E. and Proschan, F., 1981, "Statistical Theory of Reliability and Life Testing: Probability Models," To Begin With, Silver Spring, MD.
Birnbaum, Z. W., Esary, J. D., and Marshall, A. W., 1966, A stochastic characterization of wear-out for components and systems, Ann. Math. Statist., 37:816.
Cutler, R. G., 1976, Nature of aging and life maintenance processes, Interdisp. Top. Gerontol., 9:83.
Jerri, A. J., 1985, "Introduction to Integral Equations with Applications," Marcel Dekker, New York.
Maynard Smith, J., 1959, The rate of ageing in Drosophila Subobscura, in: "CIBA Foundation Colloquia on Ageing, Vol. 5: The Lifespan of Animals," G. E. W. Wolstenholme and M. O'Connor, eds., Churchill, London.
Medawar, P. B., 1957, "The Uniqueness of the Individual," Basic Books, New York. (Reprinted from the essay "An Unsolved Problem of Biology," H. K. Lewis, London, 1952.)
Sacher, G. A., 1978, Longevity, aging, and death: an evolutionary perspective, Gerontologist, 18:112.
Smith, C. O., 1983, "Introduction to Reliability in Design," Robert E. Krieger, Malabar, FA.
Williams, G. C., 1957, Pleiotropy, natural selection, and the evolution of senescence, Evolution, 11:398.

PROGRAMMED CELL DEATH AND AGING IN DROSOPHILA MELANOGASTER

Thomas A. Grigliatti

Department of Zoology
University of British Columbia, Vancouver, British Columbia
Canada V6T 2A9

INTRODUCTION

While a variety of theories regarding the etiology of aging have
been proposed, they can be classified under two extreme models. One
general model asserts that senescence is the result of attrition caused
by normal "wear and tear", that is the cumulative deleterious effects of
environmental abuse and/or internal errors generated by all physical-
chemical processes, with death as the inevitable result. At the other
extreme is the model that posits aging as a normal part of the
developmental process and therefore that at least in part, lifespan is
genetically programmed. In their simplest form, neither model is
absolutely correct, since aging, like any phenotype, must result from the
sum of the interactions of environmental influences and genotype. The
question is not whether genotype influences longevity; it certainly
does. Rather, one might question whether lifespan is genetically
programmed or not. Do genes exist whose principal, though not sole, role
is to cause cell and organismal death? There is no strong evidence to
support or reject the notion that such genes exist. Yet this hypothesis
is testable.

Hypotheses that argue that lifespan is genetically programmed make
certain predictions, namely those genes that lead to the process of
cellular deterioration and eventually organismal death, like other
developmental processes, must be activated at a precise time. Obviously,
if such genes exist, they must be activated only after the success of the
next generation has been essentially guaranteed. Such a scenario begs
the question: how might genes responsible for cell and organismal death
be temporally regulated? Development is a well-choreographed cascade or
program of genetic events. The activation of any gene, or set of genes,
ultimately depends upon the prior action of another set of genes.
Senescence and death, as the final stage of the developmental process,
should be no exception. Hence, if genes controlling longevity exist,
they must be activated at the end of the normal developmental program and
therefore their activation presumably depends upon prior and proper
activation of another set of genes. This cascade of gene action implies
that a regular pattern of gene activity exists during the adult portion
of the life cycle. Such an hypothesis is testable in organisms such as
Drosophila.

In Drosophila adults there is virtually or no mitotic cell division[1]. The only known exceptions are the premeiotic stem cells that divide to produce gamete forming cells, and the replacement of phagocytic white blood cells and possibly the cells which line the gut. In addition, there is no obvious change in cell function during the adult stage. Therefore, it is quite possible that all genes required for normal adult function and viability are activated at about the time of eclosion of the adult form and thereafter are expressed at a reasonably static level. In fact, most of the direct biochemical measurements of gene activity, including RNA synthesis[2], protein synthesis[3,4], and activity profiles of specific enzymes[5,6] are consistent with the view that gene expression during the adult portion of the life cycle is relatively static. If this is the case, it is difficult to envision how aging and death could be genetically programmed. At the very least, the absence of an obvious pattern of gene activity in the adult severely limits the type of model one might propose in which genes determine lifespan.

How can one test whether or not a temporal pattern of gene activity exists during the adult phase of the life cycle? Previous approaches have assayed the activity of specific gene products, usually common cell enzymes. We have taken a slightly different approach to this problem. We isolated a large group of temperature sensitive (ts) adult lethal mutations. These mutations identify genes whose products are essential for normal cell function and viability. By shifting cultures between the permissive and restrictive temperatures at the appropriate intervals the temperature sensitive period (TSP) can be delimited. The TSP represents the time during the adult portion of the life cycle when the functional product of the mutant gene is required, and in most cases, approximates the time at which the gene is transcriptionally active. By identifying the TSPs of a large number of essential genes we can establish whether a temporal pattern of gene activity exists. In principle, any single gene will be required either continuously throughout the adult portion of the life cycle, or only during a discrete and defineable portion of it. The absence of a temporal pattern of sequential gene expression in the adult limits the models that can be posed in which genes, required for aging and death, are activated at the end of a developmental program.

This paper describes three classes of genes. The first class is comprised of genes that act during the larval period whose normal function limit the lifespan of the larvae. Hence genes exist in the Drosophila genome that allow organismal death in response to a genetically programmed trigger. Two groups of adult lethal mutations are described: 1) those whose products are essential during both the pre-imaginal and adult stages, and 2) those required only during adulthood. These have been mapped genetically and their lethal phases determined. The TSPs for a large subset of these mutations have been delimited.

While the primary function of most of the adult lethal mutations is unrelated to longevity, one or a few of these mutations may actually play a role in the normal aging process. Hence a subset of the ts adult lethal mutations were examined for their ability to accelerate the normal aging process under the restrictive conditions. One appears to do so.

GENES THAT ALLOW PROGRAMMED CELL DEATH

Drosophila go through two different life forms: the larva and the adult. Not only are the two forms morphologically distinct, but their method of locomotion, food ingestion, sensory input (at least light detection), as well as their response to environmental cues (geotaxis and phototaxis) differ substantially. It might be argued that the larval and adult stages represent two life forms with the larva essentially being a mobile host, or embryo, for the developing adult form. Yet both share a common genome. We examined the longevity of larvae by isolating temperature-sensitive (ts) mutations that allow development to proceed normally at 22°C, but inhibit pupation or at least delay its onset substantially in populations maintained at 29°C. One strain extends the lifespan of larvae, maintained at 29°C, from the normal 5 days to at least 17 days. In fact some larvae live for over 25 days. Many of the larvae die as third instars, although some pupate. Therefore, the absolute longevity of the larval stage is at least 3 times longer than normal. Thus, during normal development the larval tissue must be programmed to undergo cell death and histolysis in response to some genetically controlled trigger (either large doses of ecdysone, or perhaps some other ecdysone-induced gene action). Transplantation studies have shown that some larval tissues acquire the competence to undergo cell death and histolysis[7]. This competency to respond to ecdysone, or the appropriate inducer, must also be genetically controlled. Hence, genes exist in the genome of Drosophila that are capable of causing cell death in response to some trigger. Since there is no evidence for loss of genetic information in adults, it is logical to assume that these genes also exist in the adult. Whether they are used to terminate the lifespan of the adults is another matter.

TEMPERATURE SENSITIVE ADULT LETHAL MUTATIONS

Adult lethal mutations were induced on the X chromosome of Drosophila melanogaster using the chemical mutagen ethyl methane sulfonate which produces primarily missense mutations. Two different genetic screens were used to select for adult lethal mutations. One protocol allowed the recovery of adult lethal mutations that were also developmental lethals; these genes might be essential at one or more stages during both the developmental and adult portions of the life cycle. The second protocol allowed the recovery of mutations in genes whose products are essential in adults only. Each protocol was run twice (4 separate mutagenesis experiments) and 61 adult lethal mutations were recovered.

Each strain was tested for longevity at 22° (permissive temperature) and 29°C (restrictive temperature). To do this, the strains were allowed to develop at 22°C, and the adults were collected within 12 hours of eclosion, separated by sex and placed into 8 dram shell vials (10/vial) and either left at 22°C or immediately placed at 29°C. The flies were transferred to fresh vials every 3 days at 22°C and every 2 days at 29°C. To obtain survival curves, the number of living flies per vial was recorded at each transfer and the total number was summed and expressed as a percent. The mutations were induced in the highly inbred laboratory strain Oregon-R. Therefore this strain was used as a control in all experiments. Figures 1 and 2 show survival curves of Oregon-R population comparing males and females at 22 and 29°C. These survival curves show the sigmoid-shaped death phase which is characteristic of Drosophila and many other organisms. The females live longer than the males at both temperatures. In addition the lifespan of population maintained at 29°C is considerably shorter than the lifespan of those kept at 22°C, which is expected for poikilotherms.

A critical assumption for our work is that temperatures as high as 29°C have no deleterious physiological effect on the organism. To verify this, survival curves for males and females at the two temperatures were compared by plotting them on a single graph with two abscissae. The 29°C

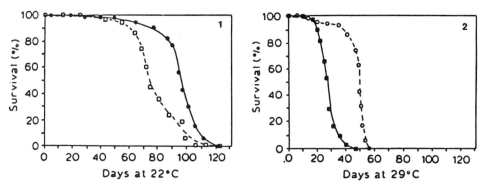

Fig. 1.   Survival curves for Oregon-R male and female adult flies
          maintained at 22°C after eclosion. Note that each survival
          curve is a composite derived from three different experiments.
          Viability measurements were made every 2-3 days, but to simplify
          presentation only a few actual data points are given. Circles
          represent females; boxes represent males.

Fig. 2.   Survival curves of Oregon-R male and female adult flies
          maintained at 29°C. Circles represent females; boxes represent
          males.

abscissa was adjusted for the difference in the rate of living at each
temperature. Conversion factors for the difference in the rate of living
at the two temperatures were calculated, separately for both males and
females, from the parameters shown in Table 1. The conversion factors
from each of these parameters were very similar, therefore an average
value was derived, of 2.65 and 2.05 for males and females, respectively;
that is, one day at 29°C is equivalent to 2.65 days at 22°C for males.
When plotted on such a graph the shapes of the survival curves for males
(Figure 3A) and females (data not shown), at the two temperatures were
identical. Thus within the range used, temperature has no effect on
aging or longevity other than to alter the rate at which events occur.
In addition, the physiological events important to longevity appear to be
affected proportionally throughout the adult lifespan. Finally, by
plotting survival curves in this way any difference in lifespan at the
two temperatures becomes obvious.

     To determine which of the 61 adult lethal mutations were
temperature-sensitive the survival curves for populations maintained at
22° and 29°C from each of the 61 mutant strains were plotted on this type
of graph. Thirty-five of the 61 mutations were temperature sensitive,
that is the longevity of both the males and females is reasonably normal
when the adults are maintained at 22°C, but is severely curtailed when
they are kept at 29°C. Examples are shown in Figure 3 B-F. The
differences in survival curves between males and females at each
temperature were minimal and typical of the differences between sexes of
wild-type strains. If anything, the female data are less variable than
the male data.

     Each of the mutations was examined for its effect on development.
To do this 500 - 600 embryos were collected over a two hour period at
22°C; these were divided into two groups (50 embryos/vial), and placed
immediately at 22° or 29°C where they were allowed to develop to
adults. Each strain was examined for the number of individuals surviving
to adulthood. Twenty of the 35 ts adult lethal mutations are also ts
developmental lethal or semi-lethal. Fifteen identify genes whose

Table 1.   Conversion Factors for Differences in Rate of Living at 22°C and 29°C

	Males	Females
$LS_{\bar{x}}$	2.7	2.0
$DP_{\bar{x}}$	2.5	2.0
DP_{onset}	2.7	1.8
D-20	2.8	2.0
D-50	2.8	2.0
D-95	2.5	2.3
DP_{end}	2.5	2.2
Final death	2.8	2.3

Each number represents the ratio of the respective 22°C and 29°C values for longevity.

products are essential only during the adult stage; thirteen of which were recovered from the screens designed to eliminate developmental lethal mutations. These findings indicate that genes whose products are essential only during the adult phase are not rare.

To date, 22 of the 61 unconditional and ts adult lethal mutations have been mapped. The results indicate that these mutations are distributed over the entire length of the X chromosome (data not shown). Ten of the mutations map within 5 centimorgans, between map positions 49 and 54. Complementation tests between these mutants indicated clear cases of allelism for 3 of them. Thus, there are a minimum of 7 cistrons located within this 5 map unit region of the X chromosome that encode functions essential for adult viability. Hence a subset of genes, whose functions are essential in the adult maybe clustered. It will be interesting to determine if they function in the same tissue type or organ.

The lethal phase (LP), or the time at which the adult dies, was determined for each of the adult lethal mutations. The relationship between the TSP and LP will take one of three patterns: 1) the TSP and LP can be virtually coincident; 2) the TSP can be discontinuous and precede the LP by a considerable period of time; or 3) the TSP can be continuous, with dysfunction of the product eventually leading to death. While the LP cannot be used to predict the TSP accurately, it obviously does define the time at which, or prior to which, the gene product is required. To be useful in determining whether or not a pattern of differential gene activity occurs during the adult portion of the life cycle, some of the ts adult lethal mutations in this collection must have LPs that occur two or more weeks after eclosion. To identify such mutations, the mean of the death phase ($DP\bar{x}$) for each of the ts adult lethal strains was calculated from the survival curve data[8]. The $DP\bar{x}$ represents the average age of individuals at death when the population as a whole is dying. With the proviso that the majority of individuals within the population die during the $DP\bar{x}$, we believe that the $DP\bar{x}$ is the most accurate indicator of longevity of any given strain[8]. The $DP\bar{x}$ was calculated for all 35 ts adult lethal mutations. Over 60% of the strains have $DP\bar{x}$ values that range between two and five weeks post-

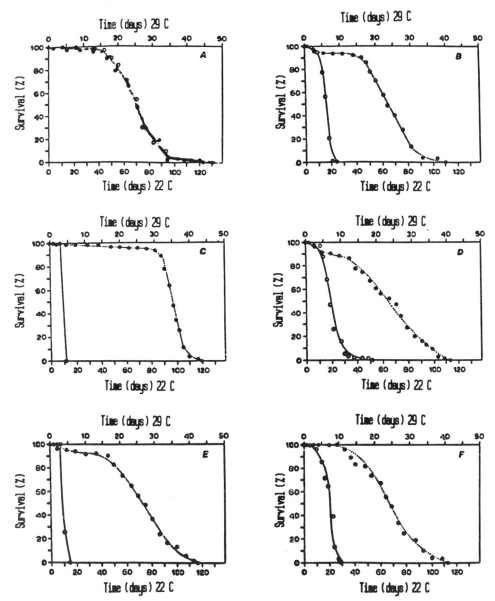

Fig. 3. Survival curves at 22°C and 29°C for adult males from wild-type and five mutant strains. All flies were raised at 22°C, collected within a day of eclosion, and immediately placed at either 22°C or 29°C. A) Oregon-R (wild-type); B) adl-2^{ts}; C) adl-4^{ts}; D) adl-13^{ts}; E) adl-14^{ts}; F) adl-16^{ts1}. Closed circles, populations maintained at 22°C: open circles, populations maintained at 29°C.

eclosion when maintained at 29°C (data not shown). Curiously, those mutations that affect the pre-imaginal as well as the adult stages, tend to have DP mean values that occur early in the adult portion of the life cycle. On the other hand, mutations that cause lethality in the adults only, appear to act later during the adult portion of the life cycle. It is unclear whether this identifies two different classes of genes or reflects differences in strengths of the mutant phenotypes. Nonetheless,

the spectrum of adult lethal phases among the mutant strains in our
collection should allow a comprehensive test of whether a pattern of
differential gene activity occurs during the adult portion of the life
cycle.

TIME OF ACTION OF ESSENTIAL ADULT GENES

The temperature-sensitive period (TSP) defines the time at which the
product of these genes are required and, for most genes, probably
approximates the time of gene action. The TSP was determined by shifting

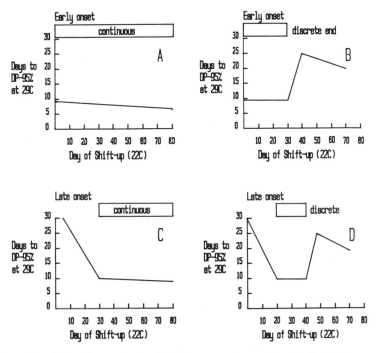

Fig. 4. The TSP of ts adult lethal mutations should fall into one of
four distinct categories.

cultures from the permissive temperature (22°C) to the restrictive
temperature (29°C) at different times during the adult portion of the
life cycle, and then measuring the longevity of the population. Each
experiment requires a large number of adults. Flies were allowed to
develop at 22°C until eclosion, collected within 24 hours separated by
sex, and placed into vials (10/vial). Groups of 100 males and 100
females were shifted up to 29°C daily for the first ten days post-
eclosion, and at three day intervals thereafter until the DP$\bar{x}$ of the 22°C
maintained populations. The 22°, and subsequent 29°C populations, were
transferred to fresh vials at 3 and 2 day intervals, respectively.
Survival was monitored at each transfer until all individuals in the
population had died. The number of days required for 95% of the
population to die (DP-95) after the shift up to 29°C, was plotted against

the age of the adults at the time of the shift. (The DP-95 usually is coincident with the end of the death phase[8]). This protocol delimits both the beginning and the end of the TSP. Four distinct categories of gene activity might be expected, and typical graphs are shown in Figure 4. These can be divided into two groups: 1) genes that are activated at about the time of eclosion, and 2) genes whose onset of activity occurs later in the adult phase. Genes activated at eclosion might be required for the duration of the adult life (continuous, Fig. 4A), or their product may only be required during the first portion of adulthood (Fig. 4B). Once active, genes with a late onset of activity, might be required continuously (Fig. 4C), or their products may be required for only a discrete period (Fig. 4D).

The TSPs of twelve mutants have been examined most of which encode products that are required throughout the adult portion of the life cycle. Examples are shown in Figure 5 A-C. Only one clear example of a gene with a late onset of activity exists (Fig. 5D). The onset of activity (gene product requirement) appears to occur about four weeks post-eclosion at 22°C (which corresponds to about day 10 or 11 in 29°C populations). Once active, this gene product is also required continuously. None of the mutations examined had a discrete period during adulthood when their products were required. Therefore, it appears that, once active, all of the genes (or their products) are required continuously; they are not inactivated.

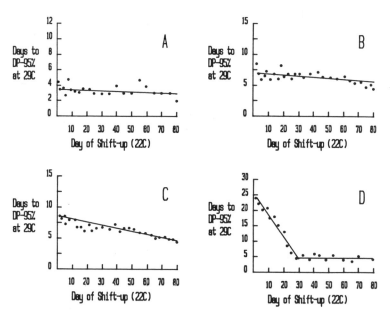

Fig. 5.   The TSPs for four ts adult lethal mutations. A) adl-19[ts], B) adl-20[ts], C) adl-3[ts]. The function of all three of these genes is required throughout the adult stage. D) adl-13[ts], the product of this gene appears to be required only in the latter part of adulthood.

Since the products of these essential adult genes are required continuously, then, in addition to delimiting the period during which the gene or its product are required, these shift-up experiments also indicate the total number of days that each strain can survive once placed at the non-permissive temperature. The mean lifespan at 29°C can be calculated from the average value of the data in the plateau phase of the shift up experiments. There is generally quite good agreement between this figure and the mean lifespan calculated from the survival curves.

Shift-down experiments (from 29° to 22°C) were done to determine whether the effects of the restrictive temperature were reversible and to delimit the minimum period of time that is required at 29°C to commit the flies to death irrevocably. The shift-down experiments were done following the same protocol as that used for the shift-up series. The number of days required for 95% of the population to die following shift-down to 22°C was plotted against the day on which the population was shifted. The minimum time at 29°C that is required to evoke a response is given by the first intercept on the graph (Fig. 6). The minimum time at 29°C that is required to commit the flies to death irrevocably is given by the second intercept. The effect of most of the mutations are completely reversible if shifted down during the first 65% of the TSP. If flies are maintained at 29°C beyond that point the effects are often non-reversible.

In summary, it appears that most of the genes that encode essential products in the adult are activated at about the time of eclosion. Once activated, the products of these genes are required continuously. A few essential genes, perhaps well after reproduction would have guaranteed enough progeny for the success of the next generation. At this point there is, at best, weak evidence for temporal patterns of gene expression in the adult. We are determining the TSPs of 8 other ts adult lethal mutations. However, our observations, taken together with data on enzyme activity, and 2D-gel analysis, suggest that if a regular cascade of gene activity occurs during the adult portion of the life cycle, it is limited to a very small subset of the genes that function in adults.

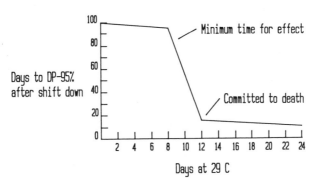

Fig. 6.   Shift-down experiments delimit the minimum time at the restrictive temperature that is required to elicit an affect on the survival of a ts adult lethal mutant. It may also define the minimum time required to commit the flies to death irrevocably.

The absence of a distinct temporal pattern of gene activity in the adult would severely limit the models one might propose in which genes play a major role in controlling lifespan. Simplified examples of some of the models that remain are as follows. One model might posit the existence of a repressor substance (or substances) which is made just prior to, or at the time of eclosion. The repressor product would be stable with a reasonably long half-life, or the gene(s) may be transcribed continuously with a reduced rate of product formation with increasing age. Once this product dropped below a certain threshold, genes that are involved in cell death would be activated. This model might be complicated by the existence of distinct repressor products in different types of cells. While the model, as stated, is overly simplistic it predicts that mutations in genes that encode such a repressor product would generally decrease longevity. An alternative hypothesis might posit that one or more genes might act as "killers". These genes would be activated early during the adult phase of the life cycle and, assuming a moderately long half-life, their products would accumulate. Once they reached a certain level in the cell or body, they either kill the cell or activate a second set of genes that eventually cause cell death. This model predicts that mutations which reduce the function of such genes would increase the longevity of the mutant strain. This second model is less attractive, since it seems likely that mutations in such "killer" genes might accumulate. Even if one postulates that a number of such genes exist, eventually all of them would be expected to accumulate mutations that cause them to dysfunction.

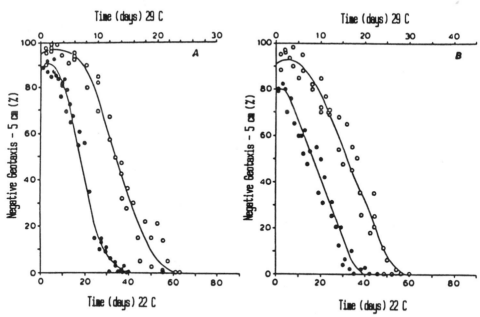

Fig. 7. Geotactic behavior of adult wild-type individuals (minimum height, 5 cm). Each value is the percent of individuals in the population that climbed to a height of 5 cm during the test interval. A sample of data points from each of three experiments are presented; thus the curve is representative of the results from each experiment. Closed circles, population maintained at 22°C; open circles, population maintained at 29°C. A) Males. B) Females.

A MUTATION THAT APPEARS TO ACCELERATE AGING

The adult lethal mutations simply identify genes whose products are essential for viability. Most of these genes probably have nothing to do with aging. Nonetheless, a small subset of them may actually play a role in the aging process, and their dysfunction might accelerate aging and lead to premature death. Mutations that actually accelerate the aging process should be distinguishable from the rest by their phenotype. Such mutations would accelerate the onset and/or progression of a set of biological landmarks (biomarkers) associated with the normal aging process. We have established that the decline and eventual loss of normal behavioral responses can serve as landmarks of physiological aging in <u>Drosophila melanogaster</u>[8]. As a population ages chronologically, the proportion of flies that are able to perform a given behavioral task within a short time interval, declines and eventually reaches zero. The behavioral tasks that we have used include phototaxis (positive), geotaxis (negative), mating behavior, and general motor activity. An example of the loss of geotactic behavior with age is shown in Figure 7. The pattern of age-dependent loss of behavior relative to longevity in populations at 22°C is shown in Figure 8.

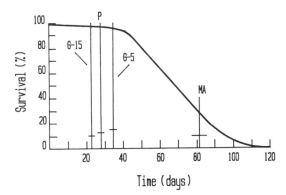

Fig. 8.   Behavior-loss relative to longevity in males maintained at
          22°C continuously. Vertical lines indicate the age at
          which the behavior is lost; horizontal lines represent 2
          standard deviations. G-15, geotaxis to a height of 15 cm;
          P, phototaxis; G-5, geotaxis to a height of 5 cm; MA,
          motor activity.

A mutation in a gene that is involved in the aging process might be expected to alter the time frame during which the pattern of behavior-loss relative to longevity is displayed, without altering either the pattern or the proportion of time between each event. Seven temperature sensitive mutations, chosen at random from our collection, were examined at both the permissive and restrictive temperatures. The pattern of age-dependent behavior loss for the mutant strains fell into four general categories: 1) abnormal behavior at 22° and 29°C; 2) normal pattern of behavior-loss at 22°C, and absence of behavior, or abnormal patterns of loss at 29°C; 3) normal behavior-loss at 22° and behavior appears normal at 29°C but flies die suddenly; 4) normal pattern of behavior-loss at 22° and 29°C relative to longevity. We observed at least one example of each category. The phenotypes of the mutant strains that fall into one of the first three categories clearly illustrates the point that mutations in genes which, in all likelihood, are not involved in the aging process usually disrupt the normal pattern of loss of behavior associated with aging in Drosophila.

The fourth category of mutations are the most interesting. They display a normal pattern of loss at both 22° and 29°C, but at 29°C, the pattern is compressed into a shorter time frame. Mutations in this class may be considered as candidates for lesions which accelerate the onset and/or rate of aging; to date, only ts adl-16 falls into this category. Rather than presenting the behavior-loss data graphically, the most pertinent aspects of these data are given in Table 2. These values represent means from three separate experiments with a minimum of 500 individuals tested. At 22°C, the pattern of behavior-loss in adl-16, and the days on which a given behavior is lost, closely resembles the pattern observed with the wild-type strain, Oregon-R, for both the males and the females[9]. In addition, the maximum levels of behavioral response attained by adl-16 and Oregon-R are comparable. In contrast, at 29°C behavior is lost much more rapidly among both males and females of the adl-16 strain than in the wild-type strain. While the actual period of time during which loss of behavior occurs in the mutant strain is drastically shortened at 29°C, both the order and the general pattern in which the behaviors are lost resembles those of wild-type. To determine if a normal pattern of behavior-loss occurs, but is simply compressed into a shorter interval when adl-16[ts1] adults are kept at 29°C, the loss of behavior relative to the longevity was examined in both the adl-16 and the Oregon-R strains at 22° and 29°C. Two sets of comparisons were made. First, the point at which the maximum level of behavior was reduced by 50% was compared to the DP$\bar{x}$ of that population. These data are shown in Table 3; in no case does the difference between the mutant

Table 2. Behavior-Loss With Age in adl-16 Adults at 22°C and 29°C

Behavior	22°C				29°C			
	Maximum %	Days	50% Loss	Minimum behavior	Maximum %	Days	50% Loss	Minimum behavior
Males								
Geotaxis-15[a]	60	1-4	12	23	80	1	3	4
Phototaxis	55	1-10	19	35	85	1	2 1/2	5
Geotaxis-5	90	1-7	22	38	95	1	3	6
Motor[b]	85	1-8	23	80	90	1-3	4	8
Females								
Geotaxis-15	55	1-6	13	25	80	1	1 1/2	3
Phototaxis	50	1-8	17	35	90	1	1 3/4	3 1/2
Geotaxis-5	80	1-7	20	40	95	1	2	4

[a]For geotaxis and phototaxis, maximum behavioral activity is given as % of individuals which display a given behvioral response during the test interval.
[b]For motor activity, maximum behavior represents the total number of lines crossed by ten individuals during the test interval.
The days during which the maximum behavioral response was maintained are also given, as are the days on which 50% behavior loss and minimum behavioral activity occurred. All behavioral data represent means from three separate experiments-that is, three separate populations subjected to the same test (n > 500).

Table 3. Proportion of Adult Life-span at Which 50% Behavior-Loss Occurs Relative to the DP$\bar{x}$ for Oregon-R and adl-16 Strains at 22°C and 20°C

Behavior	Males			Females		
	Oregon-R	adl-16	% Difference	Oregon-R	adl-16	% Difference
22°C						
Geotaxis-15	0.18	0.20	2	0.12	0.17	5
Phototaxis	0.21	0.31	10	0.22	0.22	0
Geotaxis-5	0.30	0.36	6	0.25	0.26	1
Motor activity	0.45	0.38	7			
29°C						
Geotaxis-15	0.33	0.26	7	0.23	0.22	1
Phototaxis	0.42	0.33	9	0.29	0.26	3
Geotaxis-5	0.46	0.39	7	0.36	0.30	6
Motor activity	0.63	0.53	10			

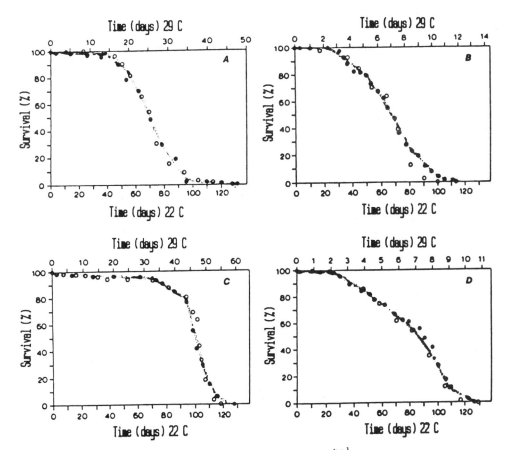

Fig. 9. Survival curves for Oregon-R and adl-16[tsl] males and females at 22°C and 29°C. A) Oregon-R males; B) adl-16[tsl] males; C) Oregon-R females; D) adl-16[tsl] females. Closed circles, 22°C; open circles, 29°C posteclosion.

205

and wild-type strain exceed 10%. Secondly, comparisons were made between the adl-16 and the Oregon-R strains for the age at which behavior-loss occurred relative to the end of the DP - that is, complete loss of the behavioral response vs. absolute longevity of the population. We found that the differences between the two strains was less than 12%[9]. The accuracy with which behavioral loss can be measured is approximately 10%[8]. Therefore, the differences noted between the two strains is negligible. Thus, the patterns of loss of behavior in both the adl-16 and the Oregon-R strains are very similar at both the permissive and restrictive temperatures, although their longevity at 29°C differs considerably. The adl-16 strain at 29°C exhibit a temporal compression proportional to the shortening of the adult lifespan. Hence, adl-16 meets the criteria of a mutation that causes premature death in adults maintained at the restrictive temperature by accelerating the rate of aging. If adl-16 acts by increasing the rate of aging at 29°C, then the shape of the survival curves at 22° and 29°C should be similar. The survival curves were plotted on a single graph with the 29°C abscissa expanded by a constant (calculated as described previously). The results for males are shown in Figure 9 (the results for females, are similar). They are consistent with the interpretation that the adl-16 mutation increases the rate at which aging occurs at the restrictive temperature. Furthermore, they suggest that all aspects of the aging process are increased proportionally. While these results are compelling, they certainly do not constitute proof that the adl-16 mutation accelerates the aging process at the restrictive temperature.

In subsequent studies, two alleles of adl-16 were recovered. The mutation adl-16^{ts2} is much stronger, it survives for about 4 days at 29°C; whereas the third allele adl-16^{ts3} survives for about 20 days at 29°C. Further genetic studies have demonstrated that each allele is a hypomorph, that is, the mutant product retains some, though limited, activity even at the restrictive temperature. The behavioral loss relative to longevity has been determined for each allele and for heterozygotes between each allele (the latter was done in females only). These studies confirm the previous data. Finally, the primary anatomical site in which the adl-16 mutation dysfunctions to cause premature death has been determined by analyzing gynandromorphs[10]. It appears that premature death results from physiological dysfunction in the central nervous system, including both the brain and the ventral ganglia. Since anatomical degeneration of the central nervous tissue is one of the generally accepted indicators of aging in Drosophila, a comparative anatomical analysis of the CNS tissue in aging populations of adl-16 and Oregon-R is planned for the near future.

ACKNOWLEDGEMENTS

The credit for the data presented in this paper must be given to several graduate and undergraduate students, and technicians. In alphabetical order these include: Kathleen Fitzpatrick, Anna Giesbrecht, Beverly Hansen, Kathy Kafer, David Leffelaar, Susan Minaker, and Murray Richter. Special thanks to my colleague and research associate Dr. Don Sinclair. The research has been supported by an NIH grant AG03088-01 and an NSERC grant A-3005.

REFERENCES

1. A. N. Bozcuk, DNA synthesis in the absence of somatic cell division associated with aging in Drosophila subobscura, Exp. Gerontol. 7:147 (1972).

2. H. V. Samis, Jr., F. C. Erk, and M. B. Baird, Senescence in
      Drosophila. I. Sex differences in nucleic acid, protein and
      glycogen levels as a function of age, Exp. Gerontol., 6:9
      (1971).
3. J. C. Hall, Age-dependent enzyme changes in Drosophila melanogaster,
      Exp. Gerontol., 4:207 (1969).
4. P. S. Chen, Amino acid pattern and rate of protein synthesis in
      aging Drosophila, in: "Molecular genetic mechanisms in
      development and aging," M. Rockstein and G. T. Baker, eds.,
      Academic Press, New York (1972).
5. S. J. O'Brien, and R. J. MacIntyre, The α-glycerophosphate cycle in
      Drosophila melanogaster. I. Biochemical and Developmental
      Aspects, Biochem. Genet., 7:141 (1972).
6. D. Armstrong, R. Rinehart, L. Dixon, and D. Reigh, Changes in
      peroxodase with aging in Drosophila, Age, 1:8 (1978).
7. D. Bodenstein, Factors influencing growth and metamorphosis of the
      salivary gland in Drosophila, Biol. Bull., 84:13 (1943).
8. D. Leffelaar, and T. Grigliatti, Age-dependent behavior loss in
      adult Drosophila melanogaster, Dev. Genet. 4:211 (1984).
9. D. Leffelaar, and T. Grigliatti, A mutation in Drosophila that
      appears to accelerate aging, Dev. Genet., 4:199 (1984).
10. Y. Hotta, and S. Benzer, Mapping of behavior in Drosophila
      mosaics, in: "Genetic Mechanisms of Development," ed., F. H.
      Ruddle, Academic Press, New York (1973).

IMMORTALITY OF THE GERM-LINE VERSUS DISPOSABILITY OF THE SOMA

Thomas B. L. Kirkwood

National Institute for Medical Research
The Ridgeway, Mill Hill
London NW7 1AA, England.

INTRODUCTION

The germ-line of species is immortal, at least in the sense that an unbroken continuity extends backwards in time to the origin of terrestrial life and forwards in time to an indeterminate future. This observation is a truism. However, when set against the fact that the bodies of higher animals are intrinsically mortal, yet composed of the same basic materials as their germ cells, the observation leads to the central puzzle of gerontology. Each new-born individual begins its life as young as did each of its ancestors but with the same certitude, if it does not meet with an earlier accident, that within a specific span of time it will arrive, through a process of steadily accelerating decrepitude, at death. The puzzle has two sides: why and how has the somatic part of higher animals come to be mortal, and how is the germ-line kept free of the progressive deterioration in the soma?

A century ago, Weismann (1890) set out his seminal view of the essential difference between mortality and immortality at the cellular level:

"The immortality of unicellular organisms, and of the germ cells of the multicellular, is not absolute but potential; it is not that they must live forever; they can die - the greater number do in fact die - but a proportion lives on which is of one and the same substance with the others. Does not life, here as elsewhere, depend on metabolism - that is to say, a constant change of material? And what is it, then, which is immortal? Clearly not the substance, but only a definite form of activity. The protoplasm of the unicellular animals is of such chemical and molecular structure that the cycle which constitutes life returns ever to the same point and can always begin anew, so long as the necessary external conditions are forthcoming. This character it is which I have termed immortality...

"If then this true immortality is but cyclical, and is conditioned by the physical constitution of the protoplasm, why is it inconceivable that this constitution should be, under certain circumstances and to a certain extent, so modified that the metabolic activity no longer exactly follows its own orbit, but after more or fewer revolutions comes to a standstill and results in death?"

Despite enormous progress in cell and molecular biology since

Weismann's time, we still cannot much improve on this. Debate in gerontology continues to center around the nature of the process which leads to "modification" in somatic cells of the "cycle of metabolic activity." Are somatic cells mortal because they accumulate random defects which result in progressively impaired function, or do they merely follow a course of genetically determined cell differentiation which leads them to death? The answer to this question will, of course, also bear on the mechanisms to ensure germ-line immortality since it will make clearer the source of somatic mortality.

Following in the spirit of Weismann's enquiry, this paper re-examines the broad theoretical issues of somatic aging and germ-line immortality in animals. Because aging means different things in the context of different species' life-histories (Kirkwood, 1985), attention is restricted to species in which there is clear segregation between germ-line and soma, and in which reproduction occurs repeatedly through life instead of in a single terminal burst. These species manifest aging of the kind most compatible with normal usage of this term. The same principles can, however, be extended with appropriate modifications to species with different kinds of body plan and life-history (Kirkwood, 1981).

THE DISPOSABLE SOMA

One way to view an organism is as an entity which takes in energy from its environment in the form of nutrients and other resources and eventually produces as output its progeny. This approach is useful in considering the evolution of species' life-histories from a physiological and ecological point of view (Townsend & Calow, 1981). Under natural selection, the genotypes most likely to survive are those which maximize the efficiency of this cycle of transformation, taking account of the constraints imposed by the species' niche.

The organism must allocate a fraction of the energy taken in to each of various somatic activities such as growth, defense, repair and maintenance activities, as well as to reproduction (Figure 1). The balance between these activities is a central part of optimizing the life-history. The greater the fraction of energy invested in one particular activity, the less will remain available for the others. While it is possible to select for an increased total intake of energy, this may not always be a viable option,

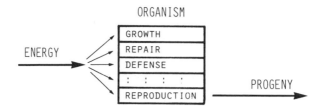

Fig. 1. Schematic representation of an organism, showing the input of energy, the partition of the energy among different activities, and the final output of progeny (from Kirkwood & Cremer, 1982).

and in any case the problem of optimal allocation will still remain even though the total which is available for subdivision may be greater. Thus, it is generally relevant to solve the problem of optimal allocation of a fixed intake.

In the context of aging, there is particular interest in the allocation of energy for the repair and maintenance of the soma as compared with the allocation to reproduction. This is because the prime object of the repair and maintenance processes is to prolong life. Repair and maintenance processes are here defined to include the full range of activities involved in guarding against and correcting defects at all somatic levels; i.e., in organs, tissues, cells, membranes, and molecules (see Kirkwood, 1981). The balance which must be reached is between the advantages on the one hand of living longer by being better able to cope with random defects, and thereby having the potential to extend reproduction over a greater span of time, and on the other hand of reproducing at a greater rate.

A measure which may be used to compare the success of different allocation strategies is the "intrinsic rate of natural increase" in a population with stable age-distribution (e.g. see Charlesworth, 1980). This is the exponential rate at which the population is growing in time and it depends directly on the schedules of average survivorship and fecundity. It is calculated by solving the integral equation

$$\int e^{-rx} \, l(x) \, m(x) \, dx = 1, \tag{1}$$

where r is the rate of natural increase, x denotes age, and l(x) and m(x) are the mean survivorship and fecundity at age x.

Varying the investment in somatic repair and maintenance will affect both l(x) and m(x). The effects to be expected from increasing the fraction of energy invested in somatic repair and maintenance are illustrated in Figure 2. For survivorship, the general effect is to raise the survival curve across all ages, assuming that the increased investment begins at birth (or earlier). For fecundity, the effect is more complex. Firstly, increased investment in repair and maintenance may cause slower growth and maturation. This is represented in the figure by delaying the age at which the fecundity curves first rises. Secondly, it will result in fewer resources being available for direct reproductive effort, so the maximum point of the fecundity curve is expected in general to be lower. Thirdly, it

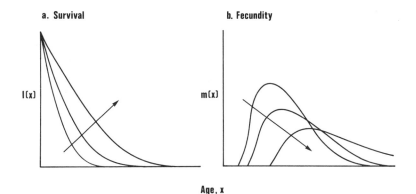

Fig. 2. Effects on a). survivorship l(x), and b). fecundity m(x), of increasing the investment in somatic repair and maintenance.

211

may retard the rate at which general physical deterioration (i.e. senescence) takes place, resulting in a less rapid fall in fecundity with advancing age.

The last comment on the fecundity curves above should not be taken to suggest that senescence is here assumed inevitable; such an assumption would defeat the object, which is to explain why the soma should be mortal. On the contrary, it needs to be assumed that there is, at least hypothetically, a critical level of investment in somatic repair and maintenance beyond which the rate at which defects arise is balanced by the rate at which they are corrected. Above this level, the soma can continue its survival indefinitely. Below this level, the soma gradually accumulates defects at a net rate which equals the difference between the rates at which defects arise and are repaired, this accumulation leading in the end to the steeply rising age-specific mortality pattern characteristic of aging (Comfort, 1979; Kirkwood, 1985). For a high enough level of investment in somatic repair and maintenance we may therefore expect the fecundity curve to remain horizontal although this situation is not represented in the figure.

Using equation (1) to calculate the intrinsic rate of natural increase, the joint effect of changing survivorship and fecundity on the evolutionary fitness of a genotype can be assessed. Figure 3 shows a plot of the intrinsic rate of natural increase against the level of investment in somatic repair and maintenance, the latter being defined on an arbitrary scale between zero (i.e. no investment) and one (maximum possible investment after the minimum essential life processes have been provided for). For illustration, it is assumed in Figure 3 that an investment of 0.8 on this scale defines the critical level at which the rate of correction of defects just matches the rate at which they arise. The range above 0.8 is therefore labelled "non-aging" and the range below 0.8 is labelled "aging." When calculation is made for any reasonable model of the dependance of l(x) and m(x) on the investment in repair and maintenance, two features of Figure 3 are found to apply generally. Firstly, the curve shows a clearly defined maximum; i.e., in a given niche there is an optimum investment in somatic repair and maintenance to which a species can be expected to evolve. Secondly, the optimum is less than the critical value required for indefinite somatic survival; in other words, the species will always evolve to a state where its soma is intrinsically mortal.

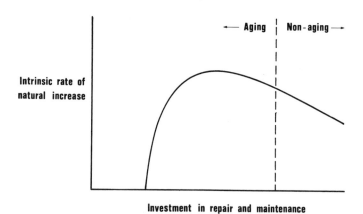

Fig. 3. Relationship between the intrinsic rate of natural increase and the level of investment in somatic repair and maintenance.

Perhaps the clearest way to appreciate the force of the latter conclusion is to suppose that there does exist a species that never ages because of a sufficient investment in repair and maintenance. Individuals of this species will nonetheless be exposed to purely random environmental mortality with an expected probability distribution of survival. For example, if the chance of dying in a year is 10% then all but 1% of individuals will die by the age of 44, and if the chance of dying is 25% all but 1% will be dead by age 16. There is therefore little advantage to be gained from investing in potential somatic immortality when in practice the return from this investment may not be realised. Taking account of the level of environmental mortality, the better course will always be to reduce the investment in somatic repair and maintenance to a level which ensures only that the soma remains in good condition through its normal expectation of life in its natural environment and to use the extra resources liberated by this action to increase reproduction. This view has been termed the disposable soma theory of aging (see Kirkwood 1977, 1981, 1985; Kirkwood & Holliday, 1979).

AGING AND DIFFERENTIATION

The disposable soma gives strong support to the view that aging occurs through random defects. An alternative view is that aging is due to differentiation; in other words, that in some way the specialization of cells which is found in higher animals is incompatible with their indefinite survival. I will not take space here to discuss the idea that aging is directly programmed into somatic cells to bring about the aging of organisms for the evolutionary good of the species. This view has been critically discussed and generally found to be wanting (e.g. see Medawar, 1952; Williams 1957; Sacher, 1978; Kirkwood & Holliday, 1979; Kirkwood, 1981, 1985). Instead, the question to be considered is whether natural selection may have favored evolution of attributes in somatic cells which have brought about aging as an indirect consequence.

The most obvious candidates for cells whose differentiation may set an intrinsic limit to somatic survivorship are post-mitotic cells; particularly those of the central nervous system. Brain growth and development is completed early in life, and apart from limited renewal and adaptation which may follow injury it appears that neurones form themselves into networks which remain largely unchanged throughout life. Such architecture imposes an inevitable mortality since individual cells will eventually fall prey to intrinsic metabolic accidents (e.g. non-repairable DNA lesions) even though there is no specifically programmed obsolescence.

The suggestion has also been made that actively proliferating cells, such as fibroblasts, may have evolved finite replicative lifespans as a protection against proliferative disorders, notably cancers. The idea is that such a limit presents one more obstacle which must be surmounted before a cell can progress into a fully malignant tumor. A difficulty with this idea is that the considerable proliferative capacity shown by normal fibroblasts calls into question whether "immortalization" is really a prerequisite for a lethal tumor. Nevertheless, the idea is compatible with evidence from in vitro and in vivo studies which suggests that immortalization may be one important step in carcinogenesis and merits further study.

An excellent general discussion on the evolution of aging by Williams (1957) provides a theoretical model to encompass the possible role of cell differentiation in aging. Williams (1957), like Haldane (1941) and Medawar (1952), pointed out that even without any intrinsic aging process the force of natural selection would be progressively attenuated with increasing age since with increasing age the fraction of individuals surviving must be smaller. Williams noted, therefore, that an attribute which conferred a survival advantage in the earlier part of the lifespan, when survivorship in the natural environment was high, would be favored by selection even if the attribute was disadvantagous at later ages when survivorship in the natural environment was low.

DAMAGE, DIFFERENTIATION, OR BOTH?

The hypothesis that cell differentiation may have lead to somatic structures which are intrinsically unsuited to immortality is not, in fact, at odds with the disposable soma theory. Taking a wide definition, one may include within the investment in somatic repair and maintenance the organization of cells and tissues so as to permit the renewal and replacement of highly specialized cells from pluripotent stem cell pools. For example, although regeneration of whole anatomical structures such as limbs is not seen in mammals, such regeneration is found among amphibians. The principle of balancing by natural selection the costs and benefits of somatic repair and maintenance, as introduced earlier, can also decide whether or not the capacity for regeneration should be retained (Kirkwood, 1981; Reichman, 1984). The same principle applies to any other feature of somatic structure and organization, and in this sense the disposable soma theory can be broadened to correspond with the more general theory of Williams (1957).

The disposable soma theory leads directly, however, to the specific prediction that whatever the organization of cellular differentiation, an accumulation of random defects should occur in all somatic cell lineages. There is, therefore, urgent need to unite both stochastic or "damage" theories with "terminal differentiation" theories in a common approach to investigating the cellular basis of aging in animals and in particular to pay close attention to the relevance of specific cell models to the aging of the soma as a whole. Theory suggests that both damage and differentiation may play a part in bringing, in Weismann's (1890) terms, the metabolic activity of somatic cells to a standstill, and the relative contributions of these causes cannot be assessed without considering both of them together.

GERM-LINE IMMORTALITY

Immortality of the germ-line requires explanation only in the sense that when a theory is put forward to explain the mortality of somatic cells, it is necessary at the same time to explain why the germ cells are in the long run unaffected. For unicellular organisms it is enough that the mechanisms of genome duplication and cell division are sufficiently faithful that each parent can, on average, produce at least one fully viable offspring. Natural selection then provides the force to winnow out defective individuals and to prevent the mean level of fitness from declining. For germ cells in a multicellular organism, the same general principles hold, but there are also some major differences. The germ cells themselves pass through distinct stages of differentiation and maturation, and several cell generations therefore elapse between successive generations of animals. In general, there is clear evidence that germ cells in animals do deteriorate to the extent that fertility declines, and the frequency of genetic abnormalities among offspring increases with both maternal and paternal age. However, apart from the increased genetic load there is no evidence that the progeny of older parents start life more aged than the progeny of young parents. A detailed review of age changes in germ cells with discussion on possible mechanisms for germ-line immortality was made recently by Medvedev (1981).

As far as the cell differentiation aspects of somatic aging are concerned, there is no problem in explaining germ-line immortality. All that is needed is that germ cells remain in a totipotent state. Thus, the issues concerning germ-line immortality all touch on mechanisms for avoidance of progressive accumulation of defects. Three broad types of mechanism can be distinguished. First, it is possible that the ongoing level of repair and maintenance is kept at a higher level in germ cells than in somatic cells, or rather, that for energy-saving reasons the level is reduced in somatic cells at some early stage of development (Kirkwood, 1977). During embryogenesis of many animal species it is observed that there is a period during which the future germ cells are physically separated from the future somatic cells, and it may be that around this time certain mechanisms for repair and maintenance are either turned off in somatic cells or switched to a lower level. Second, at key points in germ cell lineages special repair mechanisms may act to rejuvenate germ cells that otherwise accumulate damage in the same way as somatic cells. For instance, Bernstein (1977) has proposed that meiosis may provide an opportunity to remove critical DNA lesions from the germ-line. It is also suggested that during the first and second meiotic divisions there may occur a highly asymmetric partitioning of cellular defects such that damage is effectively dumped in the polar bodies, which die soon afterwards (Sheldrake, 1974). The third, and most general mechanism for germ-line immortality is selection. Selection will operate at all stages of the reproductive cycle; the production of primordial germ cells in embryogenesis, cell development, gametogenesis, inter-gametic selection at conception, selective abortion of defective embryos, and finally phenotypic selection on the progeny.

The problem for determining the mechanisms of germ-line immortality is therefore a matter of testing by experiment the extent to which these various distinct mechanisms may be used, either singly or in combination. This cannot definitively be done, however, until the nature of somatic cell mortality, in particular the role of random damage, is clarified.

IMPLICATIONS FOR EXPERIMENTAL STUDIES

Theory can be useful in two ways. It is mainly of use to the extent that it advances knowledge by suggesting experiments through which the theory may be tested. It is also of use, however, in ordering existing knowledge into a more coherent pattern. The disposable soma theory is attractive in both respects. Firstly, it makes clear predictions and defines a broad experimental path down which the causes of somatic aging may be sought. Secondly, it defines a framework within which the huge variety of observations and hypotheses about aging processes in animals can be brought together. In the latter respect it is similar to but somewhat more specific than the view offered by Williams (1957). It also extends to embrace species in which the definition of aging is not always clear (Kirkwood, 1981; Kirkwood, 1985).

The major prediction of the disposable soma theory is that somatic aging is primarily due to accumulation of stochastic defects, and so there should be a close relationship between longevity, environmental mortality, and the general level of investment in somatic repair and maintenance. The theory predicts that for a species in a niche where the environment exacts heavy mortality, the the optimum investment in somatic repair and maintenance will be comparatively small because each individual can expect to survive only a short time. By contrast, the reverse will be true for a

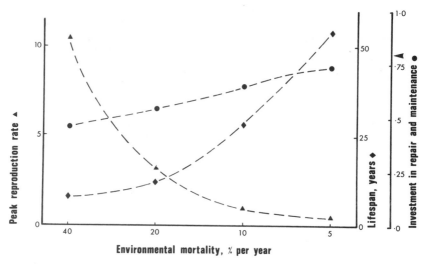

Fig. 4. Effect of varying the level of environmental
mortality on peak reproductive rate (births/
female/year), longevity (99th percentile of
lifespan distribution) and the optimum level of
investment in somatic repair and maintenance,
based on a model of Kirkwood & Holliday (1986).

species with low environmental mortality, and it will be worth investing more
in the survival of the soma, even at some cost to the rate of reproduction
(Kirkwood, 1981; Kirkwood & Holliday, 1979, 1986). Using a simple formal
model (Kirkwood & Holliday, 1986) it is possible to quantify this prediction
(Figure 4). With few assumptions and parameters the model generates curves
which define a robust pattern of correlations. One correlation in particular
which follows directly from a priori assumptions is the predicted relationship
between longevity and the level of somatic maintenance and repair (Figure 5).

The similarity of the prediction in Figure 5 to data for the excision
repair of DNA lesions induced by UV-irradiation (Hart & Setlow, 1974;
Francis et al., 1981; Treton & Courtois, 1982; Hall et al., 1984), is
striking. It suggests that a comprehensive comparative study of the levels
of somatic repair and maintenance among species of different longevities may
be illuminating. Those defects which are corrected by systems of repair and
maintenance and for which an association with longevity was discovered would
constitute prime targets for further study as causes of aging. Those which
showed no clear association with longevity would be of probable lesser
significance. It cannot be emphasized too strongly, however, that the cell
models used for such studies should be carefully validated, and that cell
cultures from different species should be controlled closely for possible
confounding variables such as culture conditions, biopsy site, and age and
sex of the cell donor.

As for mechanisms of germ-line immortality, the implications of the
disposable soma theory depend on what turns out to be the nature of somatic
cell mortality. The theory suggests as one possibility that the level of
repair and maintenance may be higher in germ cells than in somatic cells.
However, other mechanisms could act to protect the germ-line from
progressive accumulation of defects even if they arose within germ cells at
the same rate as in somatic cells. Chief among these is selection,
operating both pre- and post-fertilization. The potential for selection to
eliminate defects is entirely dependent on the degree to which competition

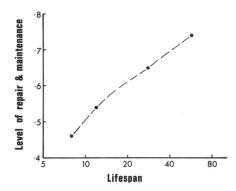

Fig. 5. Predicted correlation between species
lifespan and investment in somatic
repair and maintenance, obtained from
the data shown in Fig. 5.

is taking place. In somatic tissues, cells are restrained to be "good
neighbors" in the interests of the well-being of the soma as a whole, and
opportunities for competition are curtailed. Conspicuous exceptions occur
when cells, under the imperative of simple selection at the cellular level,
acquire adaptations which render them malignant. While there is clearly at
most only a partial correspondence between the immortalization of transformed
somatic cells and the immortality of germ cell lineages, clarification of the
difference between mortal and immortal cell cultures would be an important
step forward. In particular, close study of teratocarcinoma cells which have
infinite lifespans in culture but which spontaneously differentiate to produce
cells which have only finite lifespans (Topp et al., 1977) may help to unravel
the mechanisms by which mortal somatic cells are produced from an immortal
germ-line. Weismann would probably have approved (Kirkwood & Cremer, 1982).

REFERENCES

Bernstein, H., 1977, Germ line recombination may be primarily a
        manifestation of DNA repair processes, J. Theor. Biol., 69:371
Charlesworth, B., 1980, "Evolution in Age-Structured Populations," Cambridge
        University Press, Cambridge.
Comfort, A., 1979, "The Biology of Senescence," 3rd edition, Churchill
        Livingstone, Edinburgh.
Francis, A. A., Lee, W. H., and Regan, J. D., 1981, The relationship of DNA
        excision repair of ultraviolet-induced lesions to the maximum
        lifespan of mammals, Mech. Ageing Dev., 16:181.
Haldane, J. B. S., 1941, "New Paths in Genetics," Allen and Unwin, London.
Hall, K. Y., Hart, R. W., Benirschke, A. K., and Walford, R. L., 1984,
        Correlation between ultraviolet-induced DNA repair in primate
        lymphocytes and species maximum achievable lifespan, Mech. Ageing
        Dev., 24:163.
Hart, R. W., and Setlow, R. B., 1974, Correlation between deoxyribonucleic
        acid excision repair and lifespan in a number of mammalian species,
        Proc. Nat. Acad. Sci., U.S.A., 71:2169.
Kirkwood, T. B. L., 1977, Evolution of ageing, Nature, 270:301.
Kirkwood, T. B. L., 1981, Repair and its evolution: survival versus
        reproduction, in: "Physiological Ecology: An Evolutionary Approach to
        Resource Use," C. R. Townsend and P. Calow, eds., Blackwell
        Scientific Publications, Oxford.

Kirkwood, T. B. L., 1985, Comparative and evolutionary aspects of longevity, in: "Handbook of the Biology of Aging," C. E. Finch and E. L. Schneider, eds., Van Nostrand Reinhold, New York.

Kirkwood, T. B. L., and Cremer, T., 1982, Cytogerontology since 1881: a reappraisal of August Weismann and a review of modern progress, Hum. Genet., 60:101.

Kirkwood, T. B. L., and Holliday, R., 1979, The evolution of ageing and longevity, Proc. Roy. Soc., Lond., B205:531.

Kirkwood, T. B. L., and Holliday, R., 1986, Ageing as a consequence of natural selection, in: "The Biology of Human Ageing," K. J. Collins and A. H. Bittles, eds., Cambridge University Press, Cambridge.

Medawar, P. B., 1952, "An Unsolved Problem in Biology," H. K. Lewis, London.

Medvedev, Z. A., 1981, On the immortality of the germ line: genetic and biochemical mechanisms. A review, Mech. Ageing Dev., 17:331.

Reichman, O. J., 1984, Evolution of regeneration capabilities, Am. Nat., 123:752.

Sacher, G. A., 1978, Evolution of longevity and survival characteristics in mammals, in: "The Genetics of Aging," E. L. Schneider, ed., Plenum, New York.

Sheldrake, A. R., 1974, The ageing, growth and death of cells, Nature, 250:381.

Topp, W., Hall, J. D., Rifkin, D., Levine, A. J., and Pollack, R., 1977, The characterisation of SV40-transformed cell lines derived from mouse teratocarcinoma: growth properties and differentiated characteristics, J. Cell. Physiol., 93-269.

Townsend, C. R., and Calow, P. C., 1981, "Physiological Ecology: An Evolutionary Approach to Resource Use," Blackwell Scientific Publications, Oxford.

Treton, J. A., and Courtois, Y., 1982, Correlation between DNA excision repair and mammalian lifespan in lens epithelial cells, Cell Biol. Int. Rep., 6:253.

Weismann, A., 1890, Untitled correspondence, Nature, 41:317 (reprinted as Appendix 2 in Kirkwood, T. B. L., and Cremer, T., 1982, cited above).

Williams, G. C., 1957, Pleiotropy, natural selection and the evolution of senescence, Evolution, 11:398.

SYSTEMS ECOLOGY, OPERATIONS RESEARCH

AND GERONTOLOGY: THE MAKING OF STRANGE BEDFELLOWS

Robert R. Christian

Department of Biology
East Carolina University
Greenville, N.C.   27858-4353

INTRODUCTION

Biological gerontology is an ecclectic discipline which has drawn upon several areas of the life sciences to describe and explain aging in living systems. However, in the hierarchy of biological systems gerontologists have largely restricted their interests to the levels from the biomolecule to the population and have integrated those areas of biology which address those levels. Other areas of study that could also contribute to gerontology have received less attention. In this paper I introduce two of those areas: systems ecology and operations research. Further, I present parallels between these disciplines and gerontology and describe ways in which concepts and techniques used by them may aid gerontology. Lastly, I propose a simple model describing the interrelationship between a process or structure undergoing change with age and its effects on a system. My intent in this paper is to address the question, "In what ways is aging a characteristic of systems in general?" by applying knowledge of systems ecology, operations research and gerontology. This paper is a result of my synthesis of ideas from these three disciplines.

Strehler (1977) provided four criteria by which changes over time may be identified as an aging process: universality, intrinsicality, progressiveness, and deleteriousness. While he restricted these conditions to the description of aging in biological systems, I propose that these same criteria are justifiable for defining aging of systems in general. Strehler referred to universality as occurring "in all older members of the species." This must be extended to all older systems of the same kind. Thus a community or a factory may be considered to age. The specific mechanisms of aging would differ between the various systems, but commonality should exist in the description and analysis of aging.

While the definition of gerontology should be self-evident within the context of this symposium, the other two pertinent disciplines require definition. Systems ecology is the use of systems analysis in ecology. Systems analysis is "the process of translating physical or biological concepts about any system into a set of mathematical relationships, and the manipulation of the mathematical system thus derived" (Walters, 1971). Although systems ecology is often associated with the heirarchical levels of communities, ecosystems, biomes, and the biosphere, the study of populations may also be accomplished through systems analysis. Operations research may be defined as "the application of scientific method ... to problems involving the control of organized (man-machine) systems so as to provide solutions which best serve the purposes of the organization as a whole" (Ackoff and Sasieni, 1968). Again, operations research relies on systems analysis. The approach of systems analysis is implicit in many studies of gerontology but is explicitly recognized as such in more limited cases. Witten (1984) reviewed mathematical modeling in gerontology, and Miquel et al. (1984) explicity developed a systems approach in postulating a mechanism for cellular aging.

SIMILARITIES OF DISCIPLINES

Gerontology, systems ecology, and operations research have similarities in history, goals, and approaches. All are relatively young disciplines at least as quantitative sciences, being recognized as such within the last half century. In ecology, mathematical models of populations date back into the last century (Hutchinson, 1978), but systems ecology as a discipline largely began in the 1940's by such people as Lindeman (1942), Riley (1947), and H.T. Odum (1955). Progress was linked to the development of digital computers, and its activities intensified in the 1960's and 1970's (Odum, H.T., 1983).

Operations research began as a defined area during World War II (Ackoff and Sasieni, 1968). Teams of engineers, managers and scientists were organized to maintain efficiency of the military-industrial complexes in the United Kingdom and United States. One result was the development of this multidisciplinary approach to problem solving of human organizational structures. Both the military and industry continued to use the approach after the war, and the field has continued to develop.

These three disciplines have similar goals, but it is only in the systems' context that this may be recognized. Each discipline addresses a particular hierarchical structure of systems with each level in the hierarchy representing a system of components and a component of a larger system. Each discipline seeks to describe and explain the manner in which components interact at one level and how such interaction affects the dynamics of other levels. In gerontology, the primary characteristic of the system being studied is aging; in the other two, aging is only one of the system's characteristics.

Similarities also exist in the general approaches taken by the three disciplines. A dominant feature of each is the concern for changes or lack of them through time. None of the systems are static, and sampling and analysis invariably are time dependent. Secondly, each discipline addresses the hierarchical structure of its respective systems. Thirdly, each discipline has advanced by borrowing concepts and tools from other disciplines; the most obvious being that of systems analysis, but game theory and information theory also have been used. Tools include both those of mathematics and statistics, as well as those of physical measurement. And lastly, each discipline is striving to quantitate the structures and functions of complex and variable systems, employing models which attempt to simplify the systems to salient and workable features.

SYSTEMS ECOLOGY AND AGING

While systems ecologists have addressed time-dependent changes and age related phenomena, there is little recognition of an aging process at the hierarchical levels above the population. Communities through the biosphere change with age; these changes may be universal, progressive, and intrinsic, but whether they are deleterious is moot. Much of the debate may rest with the currency (or units of measurement) being considered. During succession from an old field to a mature forest, there are changes which occur to community structure that may be perceived as deleterious to that stage of succession. However, in considering energy flow, nutrient cycling, or general aspects of organization, the demise of an intermediate stage of succession may be better considered as a developmental change (E.P. Odum,1969). Thus, most communities or ecosystems may not age in the sense of Strehler's broadened definition. However, the global changes currently occurring in the biosphere, such as loss of energy reserves and imbalances in elemental cycling may be perceived as aging because of their deleterious nature to many living parts of the biosphere. The key to such an interpretation relies on whether or not human population growth is progressive and intrinsically irreversible, and hence the deleterious effects of human activity are progressive and irreversible.

There are two areas that have been developed in systems ecology that may be useful to the gerontologist. The first is the controversial concept of stability. The second is the use of energy circuit language, which may be applied fruitfully to the description of organismal and lower hierarchical levels.

Cutler (1984) described a mechanistic model of aging based on "dysdifferentiation." In it, he stressed that aging represents "the time-dependent drifting away of cells, cell organization, and homeostatic control from their most optimum state of function." Thus, aging represents a loss of stability of biological systems. However, he indicated that little concern has been given to the nature of stability in gerontology. In ·contrast much ecological work has been done on this topic (Holling, 1973; Webster et al., 1975; Connell and Sousa, 1983). One of the first issues is the definition of stability. One must address (1) what are the units of measure, (2) what kind of response or lack of response represents stability, and (3) to what kind of perturbation is the system considered as stable. Stability with respect to species composition within a community may be different from that for energy flow. Stability may represent constancy through time or responsiveness to perturbation. Systems which respond to a perturbation by moving away from their nominal state and then quickly returning are said to be stable by resilience. Systems that fail to move from their nominal state in the face of perturbation are said to be stable by resistance (Webster et al., 1975). Also, if response to perturbation is the mode of stability considered, a system may be stable to one kind of perturbation and not another. For example, tropical rain forests may be stable to biological but not physical perturbations. Thus ecologists have clearly defined their use of this concept. Gerontologists should consider similar rules in definitions.

In organizing one's ideas to represent a system, an early step is often to represent the system as a network of boxes and arrows. A refinement of this was introduced to systems ecology by H.T. Odum (1971) in the form of energy circuit language. Representative symbols of this language and applications to gerontological hierarchical levels are shown in Figure 1. The major improvement over a simple box and arrow diagram is that each symbol connotes a particular characteristic, so that its "vocabulary" is more exact. Also, different combinations of symbols may represent specific mathematical forms. The variety of symbols available has been enough for the depiction of most ecological systems, and gerontoligists should find the language complete enough as well. Odum (1983) is one of the few systems ecologists who has directly represented aging processes by diagramming mortality models and Strehler's energy stress model (Strehler, 1977).

The analogy between an organism's or cell's aging and the wearing out of a machine has generally been marked as being overly simplistic and unapplicable. However, there are approaches used in operations research to address the machine that may prove fruitful for the gerontologist. A major theme of this symposium involves the adaptive traits of organisms which affect longevity and the aging process. Similarly, the operations researcher may be interested in the design of a mechanical system to extend its longevity. The choices may be to: (1) use higher quality parts that may last longer, (2) ensure replacement or repair of wearing parts in a timely fashion, or

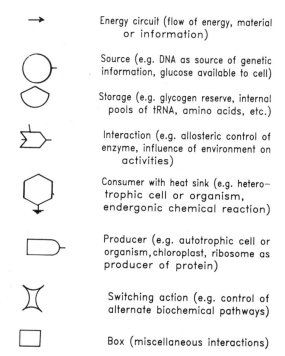

Figure 1. Representative symbols of energy circuit language and possible applications for gerontology.

(3) include redundancy of critical parts (Ackoff and Sasieni, 1968). Further, one would want to develop an analysis of each approach to maximize benefits while minimizing costs. In considering the evolution of longevity, many adaptive traits which extend longevity may be grouped into one of these three categories. Also, success of a trait is dependent on the relative costs and benefits to the organism. Although the mechanisms (genetic change and natural selection vs. a priori design) may be different, the results appear similar. Thus mathematical analyses and concepts used in operations research may be applicable to description of biological aging phenomena. In fact, similarities exist in some aging models between gerontology and operations research (Witten, 1984; 1985).

Assessment of the quality of parts may be made by analysis of the
distribution of their failure with time, namely a failure time analysis (Cox
and Oakes, 1984). In this, the probability of failure or the occurrence of
any event through time is determined. A cummulative frequency distribution
then is computed that can be used to develop a survivorship, reliability or
hazard function to describe the dynamics of the aging process. These
functions have been derived for a variety of both endogenous and exogenous
conditions that would promote failure (Sivazlian and Stanfel, 1975). Such
functions from two or more analyses then can be compared statistically to
relate effectiveness of different systems (Cox and Oakes, 1984; Muenchow,
1986). This analysis has been used in both the medical sciences and
gerontology (Elandt-Johnson and Johnson, 1980; Witten 1984).

Analysis of the second choice of ensuring replacement or repair follows
similar mathematics in defining the frequency distribution of probable
failures, but includes cost/benefit analyses for inspection and different
modes of replacement: replacement as required and group replacement (Ackoff
and Sasieni, 1968; Sivazlian and Stanfel, 1975). This is called "replacement theory" in operations research. Such analyses may be useful for eva-
luating regenerative processes. The challenge to the gerontologist is to
equate the units of measure of costs and benefits. In operations research
this is generally money, in gerontology it might be energy.

Third, there is the evaluation of redundant systems (Ackoff and
Sasieni, 1968; Sivazlian and Stanfel, 1975). Here the probability functions
of failure of each of the redundant subsystems and their joint probabilities
are analyzed with respect to how reliably the system as a whole will perform. Again cost/benefit analyses are conducted. This approach may have
direct application to tandem gene string models (Witten, 1984) or other
aging models associated with redundancy. The composite mathematics designed
to assess the way in which systems can be maintained to act effectively is
"reliability theory".

COMMON MODEL OF AGING

It is unlikely that a common mechanistic model exists to explain aging
of all systems, short of the most general one involving the second law of
thermodynamics. However, a descriptive model may be developed that
accentuates two criteria of aging: progressiveness and deleteriousness. I
present one which I hope has some applicability across disciplines and may
help to focus attention on critical aspects of aging. I consider that there
is a structure or process within a system that exists through time and may
demonstrate time-dependent and progressive change. Second, a threshold of
impairment of structural or functional integrity exists which may also be
time-dependent that if transgressed, there is has a deleterious effect on
the system. Further, I include a second (optional) threshold that denotes
failure of the system as a result of change in the original structure or
process. The degree of deleteriousness is dependent on the position of the
structure or process condition between the two thresholds. A variety of
possibilities of this model are shown in Figure 2. In Figure 2a, the
simplest case, the structural/process linearly declines with age and the
thresholds are not age-dependent. Figure 2b is a more complex case in which
the structure/process is a nonlinear function with respect to age, and the
thresholds are age-dependent with transgression being more susceptable at
younger and older ages. In Figure 2c a deleterious effect is found
immediately as the structure/process changes but failure of the system does
not occur until the structure/process reaches zero. Lastly, in Figure 2d
the structure/process is time-independent, but the thresholds are dependent
on time and intersect with the former. Thus the nature of change being both
progressive and deleterious may be derived in many ways, with these

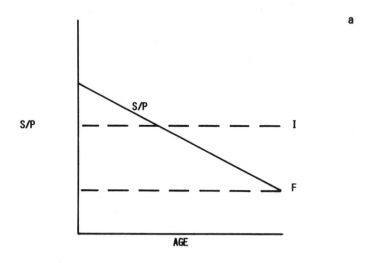

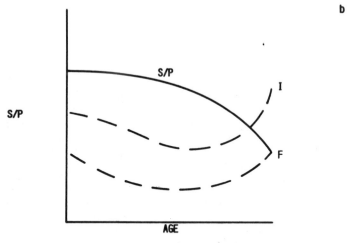

Figure 2. Examples of different modes of interaction of a structure/process (S/P) and thresholds of impairment (I) and failure (F) in aging.

224

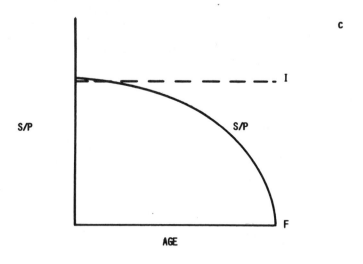

c

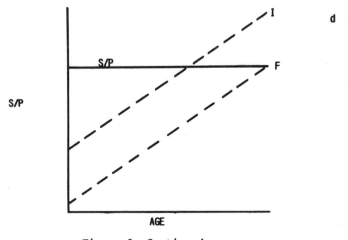

d

Figure 2. Continued.

representing only some examples. The criteria of universality and intrinsicality are implied in all examples but are not required.

In searching for a mathematical description of this diagrammatic model, I found one within systems ecology and some equation sets that I used for entirely different purposes (Wetzel and Christian, 1984; Christian et al., 1987). Wiegert (1973; 1974) and co-workers (1981) developed a mathematical approach to simulating energy or carbon flow through populations and biotic ecosystem components and population growth. The equations were designed to alleviate some of the problems inherent with the logistic and Lotka-Volterra equations. Specifically, Weigert introduced feedback terms to growth or ingestion that separately address food resource and spatial limitations. Of interest here is the food resource limitation feedback term (FB_R):

$$FB_R = (1 - ((A - R) / (A - G))_+)_+. \qquad (1)$$

where: A is the density of resource below which limitation begins.

G is the density of resource at which limitation prevents

further growth or feeding.

R is the density of resource available.

+ is the logical condition that is the value in parentheses until

that value is less than zero, then the value becomes zero.

The nature of this feedback as a function of resource density is diagrammatically shown in Figure 3a.

This feedback form can be modified for the aging model. A system's integrity function (SIF) represents the status of the system being affected by the structure/process and is normalized between 0 and 1 where 1 is the system's normal operation and 0 is system's failure. SIF, the structure/process (S/P), the threshold of impairment (I), and the threshold of failure (F) are all functions of time (t) as they may each vary with the age of the system. Thus the equation becomes:

$$SIF(t) = (1 - ((I(t) - S/P(t))/(I(t) - F(t)))_+)_+ \qquad (2)$$

An energy circuit language diagram of this is shown in Figure 4. The relationships of SIF to S/P are shown in Figure 3b which is congruent with Figure 3a. An example of the manner in which SIF may change with age relative to the interactions of S/P, I, and F is shown in Figure 5. Here, linear changes in S/P and F with age promote nonlinearity in the SIF with age.

This model has some advantages to each of the disciplines discussed but remains somewhat simplistic and subject to modification when considering other aspects of aging. The first advantage is its potential use in simulation models of aging systems. By removing the implications of universality and intrinsicality, other time-dependent systems may be modeled as well.

However, whether or not the model is incorporated into simulation, it represents a valid descriptive hypothesis of interaction associated with aging. It allows the reseacher to focus on the age-dependent nature of: (1) the structure or process (2) the threshold of impairment, (3) the threshold of system's failure and (4) the system's integrity function. Further, the interrelationship of the four may be studied. These descriptions may be used for both the evaluation of a particular system and for cross system comparisons. For example, do different species demonstrate similar SIF vs. age curves with respect to particular processes, or do different processes demonstrate similar SIF vs. age curves within a species?

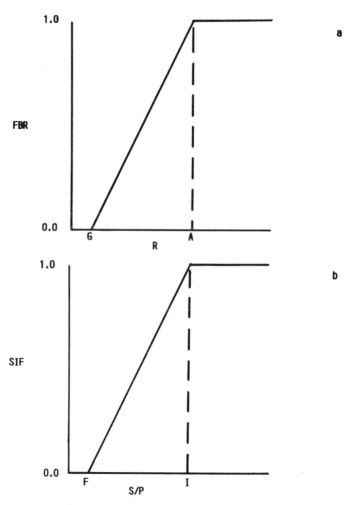

Figure 3. Relationship: (a) between resource availability (R) and limitations on feeding or growth (FBR); and (b) between a structure or process (S/P) and systems integrity function (SIF).

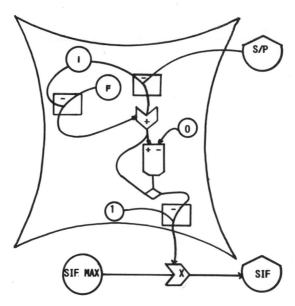

Figure 4.   Energy circuit language diagram of the SIF relationship to S/P.

There are some limitations to the model as presented. Modifications
may increase robustness and applicability. As presented, SIF is a value
between 0 and 1 inclusive. In Wiegert's model the feedback is multiplied by
a maximum ingestion rate to obtain a realized ingestion rate or by a maximum
specific growth rate to obtain a realized specific growth rate. Similarly,
the SIF could be multiplied by a measure of normal system's function to
predict the value of that function for a particular age. Also, the
relationship of resource or structure/process is linear relative to feedback
or SIF. Wiegert (1974) introduced modifications for nonlinearity that could
be made for the SIF model. For example, by squaring I,F, and S/P at each
time the effects on SIF with respect to decreasing S/P is initially more
precipitous than with the linear relationship (Fig. 6a). An alternate
relationship of S/P and SIF is shown in Figure 6b. In this, the initial
slope of effect below I is gentle and increases as S/P decreases toward F.

Thus far my approach to this model has been deterministic. However the
relationships may be considered as stochastic. If we assume some variability associated with a process, then transgression of thresholds may be related to either changes in the "accuracy" of the process or changes in its
"precision". These differences are shown in Figure 7. In Fig. 7a the
"accuracy" of the process (the ability for the process to continue without
impairment to the system) decreases with time and intersects the thresholds,
as previously described. The variance is homoscedastic throughout age, such
that the variability does not increase or decrease. In Fig 7b the process
becomes more variable with age (i.e. a heteroscedastic variance). Thus the
probability of transgressing the thresholds increases even though the mean
may remain above the thresholds. This may be viewed as a loss of
homeostatic ability. The definition of SIF must change to reflect the
probability of impairment to system's integrity. This may be achieved by
developing an SIF at some level of confidence. For example, the lower 95%

228

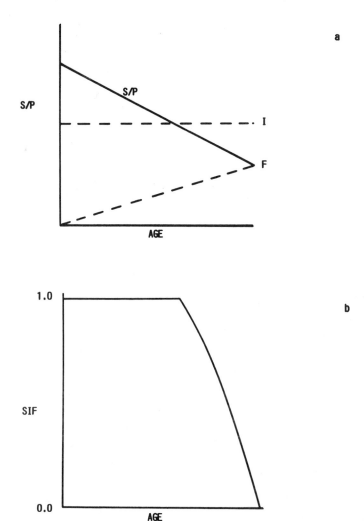

Figure 5. Conversion of interactions: (a) between S/P, I and F; and (b) between SIF and age using equation 2. See text for details.

confidence level for the process could be computed through time. This value rather than the mean would then be used to determine SIF at this level of confidence. Similarly, the variances associated with the thresholds could increase with time, and further modify the SIF calculation.

One last modification to the SIF model involves processes which increase with age and have thresholds of impairment above the initial process values. Mathematically, this modification is most easily made by transla-

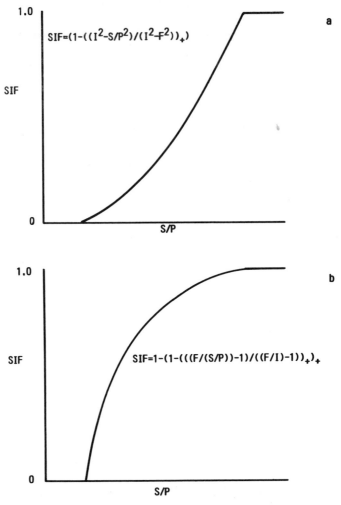

Figure 6. Two alternate mathematical forms to describe the relationship between S/P and SIF.

tion of axes such that the process and thresholds are in the negative Y, and positive X quadrant. In other words the highest value for the failure threshold becomes zero, the highest failure threshold's original value is subtracted from all other values. The subsequent mathematics are the same as in previous calculations of SIF.

I have developed a simple, descriptive model which embodies the major characteristics of an aging system with respect to how the actions of one

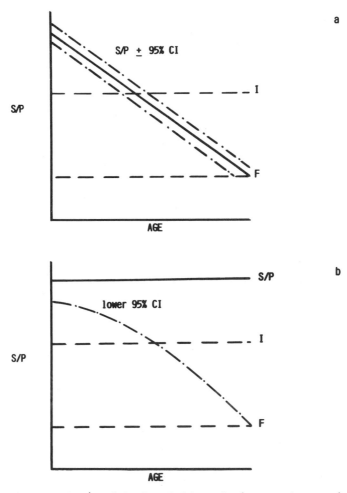

Figure 7.   Interactions of S/P with thresholds relative to changes in (a) "accuracy" and (b) "precision".

process or structure may be related to another system's atttribute. Independent of mathematical manipulations, the conceptual model focuses attention on the need to define the age-dependent relationships of the process rate or structural characteristic, a threshold of impairment, and a threshold of failure. A major challenge to the gerontologist is in describing these relationships during ages in which impairment is not normally found. This translates into measuring how the thresholds may change through time. This may require studies in which the process is altered experimentally in young systems to promote impairment or failure. In turn this may require the use of selective inhibitors of a process that do not otherwise impair the system

and measurement of effects to the system. Also, experimentation may be
necessary to project the impairment threshold beyond the point of intersec-
tion by the structure/process, by supplementing materials lost from the
declining structure or process. Then one may be able to consider other
questions about the system. For example, what is the degree of buffer that
may exist between the actions of the process and inducement of impairment or
failure of the system? Do the actions of this process or the thresholds
change most with age? Is it the "accuracy" or "precision" of events that
most affect impairment? Can one infer particular mechanisms of aging from
the relationships described?

In conclusion, I hope that I have introduced some new avenues for
exploration. Whether or not there is useful application of the model
remains to be seen. However, if nothing else is accomplished, I hope that
the gerontologist is now aware that there are at least two disciplines which
consider similar issues but on different systems. A dialog between researchers in the three disciplines may allow cross fertilization of ideas to the
benefit of each.

ACKNOWLEDGEMENTS

I thank the ecology seminar group at E.C.U. for comments on a
preliminary presentation of this work and Ms. Sheila Noe and Mr. Tim Charles
for their help in preparation of the paper.

REFERENCES

Ackoff, R.L., and Sasieni, M.W., 1968, "Fundamentals of Operations Research,"
    John Wiley and Sons, Inc., New York.
Christian R.R., Wetzel, R.L., Harlan, S.M., and Stanley, D.W., 1987, Growth
    and decomposition in aquatic microbial systems: alternate approaches in
    simple models, in: "Proceedings of Fourth International Symposium on
    Microbial Ecology", Ljubljana, Yugoslavia (In press).
Connell, J.H., and Sousa, W.P., 1983, On the evidence needed to judge
    ecological stability or persistance, Amer. Nat., 121:789.
Cox, D.R., and Oakes, D., 1984, "Analysis of Survival Data," Chapman and Hall,
    London.
Cutler, R.G., 1984, Evolutionary biology of aging and longevity in mammalian
    species, in: "Aging and Cell Function," J.E. Johnson, Jr., ed.,
    Plenum Press, New York.
Elandt-Johnson, R.C., and N.L. Johnson, 1980, "Survival Models and Data
    Analysis," John Wiley and Sons, New York.
Holling, C.S., 1973, Resilience and stability of ecological systems, Ann.
    Rev. Ecol. Syst., 4:1.
Hutchinson, G.E. 1978, "An Introduction to Population Ecology," Yale
    University Press, New Haven, Connecticut.
Lindeman, R.L., 1942, The trophic-dynamics aspect of ecology, Ecology 23:399.
Miquel, J., Economos, A.C., and Johnson, J.E., Jr., 1984, A systems
    analysis - thermodynamic view of cellular and organismal aging, in:
    "Aging and Cell Function," J.E. Johnson, Jr., ed., Plenum Press,
    New York.
Muenchow, G., 1986, Ecological use of failure time analysis, Ecology, 67:246.
Odum, E.P., 1969, The strategy of ecosystem development, Science, 164:262.
Odum, H.T., 1955, Trophic structure and productivity of Silver Springs,
    Florida, Ecol. Monogr., 27:55.
Odum, H.T., 1971, An energy circuit language for ecological and social systems,
    its physical basis, in: "Systems Analysis and Simulation in Ecology,
    Vol.2", B. Patten, ed., Academic Press, New York.
Odum, H.T., 1983, "Systems Ecology: an Introduction," John Wiley and Sons,
    New York.

Riley, G.A., 1947, A theoretical analysis of the zooplankton population of Georges Bank, J. Mar. Res. 6:104.

Sivazlian, B.D., and Stanfel, L.E., 1975, "Analysis of Systems in Operations Research," Prentice-Hall, Inc., Englewood Cliffs.

Strehler, B.L., 1977, "Time, Cells, and Aging," 2nd Ed., Academic Press, New York.

Walters, C.J., 1971, Systems ecology: the systems approach and mathematical models in ecology, in: "Fundamentals of Ecology," E.P. Odum, ed., W.B. Saunders Co., Philadelphia.

Webster, J.R., Waide, J.B., and Patten, B.C., 1975, Nutrient recycling and the stability of ecosystems, in: "Mineral Cycling in Southeastern Ecosystems," F.G. Howell, ed., ERDA Symposium Series, Conf. 740513. Energy Research and Development Agency.

Wetzel, R.L., and Christian, R.R., 1984, Model studies on the interactions among carbon substrates, bacteria and consumers in a salt marsh estuary, Bull. Mar. Sci., 35:601.

Wiegert, R.G., 1973, A general ecological model and its use in simulating algalfly energetics in a thermal spring community, in: "Insects: Studies in Population Management, Vol. 1," P.W. Geier, L.R. Clark, D.J. Anderson, and H.A. Nix, eds., Ecol. Soc. Australia, Canberra.

Wiegert, R.G., 1974, A general mathematical representation of ecological flux processes: description and use in ecosystem models, Proc. 6th Ann. SE Systems Symp. TP-2, 15 pp. Baton Rouge, La.

Wiegert, R.G., Christian, R.R., and Wetzel, R.L., 1981, A model view of the marsh, in: "The Ecology of a Salt Marsh," L.R. Pomeroy and R.G. Wiegert, eds., Springer-Verlag, New York.

Witten, M., 1984, Mathematics of molecular aging mechanisms, in: "Molecular Basis of Aging," A.K. Roy, and B. Chatterjee, eds., Academic Press, Orlando.

Witten, M., 1985, A return to time, cells, systems, and aging: III. Gompertzian models of biological aging and some possible roles for critical elements, Mech. Ageing Dev., 32:141-177.

DEMOGRAPHIC CONSEQUENCES OF NATURAL SELECTION

George C. Williams

Ecology and Evolution, State University
Stony Brook, NY 11794

Peter D. Taylor

Mathematics and Statistics, Queen's University
Kingston, Ontario K7L 3 N6

> . . . .
> Let's have a bloody good cry.
> And always remember the longer you live,
> The sooner you'll bloody well die.
>
> (from an old Irish ballad)

INTRODUCTION

From the standpoint of most people's interests and perspectives, little need be added to the simple and elegant statement above. From the special perspective of a student of evolution, the statement seems a trifle parochial, and some qualifications and additions seem justified. It seems parochial in three respects, which we will call the dimensional, the ontogenetic, and the phylogenetic.

By dimensional parochialism we mean that the usual view of mortality rates focuses on those pertaining to animals of the order of 10^1 to 10^2 kg. Variation in this narrow range is trivial compared to that between the sizes over which organisms vary, from less than a nanogram to hundreds of tons. Over these many orders of magnitude there is a simple relationship between size and the death rates and birth rates that jointly determine demography: the smaller the size the greater the rates. The exact relation can be read from data summarized by Bonner (1957) and Sheldon, Prakash, and Suttcliffe (1972), who documented the size dependence of productivity. Their data show that the potential doubling time for an organism, with mass ($\underline{m}$) measured in grams is about $100m^{.25}$ days. Since all such populations, in fact, remain finite, we assume that their environments have the capability of removing them as fast as they are produced, removing the small organisms faster than the large. A formulation for population doubling time must work equally well for cohort half life.

The immense diversity in sizes and attendant mortality rates of organisms were produced by evolution. Natural selection almost always favors lower mortality, but at any given moment in the history of life, it favored larger size for some organisms, smaller for others. We assume that this is the main way in which natural selection has shaped rates of birth and death, as an incidental consequence of selection for size. The prevailing average rates at particular sizes are scaling problems resolvable by physical principles such as surface-volume relations. It is for variation within a size category that we need the biological principle of natural selection.

The usual view of human mortality is ontogenetically parochial in its adult chauvinism. Children, at least in their early years, currently have higher mortality rates than adolescents or young adults. With the markedly higher mortality at all ages, which prevailed for most of human evolution, almost no one would survive to adult ages of higher mortality than those of the first few years. Mean or median life expectancy for a two-year-old could be greater than for either a newborn or a patriarch. The truth of our opening statement, on the relation between length of life and imminence of death, may be technically questionable even for modern populations. We suspect that if we gathered the necessary data and calculated an annual mortality rate for the first ten minutes of life, we might find it higher than that of centenarians. If you are a baby in your first minute of extra-uterine life, the longer you live the more remote your death is likely to be.

Perspectives are often phylogenetically parochial in their concentration on a single species. Ours is a species much closer to the upper than the lower end of the size scale. Our intuitive perspective relates to large organisms, with life expectancies in years, rather than the hours or days characteristic of much of the size spectrum. We are also an unusual species in the close similarity of size, and therefore mortality, of young and adult. The 15-fold increase in size between neonate and adult is trivial compared to the size contrast in other organisms between different stages in the development of a single individual. Consider the difference between a redwood seed and the mature tree. Among unitary animals (those without vegetative proliferation), it may be that the bluefin tuna is an extreme example of ontogenetic size change. A large adult may have about a billion times the mass of a newly hatched larva. Ontogenetic size changes imply ontogenetic changes in the mortality rates characteristic of the sizes of the different stages. Students of marine fish populations commonly find per-day losses among larvae that exceed per-year losses among adults. The narrowly limited size change in human development means that we experience only a narrow range of mortality rates, compared to such organisms as the redwood or tuna.

AGE AND MORTALITY AMONG HUMAN ADULTS

The rest of this presentation will be dimensionally, ontogenetically, and phylogenetically parochial. From adolescence on, a human age cohort experiences an ever rising mortality rate, and our intent here is to explore the possibility of deducing, from basic evolutionary postulates, a quantitative description of this change. Medawar's (1952) was the first valid statement of the relationship between age and selection for the maintenance of viability. We believe that the validity and fruitfulness of Medawar's theory was convincingly established by comparative evidence cited in his paper and later in Williams (1957). Experimental work has more recently added new confirmation (Bell, 1984; Charlesworth, 1984; Luckinbill et al, 1984; Rose, 1983).

The logic of the theory got detailed mathematical development by Hamilton (1966), but neither he nor anyone else has produced a conclusion in the form of an explicit $\mu = f(x)$, with μ being the mortality rate and x being age. We think it unlikely that any such formulation will be derived, because of mathematical difficulties that circumvent any attempt to use the theory in an axiomatic way. It may still be possible to use the theory to generate theoretical demographies by computer simulation. Theoretical age structures would be of value, because it is normal scientific practice to compare expectations with observations, in order to check the validity of the reasoning used in generating the expectations.

The observations needed, for checking the theorizing below, would be detailed and accurate demographic data on Stone-age populations. Such observations are not available, but we hope that our project can be rescued to some extent by a contrived alternative. Hamilton (1966) published demographic data on Chinese women living in Taiwan about 1906 to illustrate his account of the evolution of senescence. The data as published depart from average Stone-age demography in one conspicuous respect: the population was growing at a rapid rate, despite what would be considered heavy mortality by current standards. The mean condition for the Stone Age must have averaged very close to zero growth, or human numbers would not have stayed finite for so long. A growth rate of one percent per century would suffice for replacing the present population of the earth from a single pair in less than a quarter of the Pleistocene.

We presume that Stone-age mortality rates averaged greater than those of the Taiwan population, and fertility rates lower. Lower fertility may have resulted from the same sorts of stresses that caused mortality, but also from the apparent tendency for mothers in hunter-gatherer societies to nurse their babies to a greater age than in agricultural societies. The Taiwan population would conform to the zero growth requirement if it had about a 0.239 increase in mortality rate and a 0.239 decrease in birth rate at all ages (Figure 1). With this demographic schedule, girls at birth would have an average expectation of living to produce one daughter. At adolescence (age 15) about half would have died, and the remainder would now have an expectation of producing two daughters before the termination of reproduction by death or menopause or obstetrical malfunction. We would welcome suggestions as to what might be better than our derived curve (Figure 1) for use as data on Stone-age demography.

The simplest plausible expectation for a schedule of mortality rates expected from natural selection would have mortality vary inversely according to each age's importance to fitness. Using x for age, l_x for the probability of survival to x, V_x for reproductive value at x, and μ_x for instantaneous mortality at x, the expectation is that

$$\mu_x = k / l_x V_x$$

Reproductive value at age x measures the mean future reproductive output for individuals of that age. The formulation implies some genetic assumptions, in particular that proportionately equal increases in mortality are equally likely to arise by mutation. A stage with a mortality rate of 0.010 per year would be as likely to change to 0.011 by mutation as one with 0.10 would be to change to 0.11. The same must hold for decreases, although the rate of occurrence of a given decrease is expected to be much less than that of a proportionately similar increase. Under these conditions the formulation describes an Evolutionarily Stable Strategy (ESS), a state which, once attained, could not be altered by selection for a different state. A different assumption on the nature of the genetic variation may lead to a different ESS. For example, if mutational changes of equal absolute magnitude were equally frequent, the population would evolve semelparity, with a single bout of reproduction followed by death.

There are several levels of difficulty in using the equation above for deriving the equilibrium demography expected from natural selection. The first is mathematical and results from complex recursive dependencies among the terms. Survival (l) at age x depends on all previous values of μ, which in turn are functions of previous l-values. Reproductive value depends on all

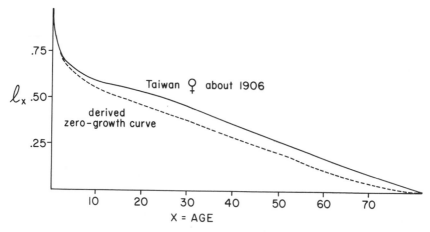

Fig. 1. The solid line shows cohort attrition over time for Chinese women in
Taiwan about 1906 (from Hamilton, 1966). The dashed line shows the
result of dividing observed mortality rates and multiplying birth
rates by 0.761. This change results in zero population growth and is
proposed as an approximation to Stone-age demography.

future mortality and birth rates. We see no hope for any precise analytical
derivation of a theoretical age structure. A still more serious difficulty
lies in the evolutionary irrelevance of any facile measure of reproductive
value. A demographer normally measures the fertility of an age class by
counting the number of babies that it produces. Human reproduction requires
that babies not only be produced but nurtured and tended for many years. A
woman past menopause is conventionally considered postreproductive, but she
may still be contributing to the welfare of her descendants and other relatives. If so she is acting in a way that enhances the proliferation of her
own genes. She is reproductively active from the standpoint of natural selection. We presume that it is for this reason alone that a woman may be able
live beyond menopause. By conventional measure, her V drops to zero at this
stage and the woman drops dead, according to our rule for mortality rate. The
fallacy here lies in the conventional formulation of reproductive value.

Our solution to the problem of analytical intractability is to abandon
mathematics and rely on computer simulation (Appendix). Our solution to the
problem of defining reproduction is to see what can be accomplished by guess-
work. In our simulation the reproductive value declines each year as a function of the expected fertility of the previous year, but only by a fraction
of the expected decline. In this way a woman still has some reproductive
value left at menopause, a value that represents a guess as to how effective
she then might be in enhancing the survival of her own genes represented in
relatives. If a plausible guess allows the generation of an age structure
closely similar to that of our modified Taiwan data, the exercise shows that
theory and observation are potentially compatible. If no plausible guess has
that result, the finding is more instructive. In the simulation illustrated,
we represent effects of kin selection by having the reproductive value of a
woman at menopause equal to a third of what it was at age fifteen. We think
this an extreme assumption, and believe that a smaller value would be more
realistic.

It is a simple matter, with these rules of the game, to use trial-and-
error simulations (Appendix) to produce theoretical demographies consistent
with the rules and with the   requirement of   zero   population   growth

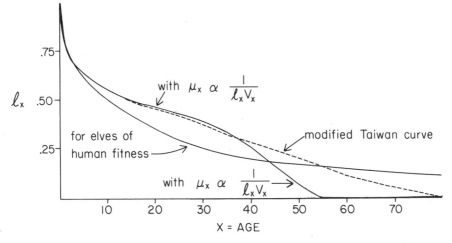

Fig. 2. The dashed line repeats the reconstruction of Stone-age demography
shown in Figure 1. The solid lines show the Stone-age demography
predicted by our theory, and the demography expected of eternal
youth purchased at the cost of developmental retardation (Tolkien's
elves).

(Figure 2). Note that senescence in the theoretical curve is much more abrupt
than in that based on the Taiwan data. A number of considerations bear on the
interpretation of this result. The theoretical curve is for a homogeneous
cohort with optimal tradeoffs of viability among ages but with all fertility
values and minimum mortality (age 15) uniformly altered from the Taiwan
values so as to achieve zero population growth. The fitness homogeneity of
the population is manifest in the low variability of life span. Any real
Stone-age human cohort would be heterogeneous in fitness. Some girls at
puberty would have great vigor of body and mind and a lofty social status.
They would be expected to have much greater than average longevity and reproductive performance. Others may be crippled or chronically ill outcasts with
little likelihood of rearing even one child.

Unfortunately, no degree of fitness heterogeneity is sufficient to ex-
cuse the discrepancy between theory and what we are using as observation
(modified Taiwan age structure). If we simulate an extreme heterogeneity by
giving half the cohort four times the fitness of the other half, but with the
total having the same mean fitness as the homogeneous cohort, we still get
only a small percentage of survivors beyond age sixty and none beyond age
sixty-six. It must also be realized that the simulation uses what we regard
as an unrealistically high reproductive value for a woman after menopause.
Lower values result in earlier and more abrupt attrition.

The outcome of our simulation is not surprising. Our formula for relating mortality to reproductive value and survival is a formula for explosive
positive feedback. Declining survival and reproductive value cause increase
in mortality rate which causes a greater decline in survival and reproductive
value in the next year and so on in an ever steeper cycle until mortality
shows a catastrophic increase in a single year and the cohort vanishes. It
should also be noted that all fertility values used in the simulation are
empirically based on the data from Taiwan. In future work we plan to simulate
fertility senescence along with viability senescence. Fertility can be expected to show the same sort of sudden collapse as viability, because it also
would have a positive-feedback relation with survival. A more sudden decline
in fertility would increase the rate of decline in viability and produce an
even steeper end to the cohort than appears in Figure 2.

We conclude that our simulation does not give a realistic picture of what we are using as primitive human demography, despite the use of numerical constants chosen to be unfairly favorable to a match between theory and observation. Either there is some flaw in our reasoning or the modified Taiwan data are grossly unrepresentative of primitive human populations. Perhaps the most probable error is conceptual, our simple assumption of an equal likelihood for proportionately equal mutational changes at different ages. This implies an absolute equivalence between developmental and absolute time, which would be clearly unrealistic for development through a broad range of sizes. Developmental processes can be expected to take place much more rapidly in the small sizes early in life than later on.

In defense of our genetic assumption we can point out that there are no important size changes in human development after age fifteen. Moreover, there are many examples of morphogenetic change at constant absolute rates during adulthood in many mammals. Those with an annual cycle of change in coat color, gonads, or secondary sexual characters would be obvious examples. We do not really view these observations as justifying the use of our simple model of the genetics of mortality rates. Our simulation (Appendix) assumes that, for instance, a mutation that lowers mortality by one percent in the tenth year only, is neither more nor less likely to arise than one that would lower it by one percent in the twentieth only. There is no reason to rule out the possibility that the twentieth and twenty-first year together would be the developmental equivalent of the tenth. Annual cycles of morphogenesis at similar rates could be exceptional, and not indicative of a general tendency for rates of development to remain uniform during adulthood. Resolution of this difficulty may have to await a more advanced understanding of developmental constraints on the evolutionary process.

DEMOGRAPHY OF TOLKIEN'S ELVES

The elves of Middle Earth, accoding to J. R. R. Tolkien in The Silmarillion and several prior works, were essentially human in most respects. A difference that Tolkien stressed was the elves' eternal youth. As adults they suffered no deterioration of adaptive performance with increasing age. This major biological advantage must have evolved at some compensating cost, otherwise they would have rapidly displaced their competitors. The co-existence of elven and human populations in approximate equilibrium for many centuries shows that neither could have had a net competitive advantage over the other.

It is clear from Tolkein's works that elves had a normal childhood in most respects, but he is silent on its duration. This raises the possibility that their freedom from senescence was purchased at the cost of developmental retardation. If this were the only cost, its magnitude must have been very nearly whatever is needed to reduce elven fitness to human fitness. The required retardation in development can be found with simulations using, throughout elven adulthood, the previously determined adolescent minimum of mortality and third-decade maximum of birth rate, with various degrees of prolongation of childhood and of childhood mortality rates. This method shows that an approximate doubling of the childhood years would give elves the required zero population growth.

The resulting elven age structure (Figure 2), after sexual maturity at about age 30, is simply determined by a constant exponential decay of each age cohort. Fertility increases gradually to its maximum after age 40 (as in the human population after age 20) and keeps this maximum value thereafter. It is clear that the elves utterly fail to conform to our postulated inverse proportionality between mortality and the product of survival and reproductive value. They may well conform to models of tradeoffs between speed of attainment of maturity and levels of adaptive performance after maturity (Taylor and Williams, 1984).

The lesson for us from this simulation of elven life history is this: If our evolution had been somehow forbidden to use fitness tradeoffs between adult ages, but had instead favored age-independent adult fitness at the cost of slower development, and had achieved the same lifetime fitness under Stone-age conditions, we would now be like Tolkien's elves. Each of us would have taken about 30 years to produce the phenotype we actually reached in 15, but we would thereafter have a 15-year-old's mortality rate. We would live until struck by lightning, appendicitis, a terrorist, or other stress that might be lethal to a fifteen-year-old.

Elves are not the only zoological example of freedom from senescence. Evolution effectively forbids senescence in any tissues that will be passed on in either sexual or asexual reproduction. So animals with limited life spans belong to potentially immortal populations, and genetically defined individuals from single zygotes can persist indefinitely in species with modular modes of development (Jackson and Coates, 1986). There may be coral colonies many millenia in age (Potts, 1984).

ACKNOWLEDGMENTS

We are grateful to Dr. Kent L. Fiala of the Department of Ecology and Evolution, State University, Stony Brook, for programming and much helpful advice.

REFERENCES

Bell, G., 1984, Evolutionary and nonevolutionary theories of senescence, Amer. Naturalist, 124:600.

Bonner, J. T., 1965, "Size and cycle," Princeton Univ. Press, Princeton.

Charlesworth, B., 1984, The evolutionary genetics of life histories, in "Evolutionary Ecology", edited by B. Shorrocks, Blackwell Sci. Publ., Oxford.

Hamilton, W. D., 1966, The moulding of senescence by natural selection, J. Theor. Biol., 12:12.

Jackson, J. B. C. and A. G. Coates, 1986, Life cycles and evolution of clonal (modular) animals, Phil. Trans. Royal Soc. London, B, 313:7.

Luckinbill, L. S., R. Arking, M. J. Claire, W. C. Cirocco, and S. A. Buck, 1984, Selection for delayed senescence in Drosophila melanogaster, Evolution, 38:996.

Medawar, P. B., 1952, "An unsolved problem in biology," H. K. Lewis, London.

Potts, D. C., 1984, Generation times and the Quarternary evolution of reef-building corals, Paleobiology, 10:48.

Rose, M. R., 1983, Theories of life-history evolution, Amer. Zoologist, 23:15.

Sheldon, R. W., A. Prakash, and W. H. Suttcliffe, 1972, The size distribution of particles in the ocean, Limnol. Oceanogr., 17:327.

Taylor, P. D. and G. C. Williams, 1984, Demographic parameters at evolutionary equilibrium, Can. J. Zoology, 62:2264.

Tolkien, J. R. R., 1977, "The Silmarillion," Houghton Mifflin, Boston.

Williams, G. C., 1957, Pleiotropy, natural selection, and the evolution of
senescence, *Evolution*, 11:398.

APPENDIX

Our Turbo Pascal program appears below. The output shown is for stone age
equal to 0.761 and cost equal to 0.666. These values give zero population
growth and the reproductive value of one (daughter) per newborn or per half
adolescent (age 15). They also give the population structure that would result from everyone having average fitness but ideal tradeoffs in viability
among adult ages. This ideal would be stabilized by natural selection if genetic variation is as explained in the text. Values for stone age other than
0.761 can be used to show the demography of groups of other-than-average fitness, but the output will be realistic only if the age-15 repr value is made
to equal the final girl sum. This compatibility can be achieved by successive
approximation. The program of course could be used as a module in a larger
program that finds the compatible pairs of values, simulates plausible
patterns of fitness variation, &c.

```
program dieoff (output);

const
  start_age = 15;
  stop_age = 65;
  start_survival = 0.5;
  Taiwan_mortality = 0.0100;
type
  age_range = start_age..stop_age;
  column = array [age_range] of real;
var
  survival, mortality, repr_value, birthrate, girls, girl_sum :
      column;  { Sons don't count here for repr_value. }
  age : integer;
  last_age : integer;
  cost : real;   { Cost would be 1.0 without aid to relatives. }
  stone_age : real; { This measures stone-age prospects, relative to
                      those of Taiwan in 1906 }
  yesno : char;
  diskout, diskopen : boolean;
  diskfile : text;

procedure init_birthrate;  { modified from Taiwan in 1906 (Hamilton, 1966) }
const
  Taiwan_birthrate : column = (        0.0036,         {15}
    0.0120, 0.0260, 0.0450, 0.0700, 0.0950,    {16..20}
    0.1170, 0.1302, 0.1640, 0.1720, 0.1733,    {21..25}
    0.1733, 0.1733, 0.1670, 0.1631, 0.1600,    {26..30}
    0.1570, 0.1552, 0.1515, 0.1494, 0.1420,    {31..35}
    0.1378, 0.1320, 0.1290, 0.1250, 0.1100,    {36..40}
    0.0930, 0.0800, 0.0600, 0.0386, 0.0320,    {41..45}
    0.0207, 0.0020, 0.0003, 0.0001, 0.0000,    {46..50}
    0.0000, 0.0000, 0.0000, 0.0000, 0.0000,    {51..55}
    0.0000, 0.0000, 0.0000, 0.0000, 0.0000,    {56..60}
    0.0000, 0.0000, 0.0000, 0.0000, 0.0000);   {61..65}
var
  age : integer;
```

```
begin {init_birthrate}
  for age := start_age to stop_age do
      birthrate[age] := stone_age * Taiwan_birthrate[age];
end; {init_birthrate}

procedure make_table;
begin {make_table}
  init_birthrate;
  survival[start_age] := start_survival;
  mortality[start_age] := Taiwan_mortality / stone_age;
  repr_value[start_age] := 1.0; { expected number of future daughters per }
  girls[start_age] := 0.0;                        { half woman at age 15 }
  girl_sum[start_age] := 0.0;
  age := start_age;
  repeat
    age := age+1;
    repr_value[age] := { approximately }
      (repr_value[age-1]) - cost * survival[age-1] * birthrate[age-1];
    if mortality[age-1] > 5.0
    then survival[age] := 0.0
    else survival[age] := survival[age-1] * exp( -mortality[age-1] );
    if survival[age] > 0.0
    then mortality[age] :=
              (mortality[age-1] * survival[age-1] * repr_value[age-1]) /
                              (survival[age] * repr_value[age])
    else mortality[age] := 1.0;
    girls[age] := survival[age-1] * birthrate[age-1];
    girl_sum[age] := girl_sum[age-1] + girls[age];
    last_age := age;
  until (age = stop_age ) or (survival[age] <= 0.0) or
        (repr_value[age] <= 0.0);
end; {make_table}

procedure write_table;
begin {write_table}
  clrscr;
  writeln('cost = ', cost:6:4, ', stone_age = ', stone_age:6:4 );
  writeln(' X      l(x)     mu(x)     V(x)      b(x)      g(x)     G(x)');
  if diskout then begin
      writeln(diskfile,'cost = ', cost:6:4, ', stone_age = ', stone_age:6:4 );
      writeln(diskfile,' X      l(x)     mu(x)     V(x)      b(x)      g(x)     G(x)');
  end;
  for age := start_age to last_age do begin
      writeln( age:2, '   ', survival[age]:6:4,
          '  ', mortality[age]:6:4,
          '  ', repr_value[age]:6:4, '  ',
          '  ', birthrate[age]:6:4, '  ', girls[age]:6:4,
          '  ', girl_sum[age]:6:4);
      if diskout then writeln( diskfile, age:2, '   ', survival[age]:6:4,
          '  ', mortality[age]:6:4,
          '  ', repr_value[age]:6:4, '  ',
          '  ', birthrate[age]:6:4, '  ', girls[age]:6:4,
          '  ', girl_sum[age]:6:4);
      if (age - start_age + 1) mod 20 = 0 then begin
          gotoxy( 20, 24 );
          write('Press any key to continue');
          repeat until keypressed;
          window(1,3,80,25); clrscr;
          window(1,1,80,25); gotoxy(1,3);
      end;
  end;
```

```
       if last_age < stop_age then begin
           writeln( 'Simulation terminated at age ',last_age:2,
                   ' because survival or repr. value reached 0.');
           if diskout then writeln( diskfile,
                   'Simulation terminated at age ',last_age:2,
                   ' because survival or repr. value reached 0.');
       end;
   end; {write_table}

   begin {main}
     diskopen := false;
     assign(diskfile,'die.out');
     repeat
       clrscr;
       write('Enter a value for "cost": ');
       readln(cost);
       write('Enter a value for "stone_age": ');
       readln(stone_age);
       write('Log this run to disk? [y/n]:');
       read(kbd,yesno);
       diskout := (yesno = 'Y') or (yesno = 'y');
       if diskout and not diskopen then begin
           rewrite(diskfile);
           diskopen := true;
       end;
       make_table;
       write_able;
       write('Do another run? [y/n]:');
       read(kbd,yesno);
     until (yesno <> 'Y') and (yesno <> 'y');
     close(diskfile);
   end. {main}
```

SAMPLE OUTPUT [X is age in years, l(x) survivorship, mu(x) mortality rate, g(x) fertility (births of daughters) and G(x) cumulative daughters.] The output is for cost = 0.666 and stone age = 0.761.

X	l(x)	mu(x)	V(x)	b(x)	g(x)	G(x)
15	0.5000	0.0131	1.0000	0.0027	0.0000	0.0000
16	0.4935	0.0133	0.9991	0.0091	0.0014	0.0014
17	0.4869	0.0135	0.9961	0.0198	0.0045	0.0059
18	0.4804	0.0138	0.9897	0.0342	0.0096	0.0155
19	0.4738	0.0142	0.9787	0.0533	0.0165	0.0320
20	0.4671	0.0146	0.9619	0.0723	0.0252	0.0572
21	0.4603	0.0152	0.9394	0.0890	0.0338	0.0910
22	0.4534	0.0159	0.9121	0.0991	0.0410	0.1320
23	0.4463	0.0167	0.8822	0.1248	0.0449	0.1769
24	0.4389	0.0177	0.8451	0.1309	0.0557	0.2326
25	0.4312	0.0189	0.8068	0.1319	0.0574	0.2900
26	0.4231	0.0202	0.7690	0.1319	0.0569	0.3469
27	0.4146	0.0217	0.7318	0.1319	0.0558	0.4027
28	0.4058	0.0233	0.6954	0.1271	0.0547	0.4574
29	0.3964	0.0251	0.6610	0.1241	0.0516	0.5089
30	0.3866	0.0270	0.6283	0.1218	0.0492	0.5581
31	0.3763	0.0293	0.5969	0.1195	0.0471	0.6052
32	0.3654	0.0317	0.5670	0.1181	0.0450	0.6502
33	0.3540	0.0345	0.5382	0.1153	0.0432	0.6933
34	0.3420	0.0376	0.5111	0.1137	0.0408	0.7342

X	l(x)	mu(x)	V(x)	b(x)	g(x)	G(x)
35	0.3294	0.0411	0.4852	0.1081	0.0389	0.7730
36	0.3162	0.0450	0.4614	0.1049	0.0356	0.8086
37	0.3022	0.0495	0.4394	0.1005	0.0332	0.8418
38	0.2876	0.0545	0.4191	0.0982	0.0304	0.8721
39	0.2724	0.0603	0.4003	0.0951	0.0282	0.9004
40	0.2565	0.0669	0.3831	0.0837	0.0259	0.9263
41	0.2399	0.0743	0.3688	0.0708	0.0215	0.9478
42	0.2227	0.0825	0.3575	0.0609	0.0170	0.9647
43	0.2051	0.0920	0.3485	0.0457	0.0136	0.9783
44	0.1870	0.1026	0.3422	0.0294	0.0094	0.9877
45	0.1688	0.1150	0.3386	0.0244	0.0055	0.9932
46	0.1505	0.1300	0.3358	0.0158	0.0041	0.9973
47	0.1321	0.1488	0.3342	0.0015	0.0024	0.9996
48	0.1138	0.1727	0.3341	0.0002	0.0002	0.9998
49	0.0958	0.2053	0.3341	0.0001	0.0000	0.9999
50	0.0780	0.2521	0.3341	0.0000	0.0000	0.9999
51	0.0606	0.3244	0.3341	0.0000	0.0000	0.9999
52	0.0438	0.4487	0.3341	0.0000	0.0000	0.9999
53	0.0280	0.7028	0.3341	0.0000	0.0000	0.9999
54	0.0139	1.4191	0.3341	0.0000	0.0000	0.9999
55	0.0034	5.8659	0.3341	0.0000	0.0000	0.9999
56	0.0000	1.0000	0.3341	0.0000	0.0000	0.9999

Simulation terminated at age 56 because survival or repr. value reached 0.

THE RELATIONSHIP OF BODY WEIGHT TO LONGEVITY WITHIN LABORATORY RODENT SPECIES

Donald K. Ingram and Mark A. Reynolds

Molecular Physiology and Genetics Section,
Laboratory of Cellular and Molecular Biology
Gerontology Research Center, National Institute on
Aging, Francis Scott Key Medical Center, Baltimore,
MD 21224

INTRODUCTION

The positive correlation of body weight (BW) to lifespan (LS) across mammalian species is well-established (Economos, 1980b; Sacher, 1959). Increases in species-representative BW are paralleled by increases in LS. According to an analysis by Economos (1980b), the correlation coefficient of log BW vs. log LS within the mammalian class as a whole is high (r = 0.79). This relation appears to hold within all mammalian orders. Within the order Rodentia, the correlation coefficient of log BW vs. log LS is even higher (r = 0.86).

In contrast to the observed positive correlation between BW and LS across mammalian species, relatively higher BW within species is thought to be associated with decreased LS. This view has long been supported by epidemiological and actuarial studies of human populations which report increased mortality associated with excess BW and obesity (Stunkard, 1983). As an example, in a study of 750,000 men and women, Lew and Garfinkel (1979) observed that mortality was about 50% higher among men and women 30-40% heavier than average. Of greater interest was their observation that the lowest mortality was experienced by those of average weight and those 10-20% below average weight. The relationship implied by these data is that relatively lower BW is associated with increased longevity within the human species.

Experimental support for the implied inverse relation between BW and LS is derived from studies of dietary restriction (DR) in laboratory rodents (Stunkard, 1983). Numerous studies have demonstrated that when the caloric content of the diet is reduced through various regimens, BW is reduced and LS is increased relative to the experience of ad libitum (AL) fed counterparts (Barrows and Kokkonen, 1977). Early studies focused on retarded development as the mechanism for the increased LS imparted by DR (McCay, 1935; McCay et al., 1939). Subsequent studies have deemphasized this hypothesized mechanism by demonstrating that LS could be enhanced in laboratory rodents when DR was imposed in adults apparently beyond the influence of development (McCay et al., 1941; Ross, 1966). Thus, other mechanisms appeared to be involved; however, the reduction of BW through DR remained as a strong correlate of the enhanced longevity associated with these treatments.

Such observations suggest that reduced BW is causally related to increased LS within rodent species. However, this conclusion would be derived primarily from inter-group comparisons. There is a risk of relying upon this type of evidence exclusively. Indeed, lower BW may be a necessary effect resulting from DR; however, reduced BW might not be the sufficient cause of increased LS that is observed with such manipulations. Lower BW may be only coincidental to the enhanced lifespan observed. Therefore, the causal relationship between reduced BW and increased longevity requires additional lines of evidence. What is implied is that if BW is linked to LS, then this postulated inverse relation should be observed when one examines the correlation between BW and LS within groups of rodents on similar diets as well as between groups undergoing various treatments that impact on BW.

Support for the inverse relationship between BW and LS was provided in the extensive studies of Ross and colleagues. Examining subgroups based on BW of rats on AL and restricted diets, Ross and Bras (1965) noted higher tumor incidence among heavier rats compared to lighter counterparts. Examining the relationship between BW and LS among rats on a self-selected diet, Ross, Lustbader, and Bras (1976) noted that significant inverse correlations occurred between the ages of 63 and 406 days with maximum coefficients of -0.46 and -0.45 for 119 and 133 days, respectively. Absolute BW appeared to be a better predictor of subsequent longevity than did measures of relative BW growth or dietary practices. However, one parameter, time to double weight of 250 gm, appeared equivalent in its positive correlation to LS as did the negative correlations for absolute BW at specified ages. No significant correlation was observed for the relationship between LS and maximum BW obtained.

Our predecessor at the Gerontology Research Center, Charles Goodrick, also provided data that appeared to support the view that BW growth should be inversely related to LS within rodent species on the same diet. Examining several strains of inbred mice from normal (Goodrick, 1978) and obese genotypes (Goodrick, 1977), he reported negative correlations between growth rate and LS within several genotype-diet groups. Goodrick (1980) reported similar negative correlations within groups of AL-fed male and female Wistar rats housed in conventional cages as well as in activity-wheel cages.

In a reanalysis of this latter study, Ingram, Reynolds, and Goodrick (1982) concluded that the growth rate parameter (maximum BW/age at maximum BW) that Goodrick had applied in his earlier studies lacked construct validity as a measure of BW growth. In fact, the reanalysis revealed no evidence of inverse correlations between LS and several conventional measures of growth rate. Instead, positive correlations between LS and growth rate were observed at ages beyond 9 months, i.e. mature rats adding weight at higher rates tended to live longer.

This alternative perspective did not conflict with other data from Goodrick's earlier studies. Goodrick (1977, 1978, 1980) had noted that maximum BW tended to be positively correlated with LS within many of the genotypes that he analyzed. The positive correlation between BW and LS in adult male Wistar rats had been reported much earlier by Everitt and Webb (1957). However, all these observations applied to rodents on AL diets and would appear to conflict with the consistent finding that DR

and, by implication, the accompanying BW loss tend to increase LS in
laboratory rodents.

The objective of the current paper is to review data from our
laboratory and others to clarify the correlation between BW and LS
between and within groups of laboratory rodents on various diets. We
have addressed this issue in several previous studies (Goodrick et al.,
1982; Goodrick et al., 1983a; Goodrick et al., 1983b; Ingram, Reynolds,
and Goodrick, 1982; Ingram, Reynolds, and Les, 1982; Ingram and
Reynolds, 1983; Reynolds and Ingram, 1984); however, the present
opportunity will permit a summary of past findings and provide a forum
for the formulation of hypotheses to address the observations. Based
upon his extensive review of the rodent research on nutrition and aging
with particular reference to studies of DR, Stunkard (1983; p. 217)
offered the following conclusion: "Almost without exception, leanness
fosters survival and there is little evidence of any favorable effects
of overweight and obesity." From our perspective as argued earlier
(Reynolds and Ingram, 1984), the relationship between BW and longevity
within rodent species is too complex to permit such a generalization.

Thus, the hypothesis to be examined is whether there exists an
inverse correlation between BW and LS within laboratory rodent species.
We will analyze several types of data that should support the following
predictions if the inverse correlation exists:

1. Inter-group comparisons:

    (a) Manipulations which reduce BW should increase LS.

    (b) Within a certain range, the increase in LS should be
         proportional to the reduction in BW.

    (c) Manipulations which increase BW should decrease LS.

    (d) Manipulations which do not affect BW should not affect LS.

2. Intra-group comparisons:

    Within a group under similar environmental/nutritional
    conditions, BW should be inversely correlated with LS.

3. Inter-strain comparisons:

    Within a species, the mean BW of specific genotypes should be
    inversely correlated with mean LS for the strains.

METHODS

Unless otherwise stated, data on rats from our laboratory will refer
to an outbred strain of male Wistar rats bred and reared in a colony
maintained by the Gerontology Research Center (Baltimore, MD). Rats
were obtained at various ages specific to the experiment and housed in a
separate vivarium dedicated to specific studies. They were housed in
pairs in standard metal suspended rat cages (Wahmann) or in
activity-wheel cages (Wahmann) which contain an outer stationary cage
and an activity wheel which is accessed through a door (see Goodrick,
1980, for additional details).

Unless otherwise stated, data on mice from our laboratory will refer to male mice from several inbred strains. Two parental strains, A/J and C57BL/6J, were used along with their F_1 hybrid, B6AF$_1$. In addition, two obese mutants on the C57BL/6J background were studied, ob/ob and A^y/a. All mice were obtained at weaning from the Jackson Laboratory (Bar Harbor, ME). Unless otherwise noted, the mice were housed in pairs in standard metal suspended mouse cages (Wahmann) and located in a separate vivarium dedicated to the experiment.

After placement in our vivaria, all animals described above were fed a NIH-07 formula diet (24% protein; 4.2 Kcal/gm). Control diets consisted of AL access to this diet placed in stainless hoppers in the cage. DR was imposed in one of two ways. Most experiments involved a comparison between the AL condition and a schedule of intermittent feeding which provided AL access to the diet every-other-day (EOD). The EOD procedure involved removing the food hoppers from the cages about 9:00-10:00 a.m. and returning them about 24 hours later. The only other regimen involved restriction (RES) in which the experimental group received daily about 50% of the amount eaten by the AL group as monitored periodically throughout the LS. These mice were housed singly and fed daily in the morning. AL access to water was provided to all animals through an automated and filtered system.

All vivaria were maintained at 22±1° C and 60-70% relative humidity. The light cycle was controlled automatically with lights on at 6:00 a.m. EST and off at 6:00 p.m. EST. The cage racks contained excrement pans filled with wood shavings that were changed three times weekly. Fresh cages and racks were provided monthly. Animals were maintained under the specified conditions until death when they were removed from the cages during daily inspections. No attempt to identify pathology was made.

Unless otherwise stated, BW measurements were obtained weekly from all groups. For DR groups, these measurements were taken on the day after feeding. For statistical analysis, LS representative estimates of BW were computed as a function of survival quartiles. Specifically, each animal's LS was divided into quartiles in order to derive BW estimates. This procedure was used to provide relative comparisons of a large number of groups representing different genotypes, ages, and treatments along an equivalent LS scale. Data on BW at specific ages (e.g., 6 and 12 months) are also provided for several analyses to compare with the analyses based on relative BW.

RESULTS

Inter-Group Comparisons of Body Weight and Lifespan

Rats; Lifespan

As observed in Table 1, the EOD regimen consistently resulted in significant increases in mean LS in male Wistar rats when compared to AL controls (Goodrick et al., 1982, 1983a, 1983b). This effect occurred when the regimen was begun at several different ages and when the animals were housed in conventional cages or in activity-wheel cages. Within groups housed in standard cages, the effect of EOD feeding on mean LS decreased as a function of age of initiation but was still effective as late as 18 months which was clearly beyond developmental influences. Within groups housed in activity-wheel cages, the age-related decrease in the effectiveness of the EOD feeding was not readily apparent. When examining the 10.5- and 18.0-month groups, the effect is apparent and similar in magnitude to that observed in the groups housed in standard cages. The relatively smaller effect of the EOD diet on mean LS when initiated at 1.5 months in activity-wheel cages reflects the beneficial singular effect of the exercise regimen on AL-fed groups. Voluntary exercise was not associated with increased LS among any diet group when begun at later ages (Goodrick et al., 1983a).

Table 1

Effect of Every-Other-Day Feeding on
Mean Lifespan in Male Wistar Rats

Housing Condition	Age of Initiation (mo)	Percent Increase in Mean Lifespan over Ad Libitum Controls
Conventional	1.5	82% *
	10.5	34% *
	18.0	11% *
Activity Wheel	1.5	21% *
	10.5	38% *
	18.0	17% *

* $p < 0.05$ compared to controls.

Rats; Body Weight

Figure 1 presents comparisons of BW loss (relative to AL groups) across LS quartiles of the various experimental groups. Data were not available for groups housed in activity-wheel cages at 1.5 months. Among those housed in standard cages, the inter-group comparisons of BW loss across the different ages of initiation parallel the LS effects. Specifically, these data support the hypothesis that the greater the BW loss, the greater the observed increase in LS.

Among the groups housed in activity-wheel cages, this relationship was not supported. While a marked difference was observed in the LS effect of the EOD regimen when begun at 10.5 and 18 months of age, no difference in the magnitude of BW loss was evident between these groups housed in activity-wheel cages. Furthermore, although there was a markedly greater relative BW loss among non-exercised, conventionally-housed 10.5-month old rats compared to exercised rats, the relative magnitude of the LS effect was similar--34% vs. 38%, respectively (Table 1).

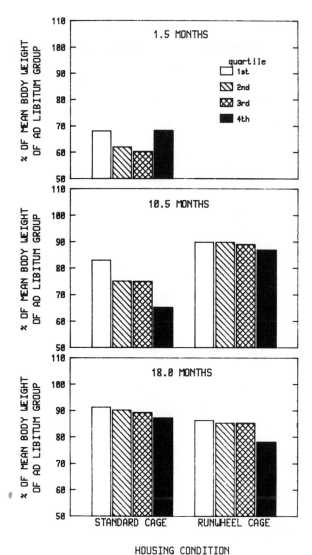

Figure 1.   Effect of every-other-day feeding on mean body weight at survival quartiles in male Wistar rats followed from three ages.

Mice; Lifespan

As observed in Table 2, the EOD regimen was also effective in increasing mean LS beyond that observed in AL groups in several mouse genotypes begun at several ages. The magnitude of the effect varied across genotypes and was again dependent upon age of initiation. When begun at 1.5 months, the EOD regimen increased mean LS in all three genotypes. The largest effect appeared among C57BL/6J mice, and the smallest effect appeared among A/J mice. Comparing groups begun on the EOD regimen at 6 months, the largest effect appeared among the B6AF$_1$ mice with no significant effect observed among A/J mice. When begun at 10 months, no significant increases in mean LS were observed among

C57BL/6J and B6AF$_1$ genotypes on the EOD regimen. In contrast, the EOD regimen decreased mean LS among A/J mice begun at this age.

Mice; Body Weight

The effect of EOD feeding on relative BW loss varied with genotype and age of initiation (Figure 2). Within the C57BL/6J genotype, the effect was fairly uniform across ages with about a 5-15% reduction in BW relative to AL-fed groups across their LS. This uniform effect on BW was not consistent with the differential effect on LS which diminished as a function of age of initiation. Thus, a 10-15% BW reduction in the 10-month old group was not associated with an increase in mean LS.

Of the three genotypes, the EOD regimen impacted on BW to the greatest relative degree among B6AF$_1$ mice. The relative BW loss was about 20-25% across the LS in all three age groups. Similar to that observed in C57BL/6J mice, there was a significant BW loss when EOD was begun at 10 months of age, but there was no significant impact on mean LS. Furthermore, in contrast to the relatively modest BW loss of C57BL/6J mice when EOD was begun at 1.5 months, the BW loss in the hybrid mice was about 10% greater but was not associated with a greater effect on LS (Table 2).

Among A/J mice, the EOD regimen had considerably less effect on BW than among the other two genotypes. In fact, when begun at 1.5 months of age, there was little effect on BW, although the regimen was associated with a significant effect on mean LS, albeit to a lessor extent than in the other two genotypes. At 6 months of age, the EOD treatment appeared to reduce BW but did not significantly affect mean LS. Finally, at 10 months of age, DR of this type impacted negatively upon survival of this genotype, yet appeared to have little effect on BW.

Table 2

Effect of Every-Other-Day Feeding on Mean Lifespan
in Three Male Mouse Genotypes

Genotype	Age of Initiation (mo)	Percent Increase in Mean Lifespan over Ad Libitum Controls
C57BL/6J	1.5	27% *
	6.0	10% *
	10.0	0%
B6AF$_1$	1.5	20% *
	6.0	19% *
	10.0	0%
A/J	1.5	12% *
	6.0	2%
	10.0	-14% *

*$p < 0.05$ compared to controls.

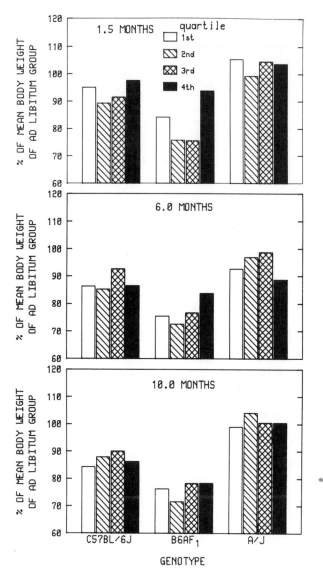

Figure 2.   Effect of every-other-day feeding on mean body weight at
survival quartiles in male mice of three genotypes followed
from three ages.

Obese Mice; Lifespan

In a separate study which applied two DR regimens to C57BL/6J mice
and two obese genotypes (ob/ob and Aʸ/a) on this genetic background, EOD
and RES· (50% below AL levels) feeding both resulted in increased mean LS
compared to AL groups as observed in Table 3.   In the normal genotype
the EOD regimen appeared more effective in increasing mean LS compared
to the RES regimen.   Among ob/ob mice, the more severe diet in the RES
group appeared more effective than the EOD diet for increasing LS.   Aʸ/a
mice were provided only the EOD regimen, which was still clearly more
effective in increasing mean LS than in the heavier ob/ob mice.

Table 3

Effect of Every-Other-Day Feeding (EOD) and Diet Restriction
(RES = 50% of Ad libitum Level) on Mean Lifespan
in Male C57BL/6J Mice and Two Obese Mutants

Genotype	Diet	Percent Increase in Mean Lifespan over Ad Libitum Controls
Normal (+/+)	EOD	56% *
	RES	36% *
Obese (ob/ob)	EOD	26% *
	RES	89% *
Obese (A^y/a)	EOD	79% *

* $p < 0.05$ compared to controls.

Obese Mice; Body Weight

As indicated in Figure 3, the data on relative BW loss among obese
genotypes generally supported the hypothesis that BW loss should be
directly related to increases in LS. Consistent with the hypothesis, the
RES regimen, which had the greatest impact on BW loss among ob/ob mice
(40%) compared to the EOD treatment (10%), also had the greatest impact
on increased LS. The EOD regimen had a greater effect on LS among A^y/a
mice than among similarly fed ob/ob mice which was also consistent with
the greater relative body loss (35%) observed among the former genotype.

Among normal C57BL/6J mice, the data relating inter-group comparisons
of BW and LS effects were inconsistent with the observations among the
obese genotypes and did not support the hypothesis. The RES regimen,
resulted in a greater relative BW loss (20-40%) compared to the EOD
regimen (5-10%), begun near weaning. However, the degree of BW loss was
opposite to the effect on LS.

Summary

Based upon this inter-group analysis of data from our laboratory, it
is evident that various regimens of DR can increase mean LS in a wide
range of genotypes when housed under different conditions and initiated
at different ages, several of which are apparently beyond developmental
influences. In many cases it is also clear that various regimens of DR
result in BW loss, but the presence and magnitude of this effect is
greatly dependent upon genotype and age of initiation. In many cases it
is also apparent that the observed degree of BW loss parallels the increase in LS. However, there are several exceptions, indeed contradictions, to the prediction that BW loss should be directly proportional
to the degree of LS extension resulting from DR within and across
different genotypes. BW loss does not appear to be a necessary nor
sufficient condition for the increased LS associated with DR in rodents.
Additional contradictions to this hypothesis are presented in the
correlational analyses which follow.

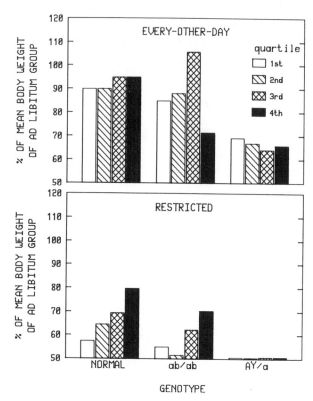

Figure 3. Effect of every-other-day and restricted (50% of control
level) feeding on mean body weight at survival quartiles in
male C57BL/6J mice and two obese mutants begun at 2.0 months
of age.

Intra-Group Correlations between Body Weight and Lifespan

Rats

Figure 4 depicts the relationship between LS and BW across survival
quartiles for male Wistar rats on both AL and EOD regimens begun at 1.5,
10.5, and 18 months of age. The analysis for animals housed in both
standard cages and activity-wheel cages have been combined; thus, the
coefficients represent partial correlations which control for any
influence of the housing condition on the relationship between BW and
LS.

Among AL groups, the only significant negative correlation between
BW and LS was observed during the first quartile for animals followed
since 1.5 months of age. This observation contrasted with the clear
pattern of positive correlations between BW and LS at virtually all
survival quartiles in all other age groups. Heavier animals, as
assessed across the LS, tended to live longer; however, the coefficients
were of low to moderate magnitudes (0.25 - 0.50).

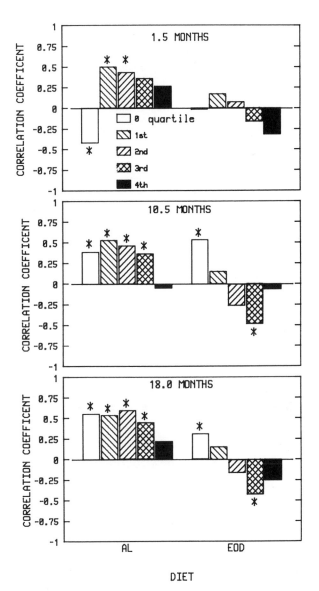

Figure 4. Pearson correlations (partial, controlling for housing
condition) between lifespan and body weight at different
survival quartiles in male Wistar rats on ad libitum (AL)
and every-other-day (EOD) feeding begun at different ages.
* $p < 0.05$

The one negative correlation deserves additional comment. Since it represents the very first estimate of BW obtained, it is the only developmental parameter presented here. Apparently a developmental pattern that moved animals from a relatively lighter BW near weaning to a relatively heavier BW during the adult period was the most beneficial to survival. This pattern might be further elucidated when the length of the BW growth period is examined in relation to LS in a later section of this paper.

Among EOD groups, the pattern of correlation between LS and BW was decidedly different to that observed among AL groups. Among animals followed since weaning, no significant correlations were observed, but there appeared to be a trend toward positive correlations early in life changing to negative correlations later in life. This pattern of low magnitude correlations would hardly be worth mentioning if it were not for the fact that it appeared to be duplicated in the other two groups in which EOD was initiated much later in life. In the 10.5-month group, initial BW was positively and significantly correlated with survival, but by the third survival quartile, the correlation was significantly negative. This exact pattern was duplicated in the 18-month group. Thus, it appeared that being relatively heavier at the outset of DR was beneficial to survival at these older ages. Also, if the restriction resulted in relatively lower BW by the third quartile, then survival also was benefited. It is noteworthy that BW near death (fourth quartile) was not significantly related to how long a rat lived within any group but was generally negative in direction.

An additional analysis was conducted in which BW at specific ages was correlated to LS. This was done because of a possible statistical confound involving correlation of LS to relative BW during developmental phases. Specifically, a positive correlation between LS and BW at early survival quartiles may be spurious because higher BW estimates for longer-lived individuals might emerge because they had been taken at relatively older ages developmentally, compared to shorter-lived individuals. Thus, we generated correlations between BW and LS at 6 and 12 months of age to assess their correspondence with the correlational analysis based upon relative BWs.

As observed in Table 4, the results of this analysis indicated partial contribution of the method by which the estimates were obtained to the magnitude of the observed correlation but do not refute the primary conclusion, i.e., no evidence was found to support a significant inverse correlation between BW and LS. In fact, no significant correlations were observed for rats. At 6 months of age, the correlations between BW and LS were negative for both AL- and EOD-fed groups. At 12 months, the direction of the correlations had changed to positive, albeit of much lower magnitude than observed in Figure 4. However, the shift from negative to positive correlation is similar to the pattern observed in the analysis involving relative BWs.

Table 4

Pearson Correlations Between Lifespan and Body Weight at Specific Ages
for Several Male Rodent Genotypes on Ad Libitum (AL) and
Every-Other-Day (EOD) Feeding Begun About 1.5-3 Months of Age

Genotype	Age (Mo)	Diet	
		AL	EOD
Wistar	6	-.13	-.16
	12	.12	.09
C57BL/6J	6	-.10	-.12
	12	.53*	.11
B6AF$_1$	6	-.10	-.20
	12	-.21	-.23
A/J	6	.23	-.39*
	12	.18	-.01
C57BL/6J (+/+)	6	.68*	.05
C57BL/6J (ob/ob)	6	-.64*	-.34
C57BL/6J (A^y/a)	6	-.10	-.03

* $p < 0.05$

Mice

Figure 5 presents the zero-order correlations between LS and BW at
individual survival quartiles for C57BL/6J, A/J, and B6AF$_1$ genotypes
that were followed from about 2 months of age. In the C57BL/6J
genotype, the correlations between BW and LS were consistent under both
AL and EOD conditions. While no significant correlations between LS and
initial and terminal (fourth quartile) BW were observed, there were
moderate to high positive correlations between LS and adult BW in this
genotype. This pattern was duplicated among A/J mice on the EOD diet.
Correlations between BW and LS were somewhat less consistent for mice of
this genotype on AL diets, but first and second quartile BWs were still
positively correlated to LS. The pattern of correlation between LS and
BW among the hybrid mice varied from that observed among the parental
strains. First quartile BW was positively correlated to LS within both
AL and EOD groups, but the pattern of correlation became negative in the
third and fourth quartiles.

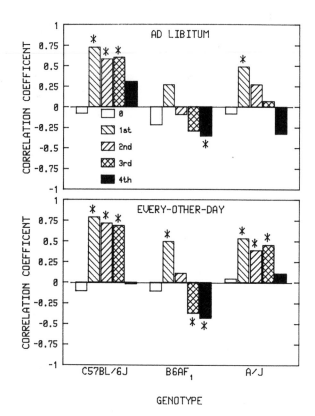

Figure 5. Pearson correlations between lifespan and body weight at different survival quartiles in male mice of three genotypes on ad libitum (AL) and every-other-day (EOD) feeding begun at 1.5 months of age. * $p < 0.05$

As had been analyzed for the rat data, Table 4 presents the correlations between LS and BW at 6 and 12 months of age for each mouse genotype on both diet regimens. The results indicate that the magnitude of some of the correlations might be influenced by the statistical confound mentioned earlier; however, the pattern of results is generally similar to that obtained for the correlational analysis based on relative BWs. For AL-fed C57BL/6J mice, a nonsignificant negative correlation is observed at 6 months of age, but the coefficient is positive and significant at 12 months. For EOD-fed mice of this genotype, the same pattern of change from negative to positive is observed between 6 and 12 months, but the correlations are nonsignificant. For B6AF$_1$ mice on both regimens, the correlational

pattern is clearly negative, but none of the coefficients were significant. For A/J mice on AL diets, the correlations were positive but
nonsignificant. For EOD-fed mice of this genotype, there was a
significant negative correlation between LS and BW at 6 months but no
significant correlation was observed at 12 months. This negative
correlation appeared to be the only major conflict between the results
of this analysis and that depicted in Figure 5.

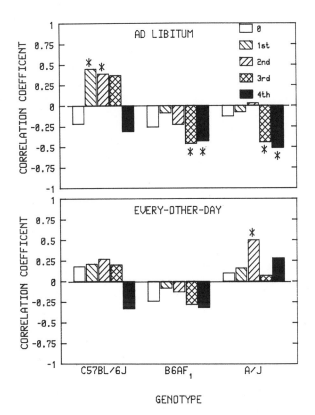

Figure 6.   Pearson correlations between lifespan and body weight at
different survival quartiles in male mice of three genotypes
on ad libitum (AL) and every-other-day (EOD) feeding begun
at 6 months of age. * $p < 0.05$

Figure 6 presents the zero-order correlations between LS and BW at individual survival quartiles for the three genotypes that were followed from 6 months of age. The pattern of correlations for the C57BL/6J mice begun at this age was similar to that observed for mice followed since weaning (Figure 5). For the AL group there were significant positive correlations between LS and BW at the first, second, and third survival quartiles. With the exception of the last quartile, the pattern of correlation for the EOD group was also positive, but none were statistically significant and were of a much lower order of magnitude than observed in Figure 5. The pattern of correlations for A/J mice was also similar to that observed for counterparts in Figure 5. For the EOD group, the pattern remained positive, but the only significant correlation occurred at the second quartile. For the AL group, however, the patterns were generally negative and somewhat unlike that observed in Figure 5. However, the significant negative correlations at the last two quartiles in this group seemed to duplicate the negative trend observed in last quartile of the AL-fed A/J mice begun at weaning. This negative trend was clearly manifested among the hybrid mice begun at this age. Negative correlations between LS and BW were observed at all quartiles in both diet groups but were significant only for the last two quartiles of the AL group. What was not observed here were the positive correlations that were seen in Figure 5 in the first quartile for this genotype.

When the three genotypes were followed from 10 months of age, the pattern of correlations between LS and BW departed still more from that observed at earlier ages. As observed in Figure 7, there were no significant correlations observed among C57BL/6J mice on AL diets; whereas, in the EOD group the pattern remained somewhat positive. Only the second quartile correlation was significant and low in magnitude. Among A/J mice on the EOD diet, the correlational pattern also remained positive with the initial and first quartile estimates showing statistical significance. Within the AL group of this genotype, the pattern appeared negative with a significant correlation observed for the second quartile. Among the EOD groups of B6AF$_1$ mice, no significant correlations were observed. Among the AL-fed hybrid mice, the pattern was definitely negative with significant correlations occurring at the last two quartiles.

Obese Mice

Figure 8 provides the correlations between LS and BW at individual survival quartiles, and Table 4 provides correlations between LS and BW at 6 months for C57BL/6J mice and the two mutant genotypes, ob/ob and A^y/a, that were on different diet regimens since about 2 months of age. For the normal mice on the AL diet, the pattern of correlation in Figure 8 is definitely positive and very similar in magnitude to that observed in Figure 5. The significant positive correlation is confirmed in Table 4 for the data obtained at 6 months. Within the EOD group of this genotype, the pattern appeared positive but was not signficantly positive as was that observed in Figure 5. A nonsignificant correlation is also observed in Table 4 for BW at 6 months. Among the RES group of normal mice, the correlational pattern was definitely positive and duplicated that observed for EOD mice in Figure 5.

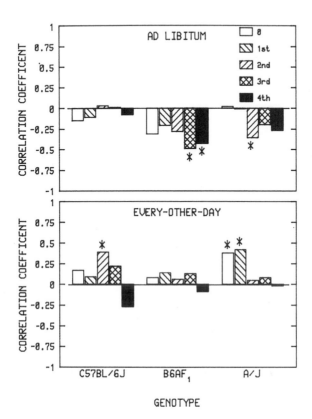

Figure 7.   Pearson correlations between lifespan and body weight at
different survival quartiles in male mice of three genotypes
on ad libitum (AL) and every-other-day (EOD) feeding begun
at 10.0 months of age.   * p < 0.05

Among ob/ob mice on the AL diet, the pattern of correlation between BW and LS was similar to that observed for B6AF$_1$ mice in Figure 5. There appeared to be a movement 'from modest nonsignificant positive correlations during the first quartile to decidedly negative correlations at the last quartiles. If these obese mice tended toward lower BW at later stages of survival, then increased LS appeared more likely. A similar pattern was observed for the A^y/a mutant on the AL diet. A low BW near death was associated with increased LS. In the other diet groups, no significant correlations were observed between LS and BW among both mutant genotypes. The pattern of correlations involving relative ages is also observed in Table 4 when BW at 6 months was analyzed. Among ob/ob mice on both diets, the correlations were negative but of higher magnitude than in the AL group. At 6 months among A^y/a mice, the correlations were low and nonsignificant in both diet groups.

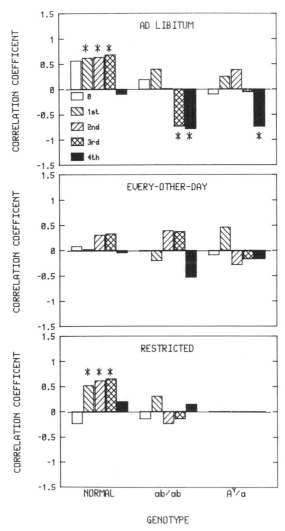

Figure 8.   Pearson correlations between lifespan and body weight at different survival quartiles in male C57BL/6J mice and two obese mutants on ad libitum, every-other-day, and restricted feeding begun at 2.0 months of age. * p < 0.05

Summary

   The analysis of intra-group correlations between LS and BW at
representative intervals yields no consistent support for the hypothesis
that lower BW is associated with longer LS. Indeed, among male Wistar
rats and C57BL/6J and A/J mice followed since weaning on AL diets, the
data suggested that relatively higher BW across the adult LS was
generally associated with longer life. Even when the diet was
restricted by EOD or RES regimens, this pattern of positive correlations
between LS and BW persisted for the C57BL/6J and A/J strains when
relative ages were analyzed. However, when BW at absolute ages were
correlated with LS, support for the positive relationship between BW and
LS was not as forthcoming. When AL groups were assessed beginning at
later ages (> 10 months), the pattern of positive correlations was very
evident for the Wistar rats--heavier rats tended to liver longer. This
pattern was also evident among AL-fed C57BL/6J mice followed since 6
months, but was lost in the 10-month group in this strain. Among A/J
mice on AL diets, the pattern became somewhat negative when followed at
6 and 10 months of age. However, among both C57BL/6J and A/J mice
placed on EOD diets at 6 and 10 months of age, the pattern clearly
tended toward the positive. The only evidence of an inverse correlation
between LS and BW was observed within groups of Wistar rats on the EOD
regimen, B6AF$_1$ mice on both the AL and EOD diets, 6-month old A/J mice
on the EOD diet, and the two obese mutants ob/ob and A^y/a mice, on AL
diets. For Wistar rats begun at all ages, for the obese mutants, and
for the B6AF$_1$ mice followed since weaning, these negative correlations
occurred toward the last survival quartiles. Moreover, among these
groups, there appeared to be a survival advantage associated with higher
BW during earlier quartiles. Thus, the data suggested that moving from
a relatively higher BW to a relatively lower BW yielded a higher
survival probability in these groups. Only among B6AF$_1$ mice followed at
later ages did the pattern of correlation between LS and BW appear more
consistently negative. Thus, this analysis documents that the direction
and magnitude of the correlations between BW and LS were greatly dependent
upon the genotype, age, and diet examined.

Inter-Strain Correlation of Body Weight and Lifespan

   In another study we examined the correlation between LS and a number
of BW growth parameters across nine inbred and six hybrid mouse
genotypes of both sexes (Ingram, Reynolds, and Les, 1983). For details
of the husbandry, the previous publication should be consulted. All
animals were fed AL (Old guilford 96WA) and were raised at the Jackson
Laboratory (Bar Harbor, ME). Data for individual mice within a cage
(4/cage) were not available; therefore, each cage was treated as an
individual with the data pooled. Thus, for each sex-genotype group,
there were 12 such estimates.

   Figure 9 provides the correlations between LS and BW at 2-3 months
and 12-13 months of age separated into inbred and hybrid groups as well
as by sex. Among male inbred and hybrid genotypes, clear positive
correlations between LS and BW emerged at 12 months of age. Heavier
strains tended to live longer. BW at 1.5 months of age was not
significantly related to LS. If one assumes that the 12-month BW might
be represented in the first and second quartile data among AL mice
depicted in Figure 5, then this pattern of correlations was similar to
that previously observed. In contrast to the positive correlations
between LS and BW for male genotypes, the pattern of correlation for
female genotypes appeared negative; however, none reached statistical
significance.

DISCUSSION

A review of findings from many other laboratories does not provide support for the hypothesized inverse correlation between adult BW and LS within laboratory rodent species as well as other taxonomic orders. This is evident when examining inter- and intra-group as well as inter-strain comparisons of the relationship within the same species.

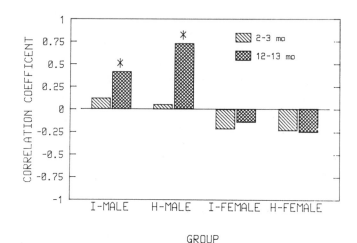

Figure 9.   Pearson correlations between lifespan and body weight at 2-3 and 12.0 months of age across nine inbred (I) and six hybrid (H) strains of male and female mice.   * $p < 0.05$

Inter-Group Comparisons of Body Weight and Lifespan

The early research of McCay and colleagues emphasized the retardation of growth as the principal mechanism by which DR promoted longevity (McCay, 1935; McCay et al., 1939). However, in their study of adult rats, it was clear that DR was still effective in increasing mean LS even when initiated beyond early developmental influences (McCay et al., 1941; Ingram and Reynolds, 1983). Furthermore, the relationship between BW and longevity was not entirely consistent with LS effects. One manipulation in this study involved reduction of dietary protein from a normal level of 20% to 8%. This reduced amount was associated with reduced BW but was not associated with a significant increase in LS (Ingram and Reynolds, 1983). Another manipulation in the McCay et al. (1939) study was daily forced exercise which appeared to increase BW in several groups but had no significant effect on LS (Ingram and Reynolds, 1983).

A marked refutation of the hypothesis was provided in the findings of Stuchlikova et al. (1976), who studied DR in rats, mice, and hamsters. The longest-lived in each species were groups that were restricted to 12 months of age and then fed AL. These groups had better survival than counterparts restricted throughout life or from 12 months of age, both of which in turn lived longer than groups fed AL throughout life. However, the longest-lived group, those under DR only during early life, were the heaviest after 12 months of age compared to all others. Nolen (1972), who studied male and female Simonsen rats, and Beauchene et al. (1986), who studied male Wistar rats, did not replicate this finding with respect to which group was the longest-lived. In the Nolen study, the group restricted throughout life lived longer than a group restricted for the first 3 months of life and then fed AL, which in turn did not differ significantly in survival to that of a group fed AL throughout life. However, the lack of significant LS differences between the latter two groups is important to note because the groups restricted early in life were lighter than AL-fed counterparts. In the Beauchene et al. study, again the group restricted throughout life experienced better survival compared to a group restricted to 12 months and fed AL thereafter and to a group fed AL to 12 months and restricted thereafter. While both of the latter groups had increased LS over that observed in a group fed AL throughout life, they did not differ significantly in survival experience. This lack of a LS effect was observed in spite of the fact that the group fed AL beyond 12 months experienced the heaviest maximum weight of all groups, a finding which matched the observations of BW in the Stuchlikova et al. study.

Other inconsistencies in the literature have also appeared which relate LS effects to manipulations that affect BW. For example, Wyndam, Everitt, and Everitt (1983) observed that AL-fed male Wistar rats reared in isolation generally weighed more than group-housed rats on AL diets, but there was no significant difference in survival. Drori and Folman (1976) reported that DR reduced BW and increased survival in male rats; however, an exercise regimen also improved survival but had no significant effect on BW. Yu et al. (1985) fed a diet composed of 12.6% protein to male F-344 rats and noted improved survival compared to a group fed 21% protein. This LS effect occurred in spite of the lack of a treatment effect on BW. In summary, findings from many studies further illustrate that reduced BW is neither sufficient nor necessary for increased LS in laboratory rodents resulting from a treatment, even DR.

Inter-Strain Comparisons of Body Weight and Lifespan

Other studies conducting inter-strain comparisons also do not consistently support the hypothesis of an inverse correlation between adult BW and LS within rodent species. Sacher and Duffy (1979) examined correlations between log LS and log BW at 6-8 months and 24-30 months among 21 strains of male inbred and hybrid mice. The respective correlations were 0.47 and 0.69. These positive correlations were also sustained when examined within strain (r = 0.40 and r = 0.46 for the young and aged BW measures, respectively). These relationships might be contaminated, however, because hybrid strains tend to be heavier and live longer than inbred strains. When we calculated the correlations between BW and LS among parental and hybrid strains separately for these data, the positive relationships held. For parental strains the correlation coefficients between LS and BW at 6-8 months and 24-30 months were 0.86 and 0.62, respectively. For hybrid strains the respective correlation coefficients were 0.34 and 0.45.

These findings were not replicated in Storer's (1967) inter-strain study. He observed nonsignificant negative correlations between LS and BW at 120 days of age among 18 inbred mouse strains of both sexes. Perhaps the early age of observation was the principal reason for this failure to replicate. As a further example of this possibility, Nash and Kidwell (1973) examined correlations between LS and BW at 26 and 60 days of age among 9 strains of inbred male and female mice and found nonsignificant positive correlations. We also did not observe significant correlations between BW and LS at 2-3 months of age in the inbred and hybrid strains examined (Ingram, Reynolds, Les, 1982). Significant correlations emerged at 12 months of age. Thus, it appears that early life BW is not as reliably correlated with LS as are measures at later ages (midlife and beyond).

Harrison, Archer, and Astle (1984) compared body weights and longevities between normal female C57BL/6J mice and a single-gene mutation that results in extreme obesity (ob/ob). Their results argue strongly against the importance of body weight and adiposity in determining lifespan. When fed AL, the obese mutant experienced drastically reduced lifespan compared to AL normal mice of the same strain. Longevity could be extended by 50% when the obese mice underwent DR from weaning. These observations support the hypothesis. However, the body weights of obese DR mice remained above those of AL-fed normal mice, yet the mutant mice had higher mean and maximum lifespans compared to normal AL-fed mice. Moreover, the degree of adiposity was much higher among restricted obese mice (fat composed about half their body weights) compared to normal AL-fed mice. Thus, these data also fail to demonstrate a clear-cut correspondence between body weight loss and increased lifespan when different rodent genotypes are compared.

Intra-Group Correlations Between Body Weight and Lifespan

Analysis of intra-group correlations by other investigators also have not found the hypothesized negative relationship between adult BW and LS. Indeed, as we observed under many experimental conditions, the most frequent significant correlation was positive in direction. In general, however, the existence and direction of significant correlation between BW and LS was dependent upon age, treatment, and genotype.

McCay et al. (1952) reported a significant positive correlation between LS and maximum BW among AL-fed rats from the Yale strain. Among AL-fed male Wistar rats, Everitt and Webb (1957) noted a significant positive correlation between LS and BW at 400 days and maximum BW. BW at other ages was not signficantly correlated with LS. Similarly, Beauchene et al. (1986) observed a significant positive correlation between LS and maximum BW among AL-fed male Wistar rats. The correlations between BW and longevity among DR rats in this study were negative but not statistically significant, which is consistent with our observations among EOD-fed rats of this strain. Goodrick (1980) also reported significant positive correlations between LS and maximum BW in AL-fed male Wistar rats housed in conventional cages. Comparable correlations in female rats of the same strain were low and nonsignificant. However, correlations between LS and BW from 3-12 months in these female rats were frequently negative in direction.

Examining the data on AL- and RES-fed male F-344 rats of Bertrand et al. (1980), we noted a positive correlation between longevity and body weights taken between 50-80% of the LS [$\underline{r}$ (12) = 0.26, p > 0.05 for AL and $\underline{r}$ (14) = 0.71, $\underline{p}$ < 0.01, for restricted]. Between 84-97% of the LS, this correlation remained positive for the AL group [$\underline{r}$ (11) = 0.20, $\underline{p}$ > 0.05] but became negative for the RES group [$\underline{r}$ (10) = - 0.57, $\underline{p}$ < 0.06]. This latter observation appeared similar to what we observed in EOD-fed Wistar rats; i.e., positive correlations in midlife converting to negative correlations late in life. When these investigators correlated maximum fat content with longevity among both diet groups, the correlations were positive and significant among RES animals but were not significant within the AL group (Masoro, 1984).

Weindruch et al. (1986) provided correlations between LS and BW at weaning, 5, 10, 15, and 22 months of age within groups of female C3B10RF$_1$ mice on AL diets and several DR regimens. The only significant correlations to emerge were positive in direction, all of which occurred beyond 5 months of age with at least one occurring at 22 months. Goodrick (1974) reported positive correlations (albeit low and nonsignificant) between LS and BW among 23-month old male and female B6AF$_2$ mice housed in conventional cages and in activity-wheel cages. In contrast, when Duffy and Sacher (1976) examined the correlations between LS and BW beyond 22 months of age within wild-type mice of two species, Mus musculus and Peromyscus leucopus, no significant coefficients were found.

In summary, age and dietary treatment are important factors in the association of BW with longevity. It is important, nonetheless, to note that no study demonstrated consistent negative correlations between LS and adult BW within AL-fed groups. As we had observed, the most prevalent significant correlation between BW and LS appeared to be positive in direction within male rodent species.

Observations from Insect Studies

Findings from studies of insect species also offer no consistent support for the hypothesized inverse correlation between adult BW and longevity. Osanai (1978) observed BW and LS within different species of silkworm moths (Bombyx mori) reared at two different environmental temperatures, 4° and 25° C. The moths raised under the lower temperature were the heaviest and lived longer than those raised under the higher temperature. Within groups, however, there were no significant correlations between LS and BW at emergence, but there were marked negative correlations between LS and BW at death. Soliman and Lints (1975) also observed no significant correlations between longevity and adult BW in flour beetle (<u>Oribolium</u> <u>castaneum</u>). In a later study of the same species, however, Soliman and Lints (1982) observed significant relationships between adult BW and longevity, but the direction was greatly dependent upon strain. In general, within lighter strains, there were significant positive correlations between LS and adult BW. However, within heavier strains negative correlations were observed. In one species of more normal weight, no significant correlations between BW and LS were observed. Thus, it appears that correlations between BW and LS emerge more frequently at the extremes of BW distribution within a species. This curvilinear relationship between BW and LS was further confirmed in <u>Drospholia</u> in a series of studies by Economos and Lints (1984, 1985). Varying environmental temperature and dietary yeast systematically, these investigators concluded that body weight did not appear to be a causative factor in determining lifespan.

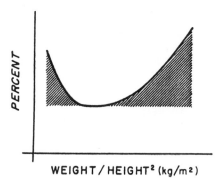

Figure 10. Relationship between body mass and percent mortality in a human population from Waaler (1984).

Relationship Between Body Weight and Lifespan in Humans

Instead of a linear correlation between BW and LS, many investigators of human populations have emphasized the curvilinear nature of the relationship as shown in Figure 10 based on a large Norwegian study (Waaler, 1984). There is abundant evidence that obesity is associated with excess morbidity and mortality. At the same time, extreme leanness is also associated with excess mortality. Large-scale epidemiological studies relying upon insurance company data have been used to construct tables suggesting ideal body weights for men and women of given heights that are associated with the lowest mortality (Build Study, 1979). Andres (1980a, 1980b, 1985) has questioned the validity of this approach which ignores age as a variable. When he examines data from a large number of studies, ideal weight, in terms of the lowest risk of mortality, increases linearly with adult age. The increase has been estimated to be about one pound per year (Andres, 1985).

Two deductions are derived from this perspective. One deduction might be that in late ages, relatively heavier persons face a lower mortality risk than lighter counterparts. One study which followed 44 men aged 65-91 years found that this relationship held (Libow, 1974). The other deduction is that gaining weight with age might reduce mortality risk. This relationship has also been supported in at least one study (Avons et al., 1983). Based on several reviews of the literature, Andres concludes that little evidence exists to support an inverse relationship between adult BW and mortality risk. Indeed, it appears that weight gain with adult age might actually decrease mortality risk.

Alternative Hypotheses

Although it can be concluded that past results offer no consistent evidence for an inverse correlation between BW and LS within a wide range of different species, the task of considering alternative hypotheses remains. What factors should be considered when attempting to provide meaning to the complexity of the relationship between LS and adult BW?

Mathematical Factors

The failure to find significant correlations in either direction within groups of rodents undergoing similar dietary treatment should be addressed. Correlational analysis is sensitive to range. Therefore, the magnitude of any existing correlation will be restricted. This might be the case when comparing the pattern of correlations between AL-fed animals and counterparts on various DR regimens. One might expect greater variability among the former and thus the greater opportunity for observing correlations. Although we did not analyze this factor systematically in our data, it should be noted that significant correlations between BW and LS were frequently observed within EOD and RES groups.

Another mathematical factor that should be considered is the reliance upon examining linear relationships only. This approach ignores the possibility of curvilinear relationships of the type observed in the human studies (Figure 10). We address this possibility in a later section.

Social Factors

Rather than BW being directly correlated with LS, it is possible that social factors confounded this relationship indirectly. Specifically, one could hypothesize that heavier rats tended to be more dominant within social groups, and that endocrinological factors associated with this form of social behavior affected the relationship with longevity more so than factors associated with BW. This criticism would hold for animals housed in groups, specifically to all of our studies of Wistar rats and all mouse studies involving EOD feeding. However, in studies in which the RES diet was employed, the mice were singly housed. This is also the case in the rat studies of Bertrand et al. (1980); Masoro, 1984; Yu et al., 1985; and the mouse studies of Weindruch et al. (1986). Therefore, significant correlations between BW and LS in these studies would not involve these hypothesized social factors.

Disease Factors

Senescent BW loss that is manifested sometime beyond 12 months of age in laboratory rodents has been associated with the incidence and progression of chronic disease (Berg and Simms, 1962; Everitt 1955). However, the precise linkage of this phenomenon to specific disease processes has not been well-established, and the validity of the relationship for all rodent species has been questioned (Duffy and Sacher 1979). Nonetheless, the problem remains that the relationship between BW and LS might be contaminated by the influence of disease particularly in late life. Specifically, one could hypothesize that a positive correlation between BW and LS exists because lighter animals are losing BW due to disease and will die sooner than heavier animals that are not losing weight.

To avoid the possible contamination of disease, we chose to conduct our correlational analysis using survival quartiles instead of only examining specific ages. By using survival quartiles, all individuals are placed on the same scale relative to LS. It should be noted that many of the positive correlations that were observed occurred before the second survival quartile. In fact, negative correlations often occurred late in the LS among RES groups and obese genotypes. Therefore, this hypothesis does not appear to be confirmed.

The question remains that for many of the groups, why should relatively heavier BW confer a survival advantage? Andres (1980a) has hypothesized that heavier BW among humans might confer a protective effect against the catabolic processes of disease when it is encountered in late life. We currently have no data to address this possibility. What is clear in our studies thus far is that at some advanced ages (beyond 24 months), BW loses its association with LS in C57BL/6J mice (Reynolds, Ingram, and Talan 1985). This is probably due to disease processes that may cause weight loss or weight gain through tumors, edema, dehydration, or other factors.

Metabolic Factors

When examined across mammalian species, the positive correlation between LS and BW is accompanied by an inverse correlation between LS and metabolic rate (Sacher, 1959). Metabolic rate declines as BW increases. This relationship concurs with the thermodynamic principle relating maintenance of heat in accordance with body surface exposure (Kleiber, 1961). Higher metabolic activity has been hypothesized to contribute to a metabolic wear factor, possibly through the increased production of oxygen radicals (Harman, 1981). Sacher (1977) hypothesized that reduction in this metabolic wear factor might be the principal mechanism involved in the increased LS associated with DR. Given this hypothesis, one would expect greater support to be found for the inverse correlation between LS and BW within species.

Sacher and Duffy (1979) examined the correlation between LS and metabolic rate (oxygen consumption per body weight) across and within 25 mouse genotypes. The hypothesized negative correlation was observed, but the best fit to the data was a quadratic function. This relationship was not confirmed in the analysis of Storer (1967), who examined LS and metabolic rate measured at 120 days across 18 inbred mouse strains. In fact, he observed a significant positive correlation between LS and metabolic rate in both males and females.

Economos (1980a) has questioned the reliability of the cross-species correlation between LS and metabolic rate. Regarding the association of DR with reduced metabolic load across the LS of rats, the studies of Masoro et al. (1982), McCarter et al. (1985), and Yu et al. (1985) have demonstrated that caloric consumption based on food intake and oxygen consumption is not different between AL and DR groups when based on a per weight basis over a lifetime. This also appears to be the case in mice on various regimens of DR; however, when based on a per animal basis, the metabolic load is reduced as a function of DR (Weindruch et al., 1986).

Other exceptions exist which do not support the hypothesis that reduced metabolic rate is necessarily associated with longevity within species. For example, Goodrick (1980) demonstrated that a regimen of voluntary exercise (housing in activity-wheel cages) increased LS, decreased BW, but also appeared to increase metabolic rate.

Body temperature (colonic) has been found to be positively correlated with BW in male C57BL/6J mice at ages ranging from 3-20 months (Talan, 1984). This relationship has also been observed within many other rodent species (Hart, 1971). Thus, the assumption that higher BW should benefit thermoregulation and thus be associated with lower body temperature and metabolic rate does not appear to hold within rodent species. Similarly, Leto et al. (1976) observed that a DR regimen of 4% protein was effective in reducing BW and increasing LS in female C57BL/6J mice compared to those on a control diet (26% protein). However, rectal temperature in the DR group was consistently higher than the control group across the LS.

In summary, similar to the complexity of the BW-LS relationship, the relation of metabolic rate to LS within rodent species is complex and has as yet to be fully clarified. Our observations on the relationship between LS and BW neither support nor refute a metabolic hypothesis.

Genotype-Environment Interaction

In the face of numerous studies which do not lend support to the hypothesis that BW should be inversely related to longevity within laboratory rodent species, it is imperative to address in detail the studies of Ross and colleagues whose findings appeared to support the hypothesis consistently. In numerous studies, BW during early development was inversely related to LS, and higher relative BW was predictive of higher incidence of a number of diseases, notably tumors (e.g., Ross and Bras, 1965; Ross et al., 1976).

Three salient features of these studies must be considered. First, these results emerged primarily from studies involving large numbers of rats housed in isolation and fed a self-selected diet. The use of a self-selected diet makes these studies unique in relation to other rodent studies discussed previously. Second, it should be noted that many of the rats became obese with average BW in excess of 700 grams and maximum BWs at late ages well over 1,000 grams in some individuals. These weights are higher than observed in AL-fed male Wistar rats. For example, we observed a mean maximum weight of less than 700 grams (Goodrick et al., 1982). In the same strain, Beauchene et al. (1986) observed mean maximum weights of less than 600 grams in male rats. Wyndam et al. (1983) reported weights among male Wistar rats in the range of 400-500 grams with isolated rats demonstrating higher weights than group-housed animals. Male F-344 rats fed AL in isolation also manifest adult BW lower than 600 gm on average (Yu et al., 1985). Thus, it is clear that the rats used in Ross's studies appeared to be from a heavier strain than used in other studies which have related BW to LS. This observation may stem from a genetic tendency toward obesity in this strain. This feature might have also been due to environmental factors; e.g., either the self-selected diet or to isolation or to the interaction of both factors within this strain.

The third and probably the most important feature bearing on the conclusions of Ross and colleagues was that their rats were from an outbred strain (COBS). Possibly this genetic heterogeneity could have confounded their correlational analysis. Specifically, the relationship of BW and other growth and dietary parameters to LS could have been coincidental. It is possible that the genetic factors regulating BW growth and longevity determinant processes were operating independently but appeared correlated. To clarify this concept, it could be deduced that rats possessed genes that influenced a lower BW compared to other members of this strain but also possessed coincidentally a separate set of genes that promoted longevity.

This criticism would also apply to all our data and those of other investigators (Beauchene et al., 1986; Everitt and Webb, 1957; Wyndam et al., 1983) pertaining to the use of outbred strains of Wistar rats for intra-group correlational analysis. It does not apply to our data involving inbred mouse strains or to those of other laboratories using inbred rats (Bertrand et al., 1980; Masoro, 1984; Yu et al., 1985) or mouse (Weindruch et al., 1986) strains where positive correlations between BW and LS were observed.

Proposed Model Relating Body Weight to Lifespan

Although little consistent support appears for the hypothesis of an inverse relationship between LS and BW within laboratory rodent strains on similar diets, the challenge remains to generate alternative

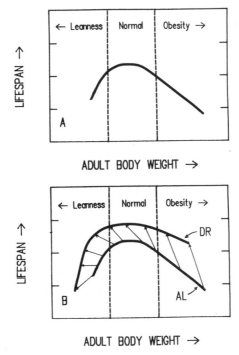

Figure 11.   Hypothetical model relating body weight to lifespan within
rodent species.

hypotheses. This is particularly difficult given the diversity of
results that appear. A simple conclusion is that the relationship
between LS and BW is greatly dependent upon genotype. This is appealing
in its simplicity but provides no order to the existing data and does
not lend itself to testing.

Therefore, as an attempt to bring some order to the apparent
diversity of results, we offer the hypothesized model presented in
Figure 11. At this point of development, the model is not data-based
but might provide some order to the observations discussed. As shown,
the relationship between BW and LS is curvilinear. It represents an
extension of the model of Economos and Lints (1984) for Drosphila and
Sacher and Duffy's (1979) perspective on this issue for mice. This also
matches the epidemiological perspective of human studies (Fig. 10).
However, it should be noted that like the criticism concerning the
analysis of the relationship within outbred rodent strains, human
analysis is also fraught with genetic heterogeneity. Thus, this model
attempts to accommodate the existence of genotypes.

The model permits several predictions. First, for genotypes prone to leanness, heavier BW should be positively correlated with LS. Second, for genotypes prone to obesity, BW should be negatively correlated with LS. It is also clear that one could shape the plateau of the curvilinear function to be sharply curved or more flat and broad. As the plateau is broadened, one might postulate the existence of genotypes in which little relationship exists between BW and LS. Another notable feature is that the slope of curve is steeper on the leaner side than on the obese side.

At present, this model might account for the correlations that we observed between BW and LS among AL-fed male Wistar rats, C57BL/6J mice, A/J mice, B6AF$_1$ mice and the two obese genotypes, ob/ob and A^y/a. In all but the B6AF$_1$ strain and the obese mice, the correlations were nonsignificant or were significantly positive. The hybrid and obese mice were heavier genotypes and thus tended toward negative correlations between LS and BW, particularly late in life. Regarding the data of Ross and colleagues, therefore, one should observe the negative correlation between BW and LS in this strain which tended toward obesity under the environmental conditions imposed upon it.

In Figure 11B we offer an extension of the model which incorporates DR. It suggests that reduced BW during DR is associated with increased LS, but again the relationship of the two parameters is very much dependent upon genotype. First, the model predicts that obese genotypes might benefit from DR differentially more with respect to gain in LS per decrement in BW when compared to leaner genotypes. Second, it indicates that among obese genotypes the inverse relationship between LS and BW still exists within a certain range. Third, within some specified range of BW, no correlation between BW and LS exists for some genotypes even when significant correlations (positive or negative) might exist under AL conditions. Fourth, among leaner genotypes the relationship between BW and LS remains positive. Finally, among the leanest genotypes it is clear that DR becomes detrimental to survival.

This model involving DR appears to hold for our data on Wistar rats and for several strains of inbred mice, including obese genotypes. What is not well handled by the model are the dynamics of weight change with age. In particular, it is difficult to account for some of the changes in correlational pattern that we observed among Wistar rats on the EOD diet; e.g., positive in early life, negative in latter life. Also, the appearance of a negative correlation between BW and LS for female genotypes does not fit well into the model unless the female genotypes that we analyzed can be considered those that tend toward obesity. Further modification of this model is clearly necessary, but it lends itself to this process.

Intra-Group Correlations Between Growth Duration and Lifespan

Thus far, the discussion has concerned the correlation between LS and BW exclusively. Final consideration should be given to a developmental parameter that appears to have proven more consistently correlated with LS than BW. This parameter is growth duration (GD), which is operationally defined as the age at which maximum BW is attained.

Table 5 presents the correlation between LS and GD obtained in several studies from our laboratory. These data are for animals on both AL and EOD regimens followed since near weaning.

Table 5

Pearson Correlations Between Life-Span and Body-Weight Growth-Duration
in Several Male Rodent Strains on Ad Libitum (AL) and
Every-Other-Day (EOD) Feeding ($\underline{n}$ = Sample Size)

Strains	Feeding Regimen			
	AL	($\underline{n}$)	EOD	($\underline{n}$)
Wistar rats	.88*	(27)	.31	(24)
C57BL/6J mice	.63*	(40)	.78*	(40)
B6AF$_1$ mice	−.08	(40)	.26	(40)
A/J mice	.28	(40)	.46*	(40)
ob/ob mice	.51	(13)	.64*	(10)
A^y/a mice	−.36	(24)	−.17	(10)

* $\underline{p} < 0.05$

The pattern of correlation is clear and consistent. Except for the A^y/a mutants and B6AF$_1$ mice on an AL diet, there is a distinct positive relationship between LS and GD. The longer the animal continues to gain BW, the longer it is likely to live even when on a DR regimen.

Similar observations have been made in our laboratory. Goodrick (1977) observed significant positive correlations between LS and GD within the C57BL/6J inbred mouse strain and within several single mutants on this background (bg and cJ) including an obese mutant (ob/ob). Consistent with our later study, the correlation for the A^y mutant was not significant although it was positive. Similarly, Goodrick (1978) observed positive correlations between LS and GD within different diet groups (4 and 26% protein) of C57BL/6J, A/J, and B6AF$_1$ strains of male mice, although again consistent with data in Table 5, the only significant correlations were for the C57BL/6J mice on both diets and the A/J and B6AF$_1$ genotypes on the restricted diet. Our observations of a positive correlation between LS and GD within different diet groups of male Wistar rats have also been confirmed in other laboratories (Everitt and Webb, 1957; Beauchene et al., 1976). There is also ample support for a positive correlation between LS and GD of adult forms of nonmammalian genotypes, including Drosphlia and Tribolium (Lints, 1985).

Therefore, a process regulating how long an individual continues to gain BW appears to be related to how long it will eventually live. This view appears to return to the McCay principle of longevity induced by retardation of development. Analyses of data from our laboratory (Ingram et al., 1982) and others (Beauchene et al., 1986) suggest that it is not the rate at which BW is gained that is the critical variable, but rather it is this time parameter which appears to manifest overriding importance. Whether the termination of BW gain signals the influence of some terminal chronic disease is still subject to debate

(Rockstein et al., 1977). Further analysis of this relationship still awaits careful pathological analysis conducted at the precise time that individuals begin this terminal weight loss. In our laboratory this terminal loss appears to be a protracted one rather than an acute phenomenon leading to rapid death.

CONCLUSIONS

A review of data from our laboratory and others has yielded little support for the hypothesis that leanness per se confers long life in laboratory rodents. It is clear that DR conducted in many and sundry studies can increase survival, markedly in many cases. But the effect of the coincidental BW loss, often but not always resulting from this treatment, is not consistently related to the LS effects. It is concluded that BW loss is neither sufficient nor necessary for effecting longevity through nutritional means or other treatments, such as exercise. Other mechanisms controlling the LS effects of DR will have to be pursued.

The most parsimonious conclusion derived from our review is that the relationship between BW and LS is complex involving the interaction of genotype (including sex), environment (notably diet), and age. If any generalization is permitted, it would be that among males of normal genotypes on the same dietary regimen, higher BW throughout adult life is associated with longevity; whereas, among females and certain obese genotypes, lower BW is associated with longevity. This genotype-environment interaction can be viewed as a curvilinear function relating BW to LS depending upon the tendancy of the genotype toward leanness or obesity within its environment. For leaner genotypes, a positive correlation between BW and LS is predicted; whereas, for obese genotypes, a negative correlation is predicted. However, for other genotypes within median ranges of BW for the species, there may be little or no relationship between BW and LS. This model fits some but not all of the data reviewed and does not attend to the dynamics of BW change with age or to a possible negative correlation between BW and LS among females. Thus, further assessment will be required.

Although lower BW does not appear to be consistently related to longevity, there does appear to be a more consistent positive correlation between GD and LS. The rate of increase in BW appears to be less important than the duration over which BW continues to increase. The linkage of this phenomenon to metabolic or disease processes remains to be determined.

In summary, extending our earlier arguments (Reynolds and Ingram, 1984), we find no basis in our data or in related literature to suggest that thinner is necessarily better for survival within species of laboratory rodents.

ACKNOWLEDGEMENTS

The authors acknowledge that most of the data herein were derived from studies conducted under the supervision of the late Charles Goodrick. We greatly appreciate the assistance of John Freeman and Edward Spangler for animal husbandry, Nancy Cider and William Richards for data analysis, Paul Ciesla for graphics, and Rita Wolferman for clerical assistance. The Gerontology Research Center is fully accredited by the American Association for the Accreditation of Laboratory Animal Care.

REFERENCES

Andres, R., 1980a, Effect of obesity on total mortality, _Int. J. Obesity_, 4:381.

Andres, R., 1980b, Influence of obesity on longevity in the aged, _in_: "Aging, Cancer and Cell Membrances," C. Borek, C. M. Fenoglio, and D. W. King, eds., George Thieme, Verlag, New York.

Andres, R., 1985, Mortality and obesity: The rationale for age-specific height-weight tables. _in_: "Principles of Geriatric Medicine," R. Andres, E. L. Bierman, W. R. Hazzard, eds., McGraw-Hill, New York.

Avons, P., Ducimetiere, P., and Rakotovao, R., 1983, Weight and mortality, Lancet. 1:1104.

Barrows, C. H., and Kokkonen, G. C., 1977, Relationship between nutrition and aging. _in_: "Advances in Nutritional Research," H. H. Draper, ed., Plenum Press, New York.

Beauchene, R. E., Bales, C. W., Bragg, C. S., Hawkins, S. T., and Mason, R. L., 1986, Effect of age of initiation of feed restriction on growth, body composition, and longevity of rats, _J. Gerontol._, 41:13.

Berg, B. N., and Simms, H. S., 1962, Disease, rather than aging, as the cause of weight loss and muscle lesions in the rat, _J. Gerontol._, 17:452.

Bertrand, H. A., Lynd, F. T., Masoro, E. J., and Yu, B. P., 1980, Changes in adipose mass and cellularity through the adult life of rats fed ad libitum or a life-prolonging restricted diet, _J. Gerontol._, 35:827.

Build Study 1979, 1980, Chicago Society of Actuaries and Association of Actuaries and Association of Life Insurance Medical Directors of America.

Driori, D., and Folman, Y., 1976, Environmental effects on longevity in the male rat: Exercise, mating, castration, and restricted feeding, _Exp. Gerontol._, 11:25.

Duffy, P. H., and Sacher, G. A., 1976, Age-dependence of body weight and linear dimensions in adult _Mus_ and _Peromyscus_, _Growth_, 40:19.

Economos, A. C., 1980a, Brain-life span conjecture. A reevaluation of the evidence, _Gerontol._, 26:82.

Economos, A. C., 1980b, Taxonomic differences in the mammalian life-span body-weight relationship and the problem of brain weight, _Gerontol._, 26:90.

Economos, A. C., and Lints, F. A., 1984, Growth rate and life span in _Drosphila_. III. Effect of body size and developmental temperature on the biphasic relationship between growth rate and life span, _Mech. Ageing Devel._, 27:153.

Economos, A. C., and Lints, F. A., 1985, Growth rate and life span in _Drosphila_. IV. Role of cell size and cell number in the biphasic relationship between life span and growth rate. _Mech. Ageing Devel._, 32:193.

Everitt, A. V., 1955, The loss of body weight in ageing rats, _Austral. J. Med. Technol._, 1:41.

Everitt, A. V. and Webb, C., 1957, The relation between body weight changes and life duration in male rats, _J. Gerontol._, 12:128.

Goodrick, C. L., 1974, Effects of exercise on longevity and behavior of hybrid mice which differ in coat color, _J. Gerontol._, 29:129.

Goodrick, C. L., 1977, Body weight change over the life span and longevity for C57BL/6J mice and mutations which differ in maximal body weight, _Gerontol._, 23:405.

Goodrick, C. L., 1978, Body weight increment and length of life: The effect of genetic constitution and dietary protein, _J. Gerontol._, 33:184.

Goodrick, C. L., 1980, Effects of long-term voluntary wheel exercise on male and female Wistar rats. I. Longevity, body weight, and metabolic rate, Gerontol., 26:22.

Goodrick, C. L., Ingram, D. K., Reynolds, M. A., Freeman, J. R., and Cider, N. L., 1982, Effects of intermittent feeding upon growth and life span in rats. Gerontol., 26:233.

Goodrick, C. L., Ingram, D. K., Reynolds, M. A., Freeman, J. R., and Cider, N. L., 1983a, Differential effects of intermittent feeding and voluntary exercise on body weight and survival in adult rats, J. Gerontol., 38:36.

Goodrick, C. L., Ingram, D. K., Reynolds, M. A., Freeman, J. R., and Cider, N. L., 1983b, Effects of intermittent feeding upon growth, activity, and lifespan in rats allowed voluntary exercise, Exp. Aging Res., 9:203.

Harman, D., 1981, The aging process, Proc. Natl. Acad. Sci., USA, 78:7124.

Harrison, D. E., Archer, J. R., and Astle, C. M., 1984, Effects of food restriction on aging: Separation of food intake and adiposity, Proc. Natl. Acad. Sci., USA, 81:1835.

Hart, J. S., 1971, in: Comparative Physiology of Thermoregulation. G. C. Whittow, ed., Academic Press, New York.

Ingram, D. K., and Reynolds, M. A., Les, E. P., 1982, The relationship of genotype, sex, body weight, and growth parameters to lifespan in inbred and hybrid mice, Mech. Ageing Devel., 20:253.

Ingram, D. K., and Reynolds, M. A., 1983, Effects of protein, dietary restriction, and exercise on survival in adult rats: A re-analysis of McCay, Maynard, Sperling, and Osgood [1941], Exp. Aging Res., 9:41.

Ingram, D. K., Reynolds, M. A., and Goodrick, C. L., 1982, The relationship of sex, exercise, and growth rate to lifespan in the Wistar rat: A multivariate correlational approach. Gerontol., 28:23.

Kleiber, M., 1961, "The Fire of Life: An Introduction to Animal Energetics," Wiley and Sons, New York.

Leto, S., Kokkonen, G. C., and Barrows, C. H., 1976, Dietary protein, life span, and biochemical variables in female mice. J. Gerontol., 31:144.

Lew, E. A., and Garfinkel, L., 1979, Variations in mortality by weight among 750,000 men and women. J. Chron. Dis., 32:563.

Libow, L. S., 1974, Interaction of medical, biologic, and behavioral factors on aging adaptation and survival. An 11-year longitudinal study. Geriatrics, 29:75.

Lints, F. A., 1985, Insects, in: "Handbook of the Biology of Aging," C. E. Finch and E. L. Schneider, eds., Van Nostrand, New York.

Masoro, E., Yu, B. P, and Bertrand, H. A., 1982, Action of food restriction in delaying the aging process. Proc. Natl. Acad. Sci., USA, 79:4239.

Masoro, E. J., 1984, Food restriction and the aging process. J. Am. Geriat. Soc., 32:296.

McCarter, R., Masoro, E. J., and Yu, B. P., 1985, Does food restriction retard aging by reducing the metabolic rate? Am. J. Physiol., 248:488.

McCay, C. M., 1935, The effect of retarded growth upon the length of life span and upon the ultimate body size. J. Nutr., 10:63.

McCay, C. M., Maynard, L. A., Sperling, G., and Osgood, H., 1939, Retarded growth, life span, ultimate body size and age changes in the albino rat after feeding diets restricted in calories. J. Nutr., 18:1.

McCay, C. M., Lovelace, E., Sperling, G., Barnes, L. L. Litt, C. H., Smith, C. A. H., Smith, C. A., and Saxton, J. A., Jr., 1952, Age changes in relation to the ingestion of milk, water, coffee, and sugar solutions. J. Gerontol., 7:161.

McCay, C. M., Maynard, L. A., Sperling, G., and Osgood, H., 1941,
    Nutritional requirements during the latter half of life. J. Nutr.,
    21:45.
Nash, D. J., and Kidwell, J. F., 1973, A genetic analysis of lifespan,
    fecundity, and weight in the mouse. J. Heredity, 64:87.
Nolen, G. A., 1972, Effect of various restricted dietary regimes on
    the growth, health and longevity of albino rats, J. Nutr.,
    102:1477.
Osanai, M., 1978, Longevity and body weight loss of silkworm moth,
    Bombyx mori, varied by different temperature treatments. Exp.
    Gerontol., 13:375.
Reynolds, M. A., and Ingram, D. K., 1984, Is thinner better? Int. J.
    Obesity, 8:285.
Reynolds, M. A., Ingram, D. K., and Talan, M., 1985, Relationship of
    body temperature stability to mortality in aging mice. Mech.
    Aging Devel., 30:143.
Rockstein, M., Chesky, J., and Sussman, M., 1977, Comparative biology
    and evolution of aging. in: "Handbook of the Biology of Aging,"
    C. E. Finch and L. Hayflick, eds., Van Nostrand Reinhold, New
    York.
Ross, M. H., 1966, Life expectancy modification by change in dietary
    regimen of mature rat. Proceed. 7th Int. Congress Nutr., 5:35.
Ross, M. H., and Bras, G., 1965, Tumor incidence patterns and nutrition
    in the rat. J. Nutr., 87:245.
Ross, R. H., Lustbader, E., and Bras, G., 1976, Dietary practices and
    growth responses as predictors of longevity, Nature, 262:548.
Sacher, G., 1959, Relation of life span to brain weight and body weight
    in mammals, CIBA Found. Coll. Aging, 5:115.
Sacher, G. A., 1977, Life table modification and life prolongation.
    in: "Handbook of the Biology of Aging," C. E. Finch and L. Hayflick,
    eds., Van Nostrand Reinhold, New York.
Sacher, G. A., and Duffy, P. H., 1979, Genetic relation of life span
    to metabolic rate for inbred mouse strains and their hybrids, Fed.
    Proc., 38:184.
Soliman, M. H., and Lints, F. A., 1975, Longevity, growth rate and
    related traits among strains of Tribolium castaneum, Gerontologia,
    21:102.
Soliman, H., and Lints, F. A., 1982, Influence of preimaginal constant
    and alternating temperatures on growth rate and longevity of adults
    of five genotypes in Tribolium castaneum, Mech. Ageing Devel.,
    18:19.
Storer, J. B., 1967, Relation of lifespan to brain weight, body weight,
    and metabolic rate among inbred mouse strains, Exp. Gerontol.,
    2:173.
Stuchlikova, E., Juricova-Horakova, M., and Deyl, Z., 1975, New aspects
    of the dietary effect of life prolongation in rodents. What is the
    role of obesity in aging? Exp. Gerontol., 10:141.
Stunkard, A. J., 1983, Nutrition, aging and obesity: A critical review
    of a complex relationship, Int. J. Obesity, 7:201.
Talan, M., 1984, Body temperature of C57BL/6J mice with age, Exp.
    Gerontol., 19:25.
Waaler, Hans Th., 1984, Height, weight, and mortality: The Norwegian
    experience, Acta Medica Scandinavica, Suppl. 679.
Weindruch, R., Walford, R., Fligiel, S., and Guthrie, D., 1986, The
    retardation of aging in mice by dietary restriction: Longevity,
    cancer, immunity, and lifetime energy intake, J. Nutr., 116:641.
Wyndam, J. R., Everitt, A. V., and Everitt, S. F., 1983, Effects of
    isolation and food restriction begun at 50 days on the development
    of age-associated renal disease in the male Wistar rat, Arch.
    Gerontol. Geriatr., 2:317.

Yu, B. P., Masoro, E. J., and McMahan, C. A., 1985, Nutritional influences on aging of Fischer 344 rats: I. Physical, metabolic, and longevity characteristics, J. Gerontol., 40:657.

IS CELLULAR SENESCENCE GENETICALLY PROGRAMMED?

James R. Smith, Andrea L. Spiering, and Olivia M. Pereira-Smith

Department of Virology and Epidemiology
Baylor College of Medicine
Houston, TX

INTRODUCTION

The limited capacity for division exhibited by normal animal cells in culture is well documented and a striking contrast to the unlimited division potential of abnormal tumor-derived or virus- or carcinogen-transformed cells. In 1965 Hayflick[1] proposed that the limited division of normal cells was a manifestation of aging at the cellular level, and we have studied normal human cells, particularly fibroblasts, as a model for in vitro aging, attempting to understand the basic mechanisms involved in normal growth control.

PROLIFERATION OF HYBRID CELLS

In an approach to the problem, we have studied the long term proliferative potential of various human somatic cell hybrids to gain an idea of the complexity of these mechanisms. We found that fusion of normal cells with a variety of immortal cell lines yielded hybrids that ceased division after as many as 70 population doublings (PD) in vitro[2]. This demonstrated that limited growth was a dominant phenotype in hybrids and, conversely, that the phenotype of immortality was recessive. This lead us to hypothesize that immortal cells arise as a result of recessive changes in the growth control mechanisms of the normal cell. If more than one such change could result in an immortal cell, since immortality is recessive, fusion of various immortal cell lines with each other should allow for complementation of the different changes and yield hybrids having limited division. We therefore fused a variety of immortal cell lines with each other. In some cases, only immortal hybrids were obtained, indicating that immortalization in the particular parents involved had occurred by the same processes. However, in other fusions we obtained hybrids that ceased division after as many as 65 PD[2], indicating that since different recessive changes had led to immortalization of the parent lines involved, complementation of these changes in the hybrids resulted in limited proliferation. To date, we have separated 22 different cell lines into 3 complementation groups (see Table 1). Cell lines have been assigned to group non-A, non-B on the basis that they complement cell lines in both groups A and B. It remains to be determined if these lines belong in group C, or whether they fall into a number of other groups. The data so far indicate the following:

1) SV40 virus induces the same recessive changes in human cells of varied origin, to cause immortalization. This is based on the observation that all hybrid clones obtained from fusions of SV40-transformed fibroblasts with each other or with SV40-transformed keratinocyte or amnion cells, are immortal.
2) Different DNA tumor viruses immortalize human cells by different processes, since the adenovirus transformed line 293 complements SV40-transformed cells 639.
3) Cell type (epithelial versus fibroblast), embroyonal layer of origin (ecto-, meso-, endodermal) and type of tumor (lung versus skin, carcinoma versus sarcoma) do not affect complementation group assignment.

Cell lines having activated H-ras, N-ras and Ki-ras oncogenes were included in this study to determine whether activation of an oncogene could be involved in the process of immortalization. All cell lines containing the active Ki-ras oncogene have been assigned a non-A, non-B status but until the assignment of group C is confirmed, a case for involvement of this oncogene in immortalization cannot be made.

Table 1.   Assignment to Complementation Groups for Indefinite Proliferation Potential

Cell line		Group assigned
GM639	SV40-transformed skin fibroblasts (IMR)*	A
GM847	SV40-transformed skin fibroblasts HPRT⁻, Lesch Nyhan)(IMR)	A
VA13	SV40-transformed lung fibroblasts (IMR)	A
wtB	SV40-transformed keratinocytes (C. Noonan)	A
A268 IV	SV40-transformed amnion (J. Fogh)	A
CMV-Mj-HEL-1	Cytomegalovirus-transformed lung fibroblasts (F. Rapp)	C
293	Adenovirus-transformed embryonic kidney (ATCC)**	Non-A, non-B
Ct1	Co-irradiated lung fibroblasts (M. Namba)	Non-A, non-B
SUSM I	4NQO-transformed lung fibroblasts (M. Namba)	Non-A, non-B
HT1080	Fibrosarcoma (N-ras$^+$) (R. Baker)	A
1080 21A	APRT⁻ clone of HT1080 (R. Baker)	A
TE85	Osteosarcoma (J. Fogh)	C
143BTK⁻	TE85 secondarily transformed by Kirsten mouse sarcoma virus (Ki-ras$^+$) (C. Croce)	C
T98 G	Glioblastoma (G. Stein)	B
HeLa	Cervical carcinoma	B
A549	Lung carcinoma (S. Aaronson)	Non-A, non-B
A2182	Lung carconoma (Ki-ras$^+$) (S. Aaronson)	Non-A, non-B
EJ	Bladder carcinoma (H-ras$^+$) (R. Kucherlapati)	A
J82	Bladder carcinoma (ATCC)	B
A1698	Bladder carcinoma (Ki-ras$^+$) (S. Aaronson)	Non-A, non-B
5637	Bladder carcinoma (ATCC)	Non-B

 * IMR = Institute for Medical Research
** ATCC = American Type Culture Collection

In order to understand the mechanisms involved in normal growth control, we extended the heterokaryon studies of Norwood et al.[3] and Stein et al[4]. These investigators had demonstrated that terminally non-dividing (senescent) normal cells could inhibit initiation of DNA synthesis in nuclei of normal and some immortal cells that were otherwise capable of synthesizing DNA. Burmer et al.[5] and we[6] independently demonstrated that cytoplasts derived from terminally non-dividing cells could inhibit DNA synthesis initiation as effectively as whole cells. We also found that treatment of senescent cytoplasts with 5 ug/ml cycloheximide or 10 ug/ml puromycin for as little as 2 hours prior to fusion eliminated the inhibitory effect of the cytoplasts[7]. We studied the kinetics of recovery of inhibitory activity in senescent cytoplasts incubated for various times after treatment with these protein synthesis inhibitors was terminated and before fusion to proliferating cells. Cycloheximide-treated cytoplasts regained their inhibitory activity within 2-3 hours after removal of the cycloheximide, and detectable levels of inhibition were observed within 1 hour of removal. Puromycin-treated cytoplasts did not regain inhibitory activity. The differential effects of these protein synthesis inhibitors can be explained by the difference in the mechanisms by which they act. Cycloheximide inhibits translocation and release of tRNA and prevents GTP dependent breakdown of polyribosomes, whereas puromycin causes premature release of the polypeptide chain from polysomes resulting in their breakdown. These results were consistent with the hypothesis that the loss of proliferative potential in normal animal cells results from the expres- sion of a new gene or a change in the expression of a gene product involved in the regulation of cell cycle. The gene product which blocks initiation of DNA synthesis appears to be a protein present in the senescent cytoplast.

To determine the localization of the inhibitory protein(s), i.e., cytosol versus cell membrane, we treated senescent cytoplasts with 0.025% twice crystallized trypsin for 1 minute at 4°C (Fig. 1).

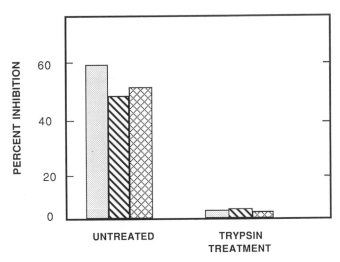

Fig. 1. Inhibition of DNA synthesis in young proliferation-competent cells by fusion with cytoplasts derived from senescent cells. Also shown is the loss of inhibitory activity by trypsin treatment. Bars show independent experiments.

Trypsin treatment eliminated inhibitory activity[8]. If the cytoplasts were allowed to recover from trypsin treatment, inhibitory activity was regained with kinetics similar to recovery from cycloheximide treatment. Since trypsin under the conditions used should preferentially affect surface membranes, the loss of the inhibitory activity indicates that the protein inhibitor(s) was present in the surface membranes of senescent cells.

Rabinovitch and Norwood[9] determined that young cells made quiescent by maintenance in low serum for 2-4 weeks exhibited inhibitory activity similar to senescent cells. We extended their observations and found that cytoplasts derived from quiescent cells also possessed the ability to inhibit DNA synthesis initiation in proliferating cells[8]. We found that the quiescent cell inhibitor (Figure 2) was eliminated by trypsin treatment, but not by cycloheximide treatment. The inhibitory activity was regained if recovery from trypsin treatment was permitted, and the kinetics of recovery were similar to that occuring in senescent cells[8].

The fact that cycloheximide treatment of quiescent cells[9] or cytoplasts[8] prior to fusion did not eliminate their inhibitory activity raised the question of whether proteins were involved in the inhibition of DNA synthesis mediated by quiescent cells and cytoplasts. We therefore treated quiescent cytoplasts with trypsin and allowed them to recover in the presence of cycloheximide. The inhibitory activity was not regained, indicating that protein synthesis must occur for the inhibitory effect and that the inhibitory activity is either a protein(s) or mediated by a protein(s) that is associated with surface membranes of quiescent cells[8]. We next isolated surface membrane enriched fractions from quiescent cells and found that fusion of 100 ug protein equivalent of surface membranes with proliferating cells resulted in DNA synthesis inhibition. Proteins extracted from these isolated membranes with 30 mM octyl- -D-glucopyranoside (OGP), a dialyzable detergent, for 30 minutes at 4°C, also inhibited DNA synthesis in cells exposed to the proteins for 24 hours in the presence of 10% fetal bovine serum (FBS).

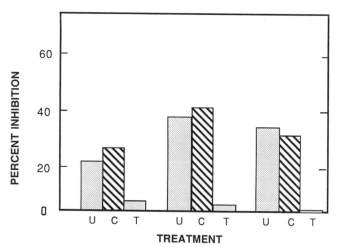

Fig. 2. Inhibition of DNA synthesis in young proliferation competent cell by fusion with cytoplasts derived from quiescent cells. Bars represent different experimental conditions: U, untreated; C, treated with cycloheximide; T, treated with trypsin. Three independent experiments are shown.

ISOLATION AND INHIBITOR PROTEIN

More recently we extracted proteins directly from the quiescent cell monolayers using 30 mM OGP for 5 minutes at 4°C. We initially concentrated our efforts on analysis of the quiescence inhibitor protein from serum-deprived (1% FBS) young human diploid fibroblasts (HDF). We found inhibitory activity in 5-week quiescent cell extracts and have determined that this inhibitory activity is dependent upon the length of time of the quiescent state. OGP extracts of monolayer cultures not deprived of growth factors (young HDF extracts) (100 ug protein/ml) shows less than 20% inhibition of DNA synthesis, 22% inhibition is obtained with 2-week quiescent cell extracts, and as much as 53% inhibition with 5-week quiescent cell extracts (Fig. 3). Maintenance of quiescent cells on low serum for more than 5 weeks does not appear to increase inhibitory activity above the level seen in extracts from cells maintained on low serum for only five weeks. That is, the presence of inhibitory activity is a response to the condition of serum deprivation, and remains constant once the quiescent state is stabilized. This apparent activation of inhibitor protein in response to serum deprivation supports the theory of a multiple step process controlling the states of quiescence and senescence, that is, the repression and/or selective expression of regulatory proteins, such as the inhibitor protein.

Attempts to further purify the inhibitor protein from quiescent HDF are complicated by the relative insolubility of this membrane-bound protein. Additionally, presence of the inhibitor is solely determined by ability to detect the inhibition of DNA synthesis in young proliferation-competent HDF. To date, coupled ammonium sulfate precipitations have allowed some degree of purification with retention of biological activity (Fig. 4). At each step, fractions were concentrated and assayed for their ability to inhibit DNA synthesis in proliferation-competent cells. Following a 10% ammonium sulfate cut in the presence of OGP, all detectable inhibitor protein was found to reside in the 10% supernatant, containing 70% of the total protein. A second ammonium sulfate cut (30%) in the absence of detergent resulted in precipitation of the inhibitor. This fraction only contained 22% of the total protein, yet all of the inhibitory activity. Corresponding extracts from young cells in the presence of 10% FBS exhibited negligible inhibition. Results through this point in the purification appear reproducible, with a 70% decrease in the fraction of cells synthe- sizing DNA observed at 100 ug protein/ml. Increasing the concentration of the quiescent extract increases the amount of inhibition in a dose-dependent manner, reaching a plateau at approximately 95% inhibition (Fig. 5). This is probably due to the portion of young cells in the substrate population which are non-synchronous, since the inhibitor affects initiation of DNA synthesis and has no effect on cells in S phase. As yet, it is not clear if the inhibitor proteins from quiescent and senescent cells are identical.

ISOLATION OF INHIBITOR mRNA

Identification of the nucleic acid sequence coding for this inhibitor protein(s) in both senescent and quiescent cells would be important in understanding the regulation of cellular senescence. As a first step in the identification of the RNA coding for this inhibitor protein, we micro-injected polyadenylated [poly(A)$^+$] RNA isolated from senescent and from young cycling human diploid fibroblasts (HDF) into proliferation-competent cells (10). Poly(A)$^+$ RNA (1 mg/ml) isolated from senescent cells inhibited DNA synthesis in proliferation-competent HDF whereas the poly(A)$^-$ RNA fraction from young cells or microinjected buffer alone caused no inhibition of DNA synthesis. The inhibitory effect of poly(A)$^+$ RNA from senescent

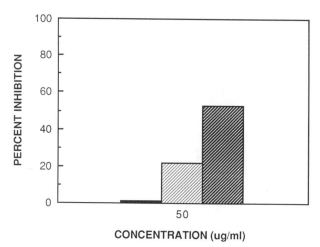

Fig. 3. Effect of duration of quiescence on inhibitor activity, ■ ,
zero time; ▨ , 2 week quiescent; ▧ , 5 week quiescent.

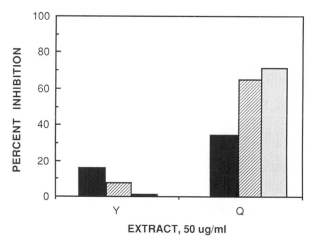

Fig. 4. Inhibition of DNA synthesis by extract from young cells (Y)
and serum-deprived quiescent cells (Q). ■ crude extract; ▧
supernatant from 10% ammonium sulfate; ▦ pellet from 30%
ammonium sulfate.

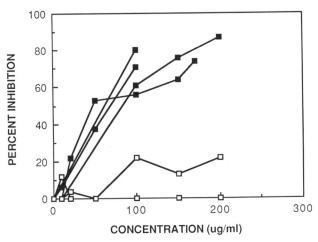

Fig. 5. Inhibition of DNA synthesis as a function of concentration of
partially purified extracts from ■ quiescent and □ young cells.

cells was lost after incubation with ribonuclease A. Thus, intact poly(A)[+]
RNA from senescent cells is responsible for inhibition of DNA synthesis.
About 10 hours after the uninjected cells began to synthesize DNA, the cells
injected with senescent cell poly(A)[+] RNA also entered S phase. We assume
that this is due to intracellular degradation of the injected RNA.

Since quiescent cells also produce a membrane-associated protein that
inhibits DNA synthesis, we determined if quiescent cells contained inhibitory messenger RNA (mRNA). Microinjections of poly(A)[+] RNA (1.7 mg/ml)
isolated from young cells that had been made quiescent by maintenance in
low serum for at least 2 weeks resulted in a significant, though consistently low, inhibition of DNA synthesis[10] (Fig. 6).

To determine the relative abundance of the senescent and quiescent cell
inhibitor mRNA's, dilution experiments were done. Quiescent cell poly(A)[+]
RNA achieved marked inhibition (57%) only at a concentration of 5 mg/ml
(Fig. 6), 160-fold greater than the concentration of senescent cell poly(A)[+]
RNA (0.03 mg/ml) that gave equivalent inhibition (Fig. 6). Control injections of young cell poly(A)[+] RNA at 5 mg/ml showed a slight inhibitory
effect. Whether this was due to competition for ribosomes or to the small
percentage (1 to 2 %) of senescent cells in young cell populations remains
to be determined. We calculated that 1/250 of a cell equivalent of poly
(A)[+] RNA from senescent cells injected into young cells resulted in significant inhibition. Thus, if 10 RNA molecules are necessary for inhibition,
each senescent cell contains approximately 2500 copies of the inhibitor mRNA
or an abundance of 0.8 percent. Similar calculations reveal that each
quiescent cell contains approximately 15 copies of the inhibitor mRNA or a
low level of 0.005 percent.

This marked difference between the copy numbers of inhibitory RNA in senescent and quiescent cells might be expected on the basis of our results from cell fusion studies. The inhibitory activity of senescent cells is rapidly lost after cycloheximide treatment[7,8], whereas the inhibitory activity of quiescent cells is stable in the presence of cycloheximide for periods of up to 24 hours[8,9]. These results indicate that the inhibitor protein from quiescent cells is very stable compared with the inhibitor from senescent cells. Our finding that inhibitory mRNA from senescent cells is 160-fold more abundant than that in quiescent cells conforms to the above data since the low turnover quiescence protein needs much less RNA to maintain an active level than the higher turnover senescence protein. These results provide strong evidence for the production of a high abundance mRNA coding for a protein that blocks initiation of DNA synthesis in senescent cells.

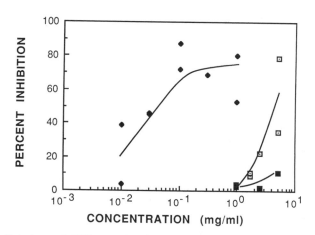

Fig. 6. Inhibition of DNA synthesis in young proliferation competent cell by injection of RNA derived from ◆, senescent cells; ▫, quiescent cells; ■, young cells.

EFFECT OF ONCOGENES ON INHIBITORY ACTIVITY

Cellular proto-oncogene and oncogene proteins have been clearly demonstrated to be positive regulators of cell growth and are potential candidates for initiators of DNA synthesis that could act antagonistically to the inhibitor(s) in senescent cells[11,12]. Since the H-ras product acts at the membrane of cells, as does the putative senescence protein(s)[13,14], we tested the ability of cloned c-H-ras DNAs to functionally reverse inhibitor activity after microinjection into senescent cells. Normal young cells that have been made nonproliferating (quiescent) by the reduction of serum growth factors also produce a membrane-associated protein inhibitor(s) of the initiation of DNA synthesis[8,9]. These cells were tested as well.

Initially, the effect of the oncogene form of c-H-ras DNAs was examined. Cloned DNA isolated from the bladder carcinoma cell line EJ[15] was injected into quiescent and senescent cells derived from the CSC303 human neonatal foreskin cell line. Cells made quiescent either by maintenance in low serum or by growth to high density were stimulated to enter DNA synthesis by c-H-ras DNA (Fig. 7). Senescent cells, however, did not respond to the c-H-ras(EJ) DNA by synthesizing DNA. Both senescent and quiescent cells expressed the p21 product of the DNA at very low levels, as detected by immunofluorescence staining with antibody Y13-259 against p21 (a gift from E. Scolnick and R.B. Stein, Merck Sharp & Dohme). Control injections of pBR322, the plasmid in which c-H-ras(EJ) DNA was cloned, did not increase the percentage of labeled nuclei over background, indicating that the microinjection procedure itself did not stimulate the cells.

Feramisco et al.[16] have reported that microinjection of the p21 protein product of oncogenic c-H-ras(T24) failed to stimulated DNA synthesis in a human fibroblast cell line H8. In contrast, Mulcahy et al.[17] demonstrated that injection of anti-p21 antibody into MRC5 cells (diploid human lung fibroblasts) resulted in a decrease in the number of cells synthesizing DNA during the time period observed, results more in agreement with our observations. Due to the apparent discrepancy with the report of Feramisco et al.[16], we examined the effect of c-H-ras(T24) DNA in our system. Another human cell line, CSC301, was also included to determine whether ras functions varied with the cell line used. In addition, both proto-oncogene and oncogene forms of c-H-ras DNA were compared to determine if the activated form of c-H-ras was more mitogenic in human cells. Cloned DNAs for the proto-oncogene (pP3) and oncogene (pT24) forms of c-H-ras were kindly provided by M. Wigler, Cold Spring Harbor Laboratory.

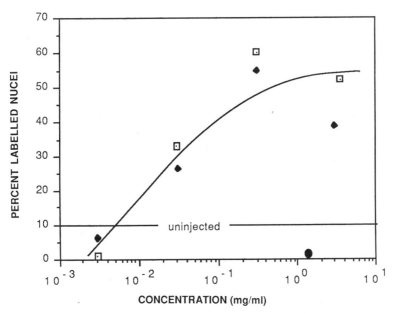

Fig. 7. Stimulation of DNA synthesis by microinjection of oncogene and proto-oncogene DNA into quiescent cells. □ proto-oncogene DNA; ◆ c-H‑ras oncogene DNA; ●, oncogene DNA injected into senescent cells.

Oncogenic c-H-ras(pT24) DNA was effective in stimulating DNA synthesis in both quiescent CSC303 and quiescent CSC301 cells. Therefore, neither the cell line used nor the sources of c-H-ras DNA affected the results. It is possible that Feramisco et al.[16] used cells at or near the end of their in vitro life span. Both the proto-oncogene and oncogene forms were equally efficient in stimulating DNA synthesis in quiescent cells, with maximal response at 0.3 mg/ml DNA and no stimulation observed at 0.003 mg/ml (Fig. 7). These results are in contrast to those obtained with rodent cells in which the oncogene form induces transformation changes at concentrations at which the proto-oncogene form has no effect.

Other laboratories have demonstrated the need for two oncogenes working in concert to convert primary rodent cells to tumorigenic cells. Oncogenes that have been shown to complement H-ras in this process are polyomavirus T antigen, the EIA region of the adenovirus genome, and c-myc[17,18]. A plasmid carrying the E1A gene (pAd12E1A, provided by R. Bernards [19]) was co-injected with the oncogene form of c-H-ras(pT24) into senescent cells. The cells did not incorporate tritiated thymidine, indicating that senescent normal cells do not respond to the mitogenic effects of a combination of oncogenes that is able to permit transformation and tumorigenic progression in primary rodent cells.

This lack of response of senescent cells to microinjected oncogenes is not due to an increased sensitivity to microinjection or to an absolute inability of the cells to synthesize DNA following any stimulus. Senescent cells can be induced to synthesize DNA following infection with the DNA tumor virus simian virus 40 (SV40) or cytomegalovirus[20-22] and following fusion to immortal human cells known to contain SV40, adenovirus, or papillomavirus sequences[23,24]. To determine if we could induce DNA synthesis in senescent cells, we microinjected a plasmid containing the entire SV40 genome (pBSV-1)[25] into senescent cell nuclei. Twenty-four hours after microinjection, 20% of the microinjected cells stained positively for SV40 T antigen by immunofluorescence. A total of 12% of the injected cells (60% of T antigen-positive cells) synthesized DNA. Senescent cells infected with 10 PFU of SV40 per cell responded comparably.

CONCLUSIONS

When normal human diploid fibroblast-like cells are fused with any one of a number of different immortal cell lines, the resultant hybrid cells behave like the normal cell parent in that they have a limited ability to proliferate in culture. This observation led us to postulate that the limited doubling potential of normal cells was due to a positive genetic program and that disruption of this program could lead to cells with indefinite division potential. This idea has been confirmed in later experiments in which we have been able to assign immortal cells into a limited number of complementation groups for finite in vitro lifespan.

If cellular aging is programmed, then what is the end project of the program? We know that the result of completing the program is the cessation of cell proliferation. We have found that senescent human diploid fibroblasts produce a protein that blocks the initiation of DNA synthesis when added to cultures of young proliferation competent cells. A similar inhibitor has been found in young human diploid fibroblasts which have been blocked in the G1 phase of the cell cycle by growth factor deprivation. The inhibitor from quiescent cells is rapidly reversible upon addition of growth factors whereas expression of the senescent cell inhibitor does not respond to growth factor stimulation.

An attractive hypothesis is that the inhibitor in young quiescent cells is inducible by growth factor deprivation but is expressed constitutively in senescent cells. If there is a program for cellular aging, then it must "play out" over a period of 100-200 cell divisions in normal human cells and it must function in hybrid cells between normal and immortal cells.

At present we do not know the molecular mechanisms controlling the expression of this program, but isolation and molecular cloning of the gene(s) coding for the senescent cell inhibitor will allow us to begin to study this problem.

Acknowledgements

Supported by grants from The United States Public Health Service, AG-04749, AG-05333, T32-CA-09197, and RR-05425.

REFERENCES

1. L. Hayflick, The limited in vitro lifetime of human diploid cell strains, Exp. Cell Res., 37:614 (1965).
2. O. M. Pereira-Smith and J. R. Smith, Evidence for the recessive nature of cellular immortality, Science, 221:964 (1983).
3. T. H. Norwood, W. R. Pendergrass, C. A. Sprague and G. M. Martin, Dominance of the senescent phenotype in heterokaryons between replicative and post replicative human fibroblast like cells, Proc. Natl. Acad. Sci, USA, 71:223 (1974).
4. G. H. Stein and R. M. Yanishevsky, Entry into S phase is inhibited in two immortal cell lines fused to senescent human diploid cells, Exp. Cell Res., 120:155 (1979).
5. G. C. Burmer, H. Motulsky, C. J. Ziegler and T. H. Norwood, Inhibition of DNA synthesis in young cycling human diploid fibroblast like cells upon fusion to enucleate cytoplasts from senecent cells, Exp. Cell Res., 145:79 (1983).
6. C. K. Drescher-Lincoln and J. R. Smith, Inhibition of DNA synthesis in proliferating human diploid fibroblasts by fusion with senescent cytoplasts, Exp. Cell Res., 144:455 (1983).
7. C. K. Drescher-Lincoln and J. R. Smith, Inhibition of DNA synthesis in senescent-proliferating human cybrids is mediated by endogenous proteins, Exp. Cell Res., 153:208 (1984).
8. O. M. Pereira-Smith, S. F. Fisher and J. R. Smith, Senescent and quiescent cell inhibitors of DNA synthesis: membrane-associated proteins, Exp. Cell Res., 160:297 (1985).
9. P. S. Rabinovitch and T. H. Norwood, Comparative heterokaryon study of cellular senescence and the serum deprived state, Exp. Cell Res., 130:101 (1980).
10. C. K. Lumpkin, Jr., J. K. McClung, O. M. Pereira-Smith and J. R. Smith, Existence of high abundance antiproliferative mRNA's in senescent human diploid fibroblasts, Science, 232:393 (1986).
11. J. M. Bishop, Viral oncogenes, Cell, 42:23 (1985).
12. T. Hunter, Oncogenes and proto-oncogenes: how do they differ?, JNCI, 73:773 (1984).
13. B. M. Sefton, I. S. Trowbridge, J. A. Cooper and E. M. Scolnick, The transforming proteins of Rous sarcoma virus, Harvey sarcoma virus and Abelson virus contain tightly bound lipid. Cell, 31:465 (1982).
14. M. C. Willingham, I. Pastan, T. Y. Shih and E. M. Schonick, Localization of the src gene product of the Harvey strain of MSV to plasma membrane of transformed cells by electron microscopic immuno-cytochemistry, Cell, 19:1005 (1980).
15. C. Shih and R. A. Weinberg, Isolation of a transforming sequence from a human bladder carcinoma line, Cell, 29:161 (1982).
16. J. R. Feramisco, M. Gross, T. Kamata, M. Rosenberg and R. W. Sweet, Microinjection of the oncogene form of the human H-ras (T-24) protein results in rapid proliferation of quiescent cells, Cell 38:109 (1984).

17. L. S. Mulcahy, M. R. Smith and D. W. Stacey, Requirement for ras proto-oncogene function during serum stimulated growth of NIH3T3 cells, *Nature* (London), 313:241 (1985).

18. E. Taparowsky, Y. Suard, O. Fasano, K. Shimizu, M. Goldfarb and M. Wigler, Activation of the T24 bladder carcinoma transforming gene is linked to a single amino acid change, *Nature* (London), 300:762 (1982).

19. R. Bernards, A. Houweling, P. I. Schrier, J. L. Bos and A. J. van der Eb, Characterization of cells transformed by Ad5/Ad12 hybrid early region I plasmids, *Virology*, 120:422 (1982).

20. S. D. Gorman and V. J. Cristofalo, Reinitiation of cellular DNA synthesis in BrdU-selected nondividing senescent WI-38 cells by simian virus 40 infection, *J. Cell. Physiol.*, 125:122 (1985).

21. T. Ide, Y. Tsuji, S. Ishibashi, Y. Mitsui and M. Toba, Induction of host DNA synthesis in senescent human diploid fibroblasts by infection with human cytomegalovirus, *Mech. Ageing Dev.*, 25:227 (1984).

22. Y. Tsuji, T. Ide and S. Ishibashi, Correlation between the presence of T antigen and the reinitiation of host DNA synthesis in senescent human diploid fibroblasts after SV40 infection, *Exp. Cell Res.*, 144:165 (1983).

23. T. H. Norwood, W. R. Pendergrass and G. M. Martin, Reinitiation of DNA synthesis in senescent human fibroblasts upon fusion with cells of unlimited growth potential, *J. Cell Biol.*, 64:551 (1975).

24. G. H. Stein, R. M. Yanishevsky, L. Gordon and M. Beeson, Carcinogen-transformed human cells are inhibited from entry into S phase by fusion to senescent cells but cells transformed by DNA tumor viruses overcome the inhibition, *Proc. Natl. Acad. Sci. USA*, 79:5287 (1982).

25. R. E. Lanford and J. S. Butel, Construction and characterization of an SV40 mutant defective in nuclear transport of T antigen, *Cell*, 37:801 (1984).

INFORMATION CONTENT OF BIOLOGICAL SURVIVAL CURVES

ARISING IN AGING EXPERIMENTS: SOME FURTHER THOUGHTS

Matthew Witten

Dept. of Community Health, University of Louisville
Louisville, KY 40292 USA

INTRODUCTION

The biology of aging can be investigated at a variety of complexity levels; from the molecular level of organization to the population(demographic) level of organization. At the demographic level of organization, one of the easiest measurements(or observations) to make is the number of individuals $N(t)$ that are alive at a given time t (Observe that this is equivalent to knowing a lifespan distribution). If the population is closed to the outside world(no migration, etc.), then the only force for change, in the population, is birth and death. Further, given that the population is unisexual, we may eliminate population changes due to reproduction. Thus, we end up with death as the only force for change in our population under observation. Such populations, as I have just described, are standard in most aging experiments, such as diet restiction experiments.

Given that we know N_0 the initial number of individuals in the population, and given that we have a nonreproducing, closed population, then the fraction of the population that survives until a given time t , denoted $S(t)$ the *survival fraction*, is given simply by the ratio of the individuals alive at time t to the initial number of individuals in that population. That is,

$$S(t) = \frac{N(t)}{N_0} \tag{1}$$

The *percent survival*, denoted $\%S(t)$, is given by

$$\%S(t) = 100 \times S(t) = \frac{100 \times N(t)}{N_0} \tag{2}$$

In the engineering sciences, the term $S(t)$ is often called the *reliability* of the system, and it is usually denoted by the symbol $R(t)$. As a quick remark, observe that $S(t)$ is also a probability distribution(In fact, it is a cumulative probability distribution describing the cumulative probability of surviving until a given time t

This is so as, at most, N_0 of the organisms might be alive yielding

$$S(t) = \frac{N_0}{N_0} = 1 \tag{3}$$

Further, none of the organisms might be alive; yielding $S(t) = 0$. Hence, $S(t)$ satisfies the following relationship: $0 \leq S(t) \leq 1$. Additionally, S(t) is always a positive number. These conditions tell us that $S(t)$ is some type of probability distribution. Figure 1 illustrates a hypothetical survival curve. Observe that such a survival curve may be interpreted as the probability of being alive until at least time t . The probability of not surviving until time t (of having lifespan less than time t) is called the *failure distribution*. This distribution is denoted by the symbol $F(t)$ (U(t) in engineering as it is thought of as the *unreliability*) and it is given by

$$F(t) = 1 - S(t) \tag{4}$$

Figure 2 illustrates the failure distribution for the survival distribution illustrated in Figure 1 .

If, as we mentioned earlier, we consider a closed population, then the *growth rate* of the population, at time t , is just the rate of change of the number of individuals $N(t)$ at time t . This rate of change is just the derivative

$$\frac{dN(t)}{dt} \tag{5}$$

Observe that if I scale this derivative by N_0 , I have the following relationship between the rate of change of $N(t)$ and the survival curve $S(t)$

$$\frac{1}{N_0}\frac{dN(t)}{dt} = \frac{d}{dt}\left(\frac{N(t)}{N_0}\right) = \frac{d}{dt}S(t) = \frac{dS(t)}{dt} \tag{6}$$

That is, modulo a scale factor, the growth rate of the population is related to the rate of change of survival. Let us go one step further. The *per capita growth rate*, of a population, is given by $r(t)$ where

$$r(t) = \frac{1}{N(t)}\frac{dN(t)}{dt} \tag{7}$$

In general, $r(t)$ is defined to be the difference between two per capita growth rates

$$r(t) = b(t) - \lambda(t) \tag{8}$$

where $b(t)$ is the per capita birth rate and $\lambda(t)$ is the per capita death rate. However, in our population, there are no births. Hence, the per capita growth rate $r(t)$ simplifies to

$$r(t) = -\lambda(t) \tag{9}$$

Combining equations(7) and (9), we see that the per capita death rate may be written as follows.

$$\lambda(t) = -\frac{1}{N(t)}\frac{dN(t)}{dt} \tag{10}$$

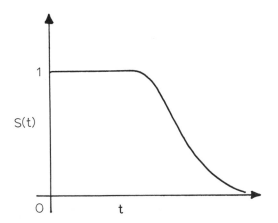

Fig.1. An illustration of an hypothetical survival curve

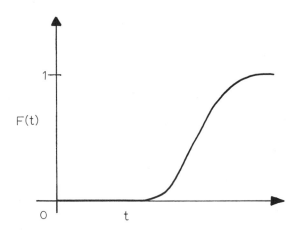

Fig.2. An illustration of the failure curve associated with Fig.1.

That is, the per capita death rate is just the negative of the per capita rate of change of the population distribution. Suppose that I now divide and multiply equation(10) through by N_0 as follows

$$\frac{N_0}{N_0}\lambda(t) = -\frac{N_0}{N_0} \cdot \frac{1}{N(t)}\frac{dN(t)}{dt} \tag{11}$$

We may rearrange equation(11) to look as follows

$$\lambda(t) = -\left(\frac{N_0}{N(t)}\right) \cdot \frac{d}{dt}\left(\frac{N(t)}{N_0}\right) \tag{12}$$

(remember that N_0 is a constant so that I can factor it in and out of taking the derivative). A quick look at equation(1) shows us that equation(12) may be rewritten as

$$\lambda(t) = -\frac{1}{S(t)}\frac{dS(t)}{dt} \tag{13}$$

That is, $\lambda(t)$ is a per capita rate of change of survival. In engineering jargon, $\lambda(t)$ is called the *instantaneous failure rate*; the biological equivalent is the *mortality rate*. We may interpret $\lambda(t)$ as the probability of surviving until time $t + \Delta t$ given that we have survived until a time t (Hence, $\lambda(t)$ is a *conditional probability*).

From equation(4)(taking the derivative of both sides), we have

$$\frac{d}{dt}S(t) = \frac{d}{dt}(1 - F(t)) = -\frac{dF(t)}{dt} \tag{14}$$

or

$$\frac{dF(t)}{dt} = -\frac{dS(t)}{dt} \tag{15}$$

However, the lefthandside of equation(15) represents the density function for the failure distribution. That is, if we let $m(t)$ be the density function, then

$$F(t) = \int_0^t m(\tau)d\tau \tag{16}$$

From this, we see that the probability of having a lifespan less than t is the integral of the function $m(t)$. The function $m(t)$ is called the *mortality* of the population at time t. Figures 3–4 illustrate our mortality and mortality rate curves for our hypothetical example.

POSSIBLE FUNCTIONAL FORMS FOR THE MORTALITY RATE

When considering possible forms for the mortality rate function $\lambda(t)$, there are a wide variety of possibilities. Some of these possibilities are based upon biological data, some upon intuition, and others upon conjecture. Among the most widely used functional forms are the following:

$$\lambda(t) = \eta t^{\beta-1} \tag{17a}$$

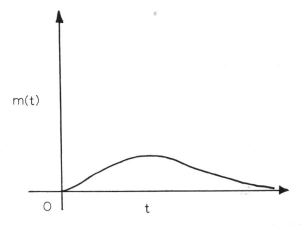

Fig.3. An illustration of the mortality curve associated with Fig.1.

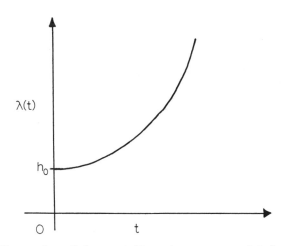

Fig.4. An illustration of the mortality rate curve associated with Fig.1.

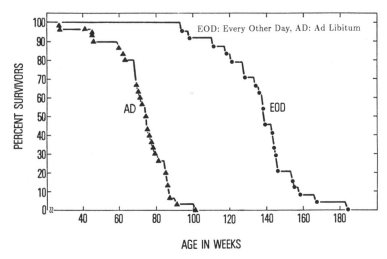

Fig.5. An illustration of sample survival curves from Goodrick et al.[8]

This two parameter mortality rate gives rise to the Weibull survival distribution having the functional form

$$S(t) = \exp\left(-\frac{\eta}{\beta}t^{\beta}\right) \tag{17b}$$

If we were to choose a mortality rate function of the form,

$$\lambda(t) = h_0 e^{\gamma t} \tag{18}$$

we would find that this mortality rate form gives rise to the Gompertz distribution(see equation(21) below). The mortality rate function

$$\lambda(t) = h_0 e^{\gamma t} + C \tag{19}$$

gives rise to the Gompertz–Makeham distribution. Finally, the constant mortality rate function

$$\lambda(t) = h_0 \tag{20a}$$

gives rise to the simple exponential survival distribution

$$S(t) = e^{-h_0 t} \tag{20b}$$

A discussion of how each of these distributions arise, in a biological context, may be found in Witten[1–6] and in Finch and Witten[7].

Historically, for aging experiments, the survival distribution of choice has been the Gompertzian survival distribution. The Gompertz survival distribution is given, mathematically, as follows

$$S(t) = \exp\left[\frac{h_0}{\gamma}\left(1 - e^{\gamma t}\right)\right] \tag{21}$$

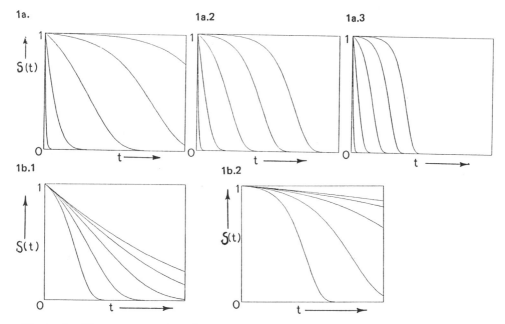

Fig.6. An illustration of the effect of varying the two Gompertz rate parameters

where h_0 is the *age–independent* mortality rate coefficient and γ is the *age–dependent* mortality rate coefficient. One can show(with a little calculus), that as γ goes to zero, equation(21) reduces to the exponential(or wild) type survival distribution. Thus, the exponential distribution is a special case of the Gompertz survival distribution; the case in which there is no age–related force of mortality. Figure 5 illustrates sample survival and mortality rate curves from the studies of Goodrick et al.[8]. Figure 6 illustrates the effect of varying the two Gompertz rate parameters h_0 and γ on the form of the Gompertz survival distribution.

Other survival distributions have been used to model aging processes. Among these are the Weibull and the truncated Gaussian distribution. We will examine these distributions at a later point in the discussion.

MIXTURE MODELS I

Many investigators have voiced the opinion that the Gompertz distribution is not accurate in the neonatal portion of the lifespan(Figures 7–8). This issue has been addressed in Witten[5].

In order to correct this problem, Witten[5] constructed a mixture of two distributions(or population survival curves); an exponential survival curve to model the neonatal failure and a Gompertz survival curve to model the non–neonatal component of the population. This is not an unrealistic approach as one either dies in the neonatal years(group 1 member) or one does not die in the neonatal years(group 2 member). Hence, we can consider a population as being composed of two components: the neonatal failures and the non–neonatal failures.

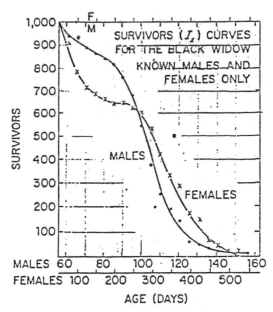

Fig.7. An illustration of non–Gompertzian survival in spiders

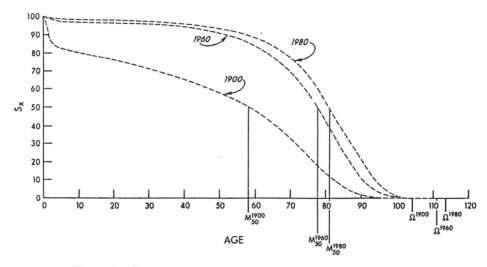

Fig.8. An illustration of non–Gompertzian survival in humans

Let $F(t)$ be the *cumulative failure distribution function* that is given by the following

$$F(t) = 1 - S(t) \tag{22}$$

Suppose that our population is comprised of the two aforementioned groups; each having independent failure distributions. That is, a failure(death) in group 1 affects nobody in group 2 and vice versa. Assume that group 1 comprises proportion p of the total population and that it has failure distribution $F_1(t)$. Hence, group 2 comprises proportion $(1 - p)$ of the population and has failure distribution $F_2(t)$. Consequently, we may express the total failure distribution $F(t)$ of the population as the weight(by their representative fractions) sum of the two failure distributions of the component groups. This is given as follows

$$F(t) = pF_1(t) + (1 - p)F_2(t) \tag{23}$$

Let us consider how such a model might be applied to survival distributions of the type analyzed in senescence studies. Suppose that $F_1(t)$ represents the distribution describing the failure of the neonatal or weak components. Such a set of components is often described by exponential or nearly exponential survival curves. These survival curves may be written as follows

$$F_1(t) = 1 - \exp\left[-\left(\frac{t}{\alpha_1}\right)\right] \tag{24}$$

where α_1 represents the expected lifespan of the short–lived component of the population.

Our second failure distribution could then be chosen to describe the bulk of the post–weak or short–lived state. As we have been discussing biological survival, it is natural to choose a Gompertzian reliability(survival) function $S_2(t)$ where

$$S_2(t) = \exp\left[\frac{h_0}{\gamma}\left(1 - e^{\gamma t}\right)\right] \tag{25}$$

Hence,

$$F_2(t) = 1 - S_2(t) = 1 - \exp\left[\frac{h_0}{\gamma}\left(1 - e^{\gamma t}\right)\right] \tag{26}$$

Combining equations(24) and (26) yields the total failure distribution

$$F(t) = p\left[1 - \exp\left(-\left[\frac{t}{\alpha_1}\right]\right)\right] + (1 - p)\left[1 - \exp\left(\frac{h_0}{\gamma}\left(1 - e^{\gamma t}\right)\right)\right]$$

Figure 9 illustrates quantitative curves for the two group survival distribution. Figure 10 illustrates the corresponding instantaneous failure rate curves.

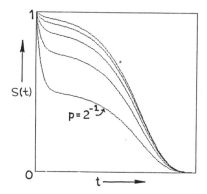

Fig.9. An illustration of the quantitative dynamics of our two–group survival model.

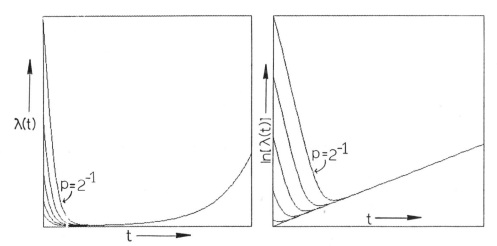

Fig.10. An illustration of the quantitative dynamics of the failure rate curves for Fig.9.

MIXTURE MODELS II:

Numerous investigators, Economos[9]; E. Masoro and B.P. Yu; and T. Johnson(personal communication) have communicated their dissatisfaction with the Gompertzian survival distribution as an adequate descriptor for the geriatric portion of the population. In general, the Gompertzian has a more rapidly decreasing geriatric tail than does the normal population that it is intended to model. Figures 11–12 illustrate sample comparisons of the actual survival versus the Gompertzian theoretical prediction. It is quite clear that the Gompertzian tail does not adequately model the geriatric decline in the illustrated population groups. It is this issue that we now wish to address. And, in doing so, we will present what we believe to be the survival distribution of choice in aging studies.

In order to construct this model, we will postulate that a closed, age–structured population is comprised of individuals of three types; a neonatal failure type, a Gompertzian failure type, and a neonatal failure type. That we make such a mixture assumption may seem surprising, as it is usually assumed that individuals in the population age according to exponential survival distributions. However, in Guess and Witten[10], we show that it is not possible to obtain Gompertzian or Weibull(with increasing mortality rate) dynamics from *any* mixture of exponential survival distributions. Therefore, it becomes crucial to assume that the population is composed of a mixture of individuals whose survival curves form a mixture of distributions; some of which are not the exponential distribution. Hence, we have that the overall failure rate of the population is a combination of the failure rates of all three subgroups of the population. It is important to realize that, while we postulate the existence of these three population subgroups, statistical analysis must verify the significance of the population(mixture) proportion coefficients. Should a population proportion coefficient be statistically insignificant, then this would imply that the corresponding mixture component of the population is not significant in contributing to the survival dynamics of the given data set.

It will also be of interest to examine how transitions from the various population subgroups might affect the shape of the survival curve. Hence, as we build the new model, we will generalize it in such a manner as to allow myself the ability to study such transitions. The allowed transitions are illustrated in Figure 13 .

With these requirements in mind, let me now discuss the new survival model.

Let me suppose that we have a closed population which, at time $t = 0$ (start time), is composed of three types of individual; N_1 the total number of short–lived individuals, N_2 the total number of Gompertz–like individuals, and N_3 the total number of long–lived individuals. It then follows that the total number of individuals in the population(at the start time) is given by the following equation.

$$N_T^{(0)} = N_1^{(0)} + N_2^{(0)} + N_3^{(0)} \tag{27}$$

where $N_T^{(0)}$ is the total number of individuals in the population at time $t = 0$ (indicated by the superscript (0)). In terms of the fractions of each group in the population, we may write equation(27) as follows.

$$1 = p_1^{(0)} + p_2^{(0)} + p_3^{(0)} \tag{28a}$$

where $p_i^{(0)} = N_i^{(0)}/N_T^{(0)}$ $i = 1, 2, 3$ is the fraction of the ith group in the population at time $t = 0$. Thus, if $F_i(t)$ is the *failure distribution* for the ith

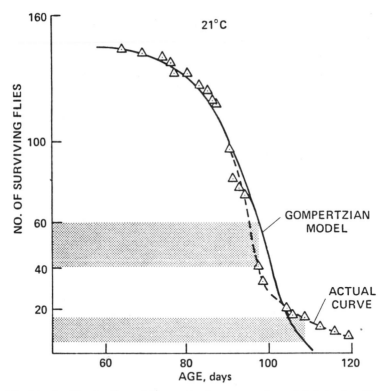

Fig.11. An illustration of theoretical vs. experimental data for flies.

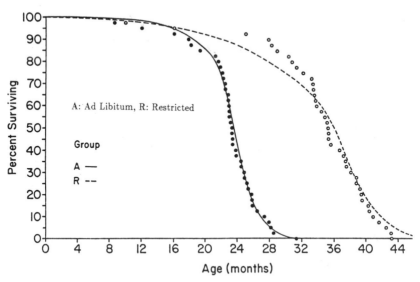

Fig.12. An illustration of theoretical vs. experimental data for rats.

subgroup of the population, then the total failure distribution of the population is
given by the following equation.

$$F(t) = p_1 F_1(t) + p_2 F_2(t) + p_3 F_3(t) \tag{28b}$$

(see Witten[5] for a discussion on how one would construct equation(28b)). We also
wish to be able to determine the various effects of transitions, from groups 1 and
2 to group 3 , on the survival curve of the whole population.

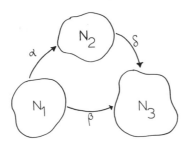

Fig.13. An illustration of the allowed transitions in the three–group survival model.

Without excessive details(see Witten[11–12]), we may show that the three group
model can be defined in terms of the following three transition fractions

δ : fraction of N_2 that become N_3

α : fraction of N_1 that become N_2

β : fraction of N_1 that become N_3

and the three initial population fractions $p_i^{(0)}$. Given prior knowledge of these
parameter values, we may define a three group population failure distribution by
the following function.

$$F(t) = \left[(1 - \alpha - \beta)p_1^{(0)}\right] F_1(t) + \left[(1 - \delta)p_2^{(0)} + \alpha p_1^{(0)}\right] F_2(t)+$$

$$\left[1 - (\beta - 1)p_1^{(0)} + (\delta - 1)p_2^{(0)}\right] F_3(t) \tag{29}$$

If we now wish to study the survival of a population, comprised of particular proportions $p_i^{(0)}$, we simply set all of the transition fractions $\alpha = \beta = \gamma = 0$. Then,

for a given set of population proportions, we can determine the total population survival function.

In order to make use of a model of the type that we have been discussing, it is important to define the survival functions for the various groups in the population. In Witten[5], we discussed how the neonatal component of the population might be modeled by an exponential survival distribution. This survival distribution has the form

$$R_1(t) = \exp\left[-\frac{t}{\tau_e}\right] \tag{30a}$$

The failure(non-survival) distribution is given by the following equation.

$$F_1(t) = 1 - R_1(t) = 1 - \exp\left[-\frac{t}{\tau_e}\right] \tag{30b}$$

where τ_e is a time constant that tunes how rapidly the survival curve describing the neonatal component of the population decays. In this same paper(Witten[5]), we discussed how the $(i = 2)$ group might be modeled by a Gompertzian distribution having the form

$$R_2(t) = \exp\left[\frac{h_0}{\gamma}\left(1 - e^{\gamma t}\right)\right] \tag{31a}$$

and which has a failure distribution given by

$$F_2(t) = 1 - \exp\left[\frac{h_0}{\gamma}\left(1 - e^{\gamma t}\right)\right] \tag{31b}$$

I demonstrated how this new model correctly embedded the dynamics of neonatal population elements into the biological survival curve.

I now wish to model the $(i = 3)$ geriatric or long–lived portion of the population. In Witten[11–12] we discussed the problem with the Gompertz distribution's not modeling the experimental survival tails in an adequate manner. In that same paper, we introduced the time t_{infl} at which the Gompertz distribution $R_2(t)$ is linear. That is, t_{infl} is the time point at which $R_2(t)$ may be truly approximated by a straight line. One can show that t_{infl}, being an inflection point of the curve, must satisfy the following requirement on the second derivative.

$$\frac{d^2 R_2(t_{infl})}{dt^2} = 0 \tag{32a}$$

After some algebra, it is relatively straightforward to show that t_{infl} must be given by the following equation.

$$t_{infl} = -\frac{1}{\gamma}\ln\left(\frac{h_0}{\gamma}\right) \tag{32b}$$

Of obvious interest is the fact that the inflection time is independent of any percentile boundary and is soley a function of the Gompertzian parameters h_0 and γ. Table 1 illustrates various estimates for h_0, γ, and t_{infl} for a variety of experimental datasets.

In order to obtain a more qualitative understanding of how the inflection time changes with the various changes in h_0, let us consider the following sequence of figures 14–15 (already illustrated in Witten[4]). In Figure 14, we show the Gompertzian survival distribution for fixed age–dependent mortality coefficient γ and

TABLE [1]

This table illustrates Gompertzian survival curve parameters for various species, as estimated from the experimental survival curves.

ORGANISM	INVESTIGATOR	h_0	γ	τ_{infl}
C. elegans(m)	T. Johnson	0.000564	0.307	20.52
C. elegans(h)	T. Johnson	0.00535	0.153	21.92
Aplysia	Hirsch and Peretz	0.000897	0.0189	161.26
Aplysia (different estimate procedure)	Hirsch and Peretz	0.00134	0.01625	153.38
Mice	Liu et al.	0.1428	0.0097	140.35
Rats (Group 1)	Yu et al.	0.00000598	0.0099	746.16
Rats (Group 2)	Yu et al.	0.00000211	0.00727	1119.48
Rats (Group 3)	Yu et al.	0.00000223	0.0098	855.31
Rats (Group 4)	Yu et al.	0.00001596	0.0057	1026.23

The data presented above is a sample of estimates from over 155 different data sets, covering 13 different species. Our studies show that the relationship $h_0/\gamma \leqslant 1$ is satisfied for every dataset. This relationship is of interest as it is predicted by the requirement that the inflection time $t_{infl} \geqslant 0$.

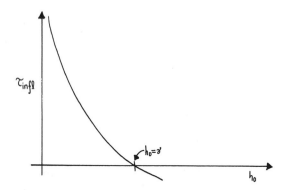

Fig.14. An illustration of how the inflection time varies with varied h_0 .

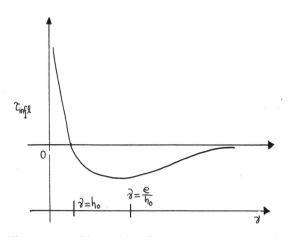

Fig.15. An illustration of how the inflection time varies with varied γ .

varying age–independent mortality coefficient h_0 . Superimposed upon this figure is the changing inflection time. Figure[15] repeats this illustration for fixed age–independent mortality coefficient h_0 and varying age–dependent mortality coefficient γ .

In order that an individual in the population be considered as part of the geriatric component of the population, we will assume that the given individual must survive until a time $t = t_{infl}$. We make this assumption for two reasons. First, because one must have some marker for a geriatric element of the population, some timepoint must be chosen as the delineation point. Thus, while any point might be chosen, such as the t_{90} boundary point, we might equally well choose our inflection time. Second, because of the nature of the inflection time in that it is only dependent upon the Gompertzian parameters, it seems that such independence might serve as a possible signal in terms of choosing which timepoint should be utilized as the geriatric demarkation point. Again, we emphasize that the importance of the inflection point lies in the fact that it is an *investigator unbiased* point in time. And, as such, is of experimental value. I will further assume that an exponential decrease occurs, in the survival distribution, after the geriatric boundary point. These assumptions are consistant with the discussion of Economos[9], in which he points out that *"the data available today show that Gompertz's law is an approximation. For most species, the force of mortality and probability of death cease to increase exponentially with age, after a certain species characteristic age, and remain on the average at a high constant rate for the rest of the lifespan."* These types of problems have been further pointed up in personal discussions with Masoro, Yu, and with Johnson.

Hence, we shall now propose a *"geriatric survival distribution"* of the form

$$R_3(t) = \begin{cases} 1 & t \le t_{infl} \\ e^{-\lambda(t-t_{infl})} & t > t_{infl} \end{cases} \tag{33a}$$

Notice that this curve, which is illustrated in Figure 9 states that one must survive until the inflection time t_{infl} before one begins to have an exponential decay in survival probability(such a distribution is called a shifted exponential survival distribution). This is akin to stating that, until one reaches a certain age, one is not yet going to age as the old component of the population would age. The failure distribution $F_3(t)$ is just

$$F_3(t) = \begin{cases} 0 & t \le t_{tinfl} \\ 1 - e^{-\lambda(t-t_{infl})} & t > t_{infl} \end{cases} \tag{33b}$$

Notice that equation(33b) says that the probability of having lifespan less than t_{infl} is zero, if you are to be considered in the *"old"* component of the population. Figures 16–17 illustrate same curves utilizing the three group model approach. Notice that they more accurately reflect the qualitative behavior of a survival curve over the complete lifespan of the population.

In order to understand the biological importance of the inflection time t_{infl} , let us consider a simple example from the literature. In Figure 18 of this paper, we reproduce Figure 2 of Lang et al.[13]. This figure illustrates the relationship of GSH content and percentage survival of the adult mosquito. Of great interest is the fact that Lang et al.[13] plot the glutathione content versus the percent survival; thereby

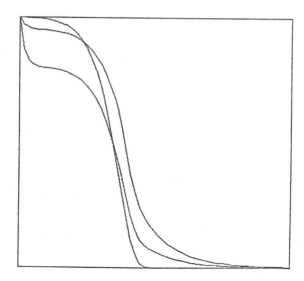

Fig.16. An illustration of the three–group survival model dynamics.

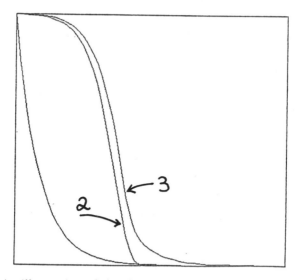

Fig.17. An illustration of the three–group survival model dynamics.

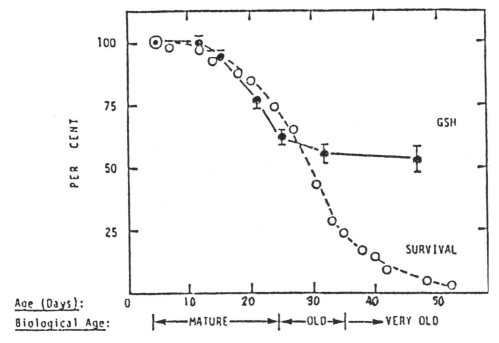

Fig.18. An illustration of the original Lang et al. data

relating a physiological observation to a survival or demographic level observation. In Figure 19 , we superimpose on the Lang figure a linear extrapolation line and we argue that this gives a qualitative location for the inflection point. From this, we may then determine the inflection time t_{infl} . Observe that the inflection time occurs in what Lang calls the *old* domain of the mosquito lifespan. Further, of interest is the fact that the glutathione level flattens out in a region very tightly described by the *inflection region* around the inflection point of linear portion of the survival curve.

A qualitative relationship of this sort can only suggest possible value, it cannot support such value. In order to further establish the value of using the *inflection time* as a population level biomarker, we turned to a larger database of information. Arking et al.[14] and Luckinbill et al.[15] have both investigated genetically long–lived *D. melanogaster* strains. Arking et al.[16] has examined the relationship between survival and drop in fertility. The detailed mathematical analysis and discussion may be found in Witten et al.[17]. Of importance to this discussion in the fact that Arking et al. determined that there was a drop in NDCL(non-density controlled long– lived group, n=13 groups) during the time interval $[44.85, 74.89]$ days. The fertility drop for the wild(short–lived) strain occured during the time interval $[17.32, 56.2]$ days(n=6 groups). Using the survival data from these groups, we were able to calculate the inflection times(using maximum likelihood estimation techniques) and determine inflection time intervals. For the NDCL group, the average inflection time was 62.31 with a standard error of 13.36 days. Notice that this falls right over the fertilty drop interval. For the R group, the average inflection time was 51.59 days with a standard error of 5.45 days. Observe that this falls over the upper end of our fertility drop interval. We believe that this discrepancy is

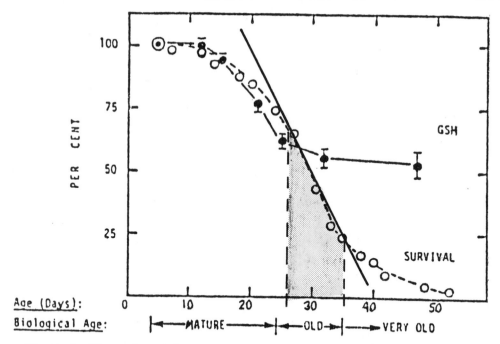

Fig.19. An illustration of the Lang data with the inflection point superimposed.

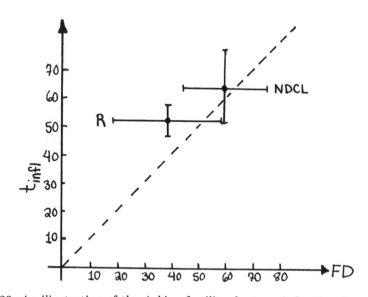

Fig.20. An illustration of the Arking fertility drop vs. inflection time data

due to the small sample size that we have for the wild group. Figure 20 illustrates a simple plot of these results.

Again, this sort of data is only suggestive and further experiments need to be done to strengthen the concept of the *inflection time*. However, we can begin to see that these results suggest that age–related changes can be seen in the region of the *inflection point* on the survival curve. Hence, if one can make a reasonable estimation of where such a point might lie, then the evidence(small though it is) suggests that investigations should look in this region for age–related changes in a given organism. From the point of view of cost–effective experimentation, such knowledge would be most useful.

ACKNOWLEDGEMENTS

Many people have contributed their time in discussion and/or data for the various phases of my research into survival distributions in aging. I cannot begin to thank them all. I would, however, like to make special mention of the contributions of the following individuals: Robert Arking, C.E. Finch, David Harrison, Tom Johnson, Calvin Lang, B.P. Yu, and Edward Masoro.

REFERENCES

1 M. Witten, A return to time, cells, systems and ageing: Rethinking the concepts of senescence in mammalian systems, Mech. Ageing and Dev. 21 :69 (1983).

2 M. Witten, Investigating the aging mammalian system: Cellular levels and beyond, Proc. 1981 Soc. For General Systems Research: 309 (1981).

3 M. Witten, A return to time, cells, systems, and aging: II. Relational and reliability theoretic approaches to the study of senescence in living systems, Mech. Ageing and Dev., 27:323 (1984).

4 M. Witten, A return to time, cells, systems, and aging: III. Gompertzian models of biological aging and some possible roles for critical elements, Mech. Ageing and Dev., 32:141 (1985).

5 M. Witten. A return to time, cells, systems, and aging: IV. Further thoughts on Gompertzian survival dynamics—The neonatal years, Mech. Ageing and Dev., 33:177 (1986).

6 M. Witten, Reliability theoretic methods and aging: Critical elements, hierarchies, and longevity– interpreting survival curves, (in) Molecular Biology Of Aging(eds.)A. Woodhead, A. Blackett, and A. Hollaender(Plenum Press, N.Y., 1985).

7 C.E. Finch and M. Witten, Mortality rates and the lifespan: Why a fly can't live as long as a man, unpublished manuscript.

8 C.L. Goodrick, D.K. Ingram, M.A. Reynolds, J.R. Freeman, and N.L. Cider, Differential effects of intermittent feeding and voluntary exercise on body weight and lifespan in adult rats, J. Gerontol., 28(1983)36-45.

9 A. Economos, A non–Gompertzian paradigm for mortality kinetics of metazoan animals and failure kinetics of manufactured products, Age 2(1979)74–76.

10 F. Guess and M. Witten, A population of exponentially distributed individual lifespans cannot lead to Gompertzian or Weibull(with increasing mortality rate) dynamics, unpublished manuscript.

11 M. Witten, Predicting maximum lifespan and other lifespan variables in lifespan studies: Some useable results and formulae, The Gerontologist, 25:215 (1985).

12 M. Witten, A return to time cells, systems, and aging: V. The geriatric years, unpublished manuscript.

13 G. Hazelton and C.A. Lang, Glutathione levels during the mosquito lifespan with emphasis on senescence(41867), Prof. Soc. Exper. Biol. and Med., 176:249 (1984).

14 R. Arking and M. Clare, Genetics of aging: Effective selection for increased longevity in Drosophila,(in) Comparative Biology Of Insect Aging: Strategies And Mechanisms, (eds.) K. Collatz and R. Sohal(Springer–Verlag, Berlin, 1986).

15 L.S. Luckinbill, R. Arking, M.J. Clare, W.C. Cirocco, and S.A. Buck, Selection for delayed senescence in Drosophila melanogaster, Evolution 38:996(1984).

16 R. Arking, Successful selection for increased longevity in Drosophila: Analysis of survival data and presentation of a hypothesis on the genetic regulation of longevity, (1986) unpublished manuscript.

17 M. Witten and R. Arking, Theoretical analysis of longevity changes in increased longevity strains of Drosophila melanogaster, in preparation.

18 B.P. Yu, E.J. Masoro, I. Murata, H.A. Bertrand, and F.T. Lynd, Lifespan study of SPF Fisher 344 male rats fed Ad Libitum or restricted diets: Longevity, growth, lean body mass, and disease, J. Gerontology 37:130 (1982).

19 P.H. Jacobson, Cohort survival for generations since 1840, Milbank Memorial Fund Quarterly, 42:36 (1964).

20 T.E. Johnson and W.B. Wood, Genetic analysis of lifespan in Caenorhabditis elegans Proc. Nat . Acad. Sci. USA, 79:6603 (1982).

21 B.L. Strehler, Time, Cells, and Aging (Academic Press, N.Y., 1977).

22 J. Smith–Sonneborn, Programmed increased longevity induced by weak pulsating current in Paramecium Bioelectrochemistry and Bioenergetics 11:373 (1983).

23 G.C. Meyers and K. Manton, Compression of mortality: Myth or Reality? The Gerontologist, 24:346 (1984).

24 National Center For Health Statistics, Vital statistics of the United States, 1980 11, Section 6, Life Tables. DHHS Publication Number (PHS)84–1104. Public Health Service, Washington. Government Printing Office. 1984.

APPENDIX I

After having typeset this manuscript, I realized that I had failed to insert a number of important points. First, I wish to acknowledge that Figure 7 of this paper came from Comfort's classic on aging. Figure 8 was given to me by K. Manton. Figure 9 is copied from reference [9] of this manuscript. Figure 10 is from Yu et al., J. Gerontology, **40**(1985)657–670. Finally, Figures[18–19] are from Hazelton and Lang, Proc. Soc. Exp. Biol. and Med., **176**(1984) 249–256.

Earlier in the discussion, I mentioned that I would discuss other survival distributions such as the Weibull distribution. Unfortunately, space limitations have eliminated that possibility. A thorough discussion of the topic may be found in Witten, Math. Modeling, (1987) in press.

In rereading the legends under some of the figures, it became clear that some explanation was due. Let me take a moment, though somewhat after the fact, to explain certain figures in more detail.

Figure 6 depicts the effect of varying the two Gompertz parameters h_0 and γ . These two parameters represent, respectively, the age–independent mortality rate coefficient and the age–dependent mortality rate coefficient. In the figures labeled 1a, the age–dependent mortality rate coefficient γ is fixed while the age–independent mortality rate coefficient h_0 is varied. In the figures labeled 1b, the reverse is true.

In Figures 7–8 it is important to observe that the survival curve has an early neonatal dip which can be interpreted as deaths due to neonatal or early life failure. Thus, it is not unnatural to assume that the population of interest is composed of two sub–populations; neonatal failures and non–neonatal failures. Figure 9 illustrates how changing the fraction of neonatal failures, in the population, can affect the survival curve shape. In this model, for the purposes of forcing the issue, we have chosen the following values for the parameters: $h_0 = 0.001$ and $\gamma = 0.25$. Further, we have let $p = 2^{-n} n = 1, 2, 3, 4, 5$. Figure[10] shows the basin–like behavior of the mortality rate function $\lambda(t)$. Finally, the second figure in Figure 10 illustrates the standard $\ln[\lambda(t)]$ curve. Notice the linear portion, in the latter portion of the curve. This reflects the Gompertzian component of the population. The decreasing portion of the curve illustrates the neonatal failure portion of the curve.

Figures 16–17 illustrate the variety of dynamics available to the new three group survival model. Observe how the tail of the newer model is more accurate in its description of the more slowly declining "geriatric" tail. This is particularly easy to see if one compares the curves labeled 2 and 3 in Figure 17 . Curve 2 is a pure Gompertz description while curve 3 incorporates the "geriatric" tail adjustment.

In Figure 19 we have drawn a tangent line to the survival curve. This line is somewhat inaccurate in that it is not quite possible to determine the actual inflection point. However, it is clear that there is a tangent or inflection region(the shaded area) which must contain the inflection time t_{infl} . This region, when projected down upon the time axis clearly shows that the region overlays the "old" section of the mosquito's lifespan. Thus, the inflection time t_{infl} must lie somewhere within the "old" portion of the mosquito's lifespan. Now, observe that the GSH curve begins to flatten out in this same region. Unfortunately, little data is available to address such questions as: What is the correlation between the inflection time and the onset or flattening of the GSH curve?

SYMPOSIUM DEBATE

THE MICROSCOPE (REDUCTIONIST) OR THE TELESCOPE (HOLISTIC)?

MODERATOR: Richard L. Sprott

                 National Institute on Aging
                 National Institutes of Health
                 9000 Rockville Pike
                 Bethesda, MD 20205

HOLISTIC: C. Ladd Prosser

                 Department of Physiology and Biophysics
                 University of Illinois
                 Urbana, IL 61801

REDUCTIONIST: Ronald W. Hart

                 Department of Health, Education and Welfare
                 National Center for Toxicological Research
                 Jefferson, AR 72079

Richard L. Sprott

     I think most of you here tonight know speakers quite well. I know
one of them extremely well, the other not quite so well. When this debate
was set up the organizers did not know that our two speakers have known
each other for 20 years and have been on opposite sides of the fence, although both have revised their points of view somewhat in the ensuing
years. C. Ladd Prosser is from the University of Illinois where he first
went in 1939. He was away from Illinois for 4 years during the war, when
he worked as a radiation biologist and during that period he met George
Sacher: he continued to have significant interaction with him over all the
ensuing years. Dr. Prosser is a self-described generalist with over 50
years involvement in physiology and he describes himself as trying to
alter the trend toward increasing specialization, which he feels is terri-
bly narrowing in its effects on biology. Our speakers first met when Ron
Hart was a student in Howard Ducoff's lab and took Dr. Prosser's comparative physiology course. Both of them want to tell me stories from those
days about an encounter that took place in the elevator. Maybe Dr. Hart
will finish that story for us.

     Dr. Prosser recently published a book, (Adaptational Biology, Mole-
cules to Organisms, John Wiley, 1987) in which, among other things, he
explores five different definitions of species. I asked Dr. Prosser what
he thought was the most important point he will make tonight and he feels
that he can present a cogent case for the advantages of a multi-faceted
approach to very complex problems like aging, which are under the control
of many genes. So he will present the holistic point of view.

Ronald Hart got his Ph.D. at Illinois in 1971. He was offered a postdoctoral Fellowship at Oak Ridge with Richard Setlow, but he also was offered the post of Assistant Professor at Ohio State University. He looked at the comparative advantages of regular pay, and finally opted for the best of both worlds. He spent the next three and a half years at both places, leaving Ohio State every Wednesday night, driving 417 miles to Oak Ridge and working there until Sunday evening, then driving back again. Dr. Hart went to the National Center for Toxicology Research in September, 1980 where he has instituted a system for rewarding good science and moving politics out of science. When I asked Ron what he thought was important about what he was going to say tonight, he summed it up by saying that real progress in the sciences always has been made through a dualistic approach, the combination of the holistic and reductionist points of view. Then he talked about the impact of computers, pointing out that we have acquired the scientific technology to generate tremendous amounts of particulate knowledge and the computer technology to look at this in ways that the human mind might think of, but never will have the time to do. Perhaps his view of the holistic approach is one that will be accomplished by computers. With that I am going to turn this debate over to Dr. Prosser.

C. Ladd Prosser

I am an outsider to this cause of aging. My only knowledge of aging comes from the fact that I think I am the oldest participant in this conference and I feel very much that I am aging in my entirety--in other words, in a holistic way. I am pleased to participate in a symposium honoring George Sacher. I was involved in hiring George in the metallurgical laboratory during the war years when he was a graduate student, and I kept in touch with him up until his untimely death. But I am an old timer in comparative physiology, and Ron is a mere stripling! What I want to do this evening, is to list some of the principles in holistic biology, in the hope that you will find ways in which some of them may be applicable to your areas of senescence.

My first figure indicates the hierarchical organization of living matter and shows that in this hierarchy, we have levels of organization all the way from molecules to tissues and cells, to various kinds of organisms and communities (Fig. 1). We could add societies, if we do not want to use the word community as equivalent to society. The first principle that I would state is that, at each level, there are certain principles, vocabulary, and terminology that does not apply at other levels. Extrapolation from one level to another is very difficult. In fact, some theoreticians believe that it is impossible to go from mitochondria, golgi apparatus, and microsomes even up to whole organisms. I think that we have to recognize this; while it is a very familiar concept to biologists, it is one that we sometimes lose sight of.

As related principle has to do with the thermodynamics of biological systems, as opposed to extreme reductionist systems, test-tube analyses of enzyme systems and molecular systems are usually made with the assumption that we are dealing with a closed system, in a thermodynamic sense. Living systems, on the other hand, are open thermodynamic systems. There is input and output, although for practical experimental purposes we cannot consider them fully as open system. Some limit must be imposed that varies, so I think that we have to recognize that this is an important difference between the reductionist and the holistic view, the difference between the closed and open system. Related to this is the problem of information content. Information, as it is contained in a biological system, is of two sorts. There is intrinsic information and

Biological systems can be arranged by level of organization as follows:

Communities
Independent individuals
Dependent (colonial and parasitic) organisms
Organs
Tissues
Cells
Organelles
Molecules
Atoms

Fig. 1. The hierarchical organization of living matter.

there is interactive information. The intrinsic information is that which
is contained within the organelle, within the molecules. The interactive
information is that the particular system interacts with other systems.
As you go from the molecular, to the organelle, to organismic levels,
there is an increase in integration, and correspondingly, the interactive
information of a component increases. At the same time, the information
content of the whole increases as elements are added, so that while the
information content of a component decreases that of the total system
increases. A corollary of that is the well-known aphorism that the information content of the whole is not equal to the information content of the
sum of its parts. If we take a watch apart, each part has an information
content which is different from its content when it is in the integrated
watch. Very much the same sort of reasoning could be applied to a living
system, when in general, the information of the whole may be greater or
less than the information content of the sum of the parts.

I would like to say a little about the problem of evolution and some
of the consequences of evolution. We have heard today that there are various strategies of evolution, in particular, of species evolution. As I
see it, the essence of evolution is to produce biological diversity at all
levels of taxonomy. I think that we have vastly overestimated the importance of the meaning of the term species, probably because of the tremendous impact of Darwin. I have taken issue with the species concept.
There are at least five different ways in which one can use the word species, in fact the word has so many meanings, that I do not like to use it
any more. We have the strict taxonomic species, we have the cladistic
species (that which is computerized), the biological species, as used
mainly by animal geneticists and evolutionists, and a modification with
plants, where there is a great deal more hybridization than with animals. Then I like to think of a physiological species, that is uniquely
adapted for a particular niche and geographic range. If we could describe
a set of populations with respect to their physiological adaptations to
the environment, we would have a true definition of a species, as seen by
natural selection. I think that each definition of species has validity,
and I would not wish to favor any particular one. We have been somewhat
misled by the notion of species.

I have had some debate with my friends who are worried about preserv-
ing certain endangered species. I agree that we must preserve diversity,
but a major form of diversity is that which the taxonomist assigns and I
think that here we may be missing a very important concept, namely that of
adaptation. By adaptation, I mean not only adaptation to the physical environment, but also to the biotic environment. We have to consider the

interaction between organisms, particularly the social interactions, as
determining the course of evolution. For many years I have been concerned with the adaptations of fishes to temperature. Many mechanisms are
involved in this type of adaptation, all of which have a genetic basis but
are responsive to environmental stresses. We are accustomed to using the
word homeostasis, that is, a term concerned with constancy of the internal
environment as used by Claude Bernard. But many animals have a varying
internal environment, and energy is available to them by a variety of metabolic pathways. Let us take an example of rate-functions in fish. If we
start with fish at some intermediate temperature, and drop them to a lower
temperature or raise them to a higher temperature, over a period of some
weeks the fish show a direct response, followed by a second acclimatory
response; for some individuals, this may require a very long time. During
these responses there is a tendency towards maintenance of a constancy of
energy output. I have suggested that we call this process homeokinesis,
as opposed to homeostasis. I think that it is important for us to distinguish, in terms of whole animals, that there are other kinds of adaptive
responses. Here we come to the genetic control of variation. Each organism has a certain capacity for acclimation or acclimatization, depending
upon whether one is dealing with laboratory conditions or with field conditions, and this capacity is limited by the genotype. I believe that
aging or senescence, while it is genetically programmed, also is dependent
upon the interaction between organism and environment.

The next characteristic of systems, from the holistic viewpoint, concerns those properties which we can observe in vivo, which we do not see
in vitro. This afternoon we saw extensive diagrams of metabolic pathways,
demonstrating that the level of activity of some of the enzymes in these
pathways may be different in vivo, and in vitro; usually the levels in the
whole animal are much lower than the levels studied in vitro. There are
many examples of such differences. I think that it is very frequently
difficult, if not impossible to extrapolate back to the intact animal from
studies of component molecules, enzyme systems. I will give two or three
examples from my own laboratory, of cases in which we have obtained results in vivo which we would never have predicted from in vitro studies.
One of my colleagues, John Zehr measures blood pressure over periods of
hours. We think of blood pressure as a value read on a monometer. However, when dogs are chronically implanted with catheters and pressure
gauges, one sees rhythms in blood pressure: there is an overall slow
rhythm with a period of several hours, and superimposed on this a faster
rhythm. The blood pressure curve follows a heart-rate curve. This will
never be seen by studying isolated strips of blood vessels and heart
muscle. This is a property of the whole animal, strictly a holistic property. In my own studies on the smooth muscle of the digestive tract (from
a cat), we find rhythms that we call slow waves. These rhythms have a pe-
riodicity of about 5 secs. We have been studying rhythms for many years
in in vitro systems, and we developed a hypothesis concerning their
nature. But when we went to the in vivo situation we found not only these
five second rhythms but, in addition, a very interesting new kind of
rhythm which occurs in bursts. These bursts go down the intestine and
occur at approximately hourly intervals. We have no idea how one goes
from a 5 sec. rhythm to an hourly rhythm. These hourly rhythms were never
seen in vitro. These are kinds of phenomena which are very imporant for
the life of the animal and could not be predicted from studying isolated
strips of muscle.

I am continually impressed by the very great number of safety factors
and redundancy that one sees in many physiological systems. For example,
control of blood pressure occurs at several levels: at the level of the
individual arteries, and at the level of the autonomic nervous system,
both parasympathetic and sympathetic. In addition, blood pressure is

322

controlled by several hormones, the renin-angiotensin system, by adrenalin, in addition to the ephinepherine from the sympathetic nervous system. In the intestinal system, which has been one of my interests, Australian researchers have identified 16 neuropeptides, that are all potential transmitters or modulators. Perhaps, parenthetically I can point out that each one of us has more neurons in our gut than we have in our spinal cord. I think that redundancy is a very real property of intact systems, and yet, the whole concept of multiple controls is rather unique to the holistic approach. Another example of redundancy has come from the experiments of Bruce Dill, who is very famous exercise/respiration physiologist. Dill gave a very interesting paper two years ago when he was 93. He measured his V_{max}, that is the maximum amount of oxygen consumed per kg per min. when he was exercising to near exhaustion. He started these measurements when he was aged 37 and, at that time, his V_{max} was 3.3, in ml of oxygen per kg per min. By age 66, he was down to 2.8 and at age 93 the value was 0.76, and was approaching his standard resting metabolism. Unfortunately Dr. Dill died this year, before it actually reached that level. My point is that here is a function of the whole animal, the whole human in this case, where the capacity to do work actually diminished in a predictive fashion.

So much for some of these examples from mammalian physiology. I want now to move into an area which certainly cannot be approached by molecular methods, neither at the present time, nor for the foreseeable future. Behavior is very important in many aspects of biology, including aging. The social impact is tremendous in aging not only in humans, but as we heard today, in the crowding of fruit flies. There is no question that many kinds of animals show social effects. I have seen it in the fish with which I work. They are highly social organisms, with some behavior patterns that are exceedingly complex. One has great difficulty in understanding how some behavior patterns could have evolved. One example is that of the courting dance of a bower bird, where the male builds a very elaborate nuptial chamber, that he decorates with flowers and colored objects. His whole purpose is to attract a female to this chamber, and he goes through an exceedingly complicated pantomime to do so. As one naturalist friend of mine said, it would be useful for every molecular biologist to watch a movie of the bower bird at least once a month. The complex behaviors of animals have a neurological basis. There are neuroanatomical characteristics of the unique features of the human brain. Brain size relative to body mass is one of them; speech areas are probably the most unique part of the brain in humans, as is the number of small neurons, and complexity of circuitry. Perhaps the most spectacular properties of the nervous systems and the most difficult to unravel at the present time have to do with its plasticity. There has been an effort to study learning from the point of view of molecular mechanisms, but this has not gotten very far. A variety of these behaviors are difficult to understand because they are strictly subjective. Sensation, for example, is not equivalent to perception. Perhaps the most difficult to understand of these is the notion of consciousness. Tolstoi said "I am as conscious of myself, the I at 81, as I was at 5 to 6." I think that this problem of consciousness is one of the most difficult to elucidate certainly from any molecular analysis.

Finally, I would emphasize that we are the product of two kinds of inheritance, biological inheritance and a cultural inheritance (Fig. 2). The biological heritage, the genotype, has two components, heredity and environment, Also, we have to take into account development and experience. But in addition, we are the result of a cultural inheritance, of general cultural characters and of very specific ones. We would not be Homo sapiens without both of these. If we consider the ranges of tolerance I am sure that you will agree that molecules, proteins, phospholipids

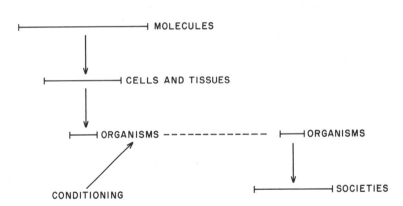

GENETIC
INHERITANCE

CULTURAL
INHERITANCE

MOLECULES

CELLS AND TISSUES

ORGANISMS ------------- ORGANISMS

CONDITIONING

SOCIETIES

Fig. 2   Diagram of ranges of genetically transmitted functional limits of
molecules, cells and tissues, and organisms, showing decreasing
ranges with integration, and of culturally transmitted functional
ranges of organisms and societies showing increasing ranges in
more complex systems.

can tolerate wide ranges of environmental conditions, such as temperature,
for example. Cells and tissues tolerate somewhat narrower ranges. When
you get to a whole organism, the range is still smaller. If we consider
humans, we have then, in parallel to this biological sequence, the organism as a biological entity, but cultural inheritance actually reverses the
trend and increases the tolerance of the organism as a whole. Therefore,
we have to recognize that the social and cultural controls are as important as biological ones in determining the nature of human beings. I
believe that social influences alter one's rate of aging and these certainly are very strictly holistic properties. The challenge of the holistic approach is to understand and relate the properties of whole organisms to evolution, and to adaptation. I have tried to indicate to you
that very frequently we do not find in vitro systems which show the same
properties that we see in vivo. Finally, I feel very strongly that we
must take into account the social and cultural inheritance which we all
share. All of these together then add up as a holistic challenge to
understand the adaptations of the total organism to its environment.

Ronald W. Hart

I think the question that one must always ask is "How does one debate
one's former mentor?" I remember very well one day when I was at the University of Illinois and I was coming up in the elevator to my third class in
comparative physiology, taught by Dr. Ladd Prosser, whom I greatly admired
and respected. I had come up with a conceptualization about how DNA repair
was important in aging, in carcinogenesis, and atherosclerosis. There I
was, making this presentation to Dr. Prosser and he turned to me and said,
"Anyone can come up with holistic concepts, but it is much more difficult to
figure out how to test them." Now I find myself on the opposite side of the
fence, arguing the reductionist approach rather than the holistic approach.
In actuality, these two approaches are not necessarily exclusive of each
other.

It is important to place this discussion within context. The use of diametrically opposed contrasting terms to aid in the organization of important conceptualizations has an ancient history. The roots of this practice are sunk deep in the intellectual past; for instance, in the classic contest between nominalism and idealism. However, this almost Manichean dualism should not blind us to the reality that each antipodal approach has value and utility. Frequently science advances as the result of tension between these dialectics, and intellectual progress is characterized by the ebb and flow of these approaches. Therefore, from the outset, I want to make it clear that this presentation simply is suggesting that emphasis be placed on a particular approach at this point in time, and I do not ignore the important role that holistic thinking has to play in the progress of science.

In his talk, and in his recent book on adaptational biology, Dr. Prosser has used holistic thinking to explain integrated phenomena, such as homeostasis and behavior, as being something different than simply the result of the properties of their components, molecules and neurons, respectively. Simplifying this complex argument, hopefully not to the point of misstating it, some key aspects can be discussed under the categories of: 1) "The whole is greater than the sum of the parts," 2) diversity, and 3) ecology. I also will discuss some aspects of reductionist thinking in aging.

The observation that the whole is greater than the sum of the parts has been the basis for much of the support of the holistic argument. An example for this "Synergism" is the function of a spring-operated watch, in which the various components, spring, cogs, gears, dial, by themselves can not denote time, but together they do.

It may be useful to consider this argument in a new context. If we consider the actual function of the watch, the spring "tells time" through the relationship of potential and kinetic energy. The function of many of the cogs is simply to regulate this release of energy to allow it to be expressed in a manner which is useful to the users of the watch, i.e., fulfill its design parameters. The watch has a primary generator, with modulators which regulate expression.

The same analysis, with modifications, can be extended to an organism. In a cell, different molecules can serve different functions. Diversity is the "primary generator," with natural selection providing the design parameters, and many modulators emerging to allow the fitting together of these parameters into a "cell watch." In a multi-cellular organism, there are a number of differently designed "cell watches" which are combined into an "organism watch" again, with design parameters provided by natural selection and the modulation of expression to fit the parameters. Unlike a simple watch, the same process, natural selection, operates at all levels simultaneously. Different circumstances may necessitate differing requirements for the cells at different times (e.g., vigorous growth, and then programmed death in the same cell). Extrapolation to assemblages of individuals of course is possible.

However, it is important to emphasize that the conditions of the environment in which the expression occurs is a factor in expression and can modify it. For instance, based on the observation that outside of a cell-like environment, a virus is not alive, an argument has been made that life can not be defined except in holistic terms. However, outside the kidney, or a kidney-like culture environment, a kidney cell loses many of the properties of life and will quickly die. As a rule the expression of modulation is very environment-dependent, and whether a system is considered alive or dead depends on the test system used to evaluate it. Using the earlier metaphor, unless one can read the dial, effectively, a watch does not tell time. In a dynamic process, an important part of the effort to understand the process is reducing the effect of environment to critical parameters for a particular test. A true reductionism considers this.

Thus, using Occam's razor, we can conceptually dispense with the holistic approach and define the whole in "the whole being greater as the sum of the parts" for organisms as a useful result of a series of molecular mechanisms modulating expression of diversity, in order to conform to design criteria imposed by natural selection at a series of levels, in terms of a particular test or milieu which requires the modulation to be obscured.

For instance, for blood pressure, if the test uses merely an aortic strip the result will be quite different than a test using an aortic strip plus a generator of patterned neurohormonal stimulation. The modulator of the effect will be different.

Diversity

The extent of diversity in biological systems provides tremendous complications to systematists. For modern systemics, imposing the requirement that members of the same species be able to reproduce upon mating reduces the definition of species to the capability of certain molecular mechanisms involved in chromosome pairing and disjunction. Although this definition creates problems it also may have some basic value since natural selection acts on this level, in sexual animals.

One problem noted is that such a criterion is impossible to measure using fossils. For extinct animals, a series of morphometric criteria are used to distinguish species, with the relationship of the different approaches, i.e., reproductive isolation and morphological differences unknown. This practice has led to arguments that definitions of concepts such as species should be in terms of global concepts, or five different definitions used.

It appears that a better way to address this problem concerning different measures is not an appeal to holistic thinking, but the detailed examination of the relationship of the morphometric approach to the non-cross-breeding one, perhaps deriving conversion parameters. For animals with other than reproductive mechanisms, other molecular criteria should be defined. If species can not be defined rigorously, it should be clearly understood as merely a temporary deficiency in technique, not an inherrent problem.

Ecology

It has been traditionally useful to take the global approach to ecology because of the lack of information on any of the components and lack of understanding of how many components interact in a system. In a sense, holistic thinking is equivalent to probabilistic thinking in which one replaces detailed descriptions with averages, because there is not enough information about the system. The advent of the supercomputers has changed this situation radically. It is possible to model large ecosystems with increasing sophistication (e.g., weather systems), and this area can only improve with time. Sharpening models with real data is an important activity in applying the models to real-time situations. Rather than throwing up one's hands, we should agree with Einstein that "God does not throw dice," and attempt to crack the complexities with our new tools.

Aging

It is becoming evident that the senescence of integration capabilities which occur in older organisms is an important determinant of aging in mammals. Loss of the ability to maintain homeostasis with age is one of the most consistent observations made in this class, although it is not clear that this factor is of the same importance in other classes. Exploration of a diverse set of senescent phenomena, such as in muscle, heat-generating metabolism, and hormonal alterations has inevitably led to the conclusion that there is a loss of integrative control, usually in the brain. The mechanisms which result in this loss are unclear. However, my candidate is the result of DNA damage in critical brain areas, influenced by the ability of various cells to repair and cope with the damage resulting from everyday metabolism, and hormone effects. Reductionism would attempt to tie the loss in homeostatic ability to the loss of cells, and the loss of cells to the loss of molecular mechanisms. Although the lack of ability to cope with damage may ultimately be influenced by some hormonal mechanism, an approach which attempts to look for the specific molecular modifications required by selection at every level, and the local environment in which these modulatory actions express themselves, is critical to understanding the process of aging and thus intervention.

Conclusion

There is a dynamic balance between reductionist and holistic thinking in the advance of biology, and both are necessary. At the present time, because of the success of the new tools of molecular biology and the advances in computers, I think we are in an era of glorious reductionism which can attack basic problems in complex systems such as organism and ecosystems which were only dreams before.

ACKNOWLEDGEMENT

The presentation given by Ronald W. Hart was a collaborative paper with Angelo Turtorro, who unfortunately was unable to be present.

DISCUSSION

Question: It seems to me that as one thinks incisively about molecules, one is thinking about ways of simplifying a complex problem down to its component parts. In a sense, therefore we are still somewhere up there with organisms and populations.

R. Hart: That is an excellent point. Over the history of population genetics, especially in the evolution of mathematics as applied to population genetics, between the early 1960's to the present time, the number of parameters being factored into the model system are increasing and becoming ever more complex. One of the questions that always faces us in toxicology is, how do you handle complex mixtures? We can make eloquent tests, compound by compound, a purely reductionist approach, in a number of different systems, but now all of a sudden we are faced with the problem, how would you handle complex mixtures? If you try to test compound by compound and use a matrix approach, suddenly you may be dealing with a mixture having a hundred components within it--a matrix of a hundred by a hundred chronic bioassays would involve a lot of mice. In toxicology we tried to approach this complex problem by using four by four matrices. But even if you try to use the house fly as a test animal, there would be so many in the experiment that the buzzing alone would drive you wacky! I am arguing that we can look at the interaction of compounds with macromolecules with something similar to a force field analysis. There, one considers what happens when a molecule interacts with a macromolecule, and next when a second molecule interacts with that same macromolecule. Does the first interaction predispose to further interaction, and if so, to how great an extent? In the past one could never approach the number of potential molecular interactions because the total number of daltons of DNA in the cell is so large. But now using a supercomputer, these interactions can be studied and questions asked about how, in complex mixtures, combinations of chemicals interact with macromolecules. From this one can make predictions about the degrees of distortion in the DNA. From some of our preliminary work we are finding that it is possible to start to predict, through a series of force field calculations, what will happen when different compounds interact with a macromolecule relative to tumor occurrence. That is a very exciting event. Many of the parameters that the people wanted to look at simply could not be factored in because there was a flood of reductionist data. I do not think that supercomputers will ever replace the human mind, but for aging research one could develop a data base, such as maximum achievable lifespan, and run correlations against that single factor. The computer can perform the analysis from a huge data base, at speeds which are far beyond any ability of a human, and at the same time can look at cross-correlations.

Question: Based upon what you just said, do you think that this modeling approach will put the use of animals out of business?

Hart: In actuality, we are just at the threshold of being able to understand things that we could never conceptualize even when I was a graduate student, as far as new data, new tools, new methods of analysis. The degree of eloquence of some of the presentations today is overwhelming compared to those of a decade ago.

Prosser: I think this is something we may have to face as experimentalists. The people advocating animal rights suggest that we go more and more toward model systems.

Question: Do you think that aging occurs in different organisms by the same mechanism? So many researchers have said that aging is under genetic control, and in every textbook there are statements to that effect. But the question arises, what kind of genes are these? What would they be controlling, and what functions would they be controlling? Do these genes produce a death hormone?

Hart: That is a fascinating question. In the simplistic fashion, and for the benefit of those who do not work on mammalian systems, it would be a delight to say that all aging is equivalent and occurs by the same mechanism regardless of species, and perhaps even regardless of whether it is a plant or animal species. Indeed, that may be the case. One cannot argue that it is not the case, because one does not know the mechanism of aging. In convergent evolution, as I learned from Dr. Prosser's course, many classes of animals have achieved the same end point by different mechanisms and means, to such an extent that they look very much the same and adapt in very much the same way under similar conditions. But they do not necessarily do so by the same mechanism. I think the argument about whether or not Drosophila, or the house-fly, or fish (I mention these organisms as I have worked on some of them) do or do not age by the same mechanism is a fascinating discussion but probably cannot be proved or disproved. Because one class of animal ages in one fashion, does not mean that all classes of animals must age in the same fashion. There are many enzymes, many proteins, and many functions to consider within any organism at all levels of structural and biological organization. However, there are certain genes which control a regulatory function for homeostatic capability, whether it is informational fidelity within DNA or replicative fidelity, and these genes have more importance relative to maintaining homeostasis, than do the genes that, for example, determine the color of one's hair. Not all genes are created equal, but at the same time, there probably are a number of genes which control homeostatic parameters at certain key functional points within an organism. Some of these may be the same between species and others may differ between classes.

Question: You distinguish between intrinsic information and interactional information and I think you implied that the intrinsic information was somehow associated with the structure of the system. I would like you to respond to this example. It is possible to take a number of living organisms, cellular and multicellular, and freeze them, stopping all the interactions cold, and then warm them up. My question is, where does the interactional information come from?

Prosser: It is there all the time, and as soon as you warm them up they become alive.

Question: I think the information is implicit in the instructional information, is it not?

Prosser: Yes.

Question: The distinction does not seem to be a fundamental one.

Prosser: Both types of information are frozen. That is, if you consider the organelle as being under the structure which is frozen, I would not make any distinction. I agree that you have suspended life as it were, and as soon as you warm up the animals, life continues with both types of information.

Question: In a sense, the implication is that all the essential information is in the structure.

Prosser: I think so.

Hart: Going back to our analogy, it would be like stopping the watch. Once the watch has wound down, that is the actual generator of time, and is based implicitly within the structure. And all the rest of the watch, its parts, are simply modulators of time.

Question: I would like to react to Dr. Prosser's emphasis that behavior transcends the organism, and take the radical approach that behavior is the unit of selection; genes are not selected for, organs are not selected for, morphology is not selected for. The animal interacts with the environment; how fast it can run, find food, find a mate, so if animals evolve, they have to evolve through their actions. Animals cannot be too far disconnected from those genes that control their behavior.

Prosser: Certainly. I think it was G.G. Simpson that emphasized over and over again that natural selection acts on the phenotype, not on genotype. I was purposely omitting the possibility that you could explain behavior alternately in molecular terms. I think that this is something for the future; at the moment, we are completely in the dark concerning the molecular basis for behavior.

Hart: I think I can give an example here, perhaps not with normal behavior but with abnormal behavior. We have been doing a series of cooperative studies with the National Institute on Drug Abuse in which we looked at the behavioral and neurological effects of the active component in marijuana. Both primates and rodents were exposed for long periods (chronic usage) and then exposure ceased. Several months later we looked at a very complex series of parameters which allows us to measure complex motor reflexes and behavioral changes within confined limits. We found large behavioral changes, and then traced them to given regions of the brain, then

329

to changes in particular brain cells. We are looking now at the chemical alterations which lead to these cellular changes and are devising strategies for medical intervention. Then we hope to show that without marijuana we can induce the same behavior patterns by altering the biochemistry of the cells. Now, that does not constitute normal behavior nor does it carry over to cognitive behavior, but it shows how abnormal behavior can be induced by an exogenous substance.

Question: The ratio of maximum life span to body weight often is used to compare longevity of species: data on bat species now has been added to previous data bases. Species with the highest ratio are bats, birds and next, humans. These findings motivate a speculation on connective fibre maintenance and its possible effects on longevity.

Maintenance of elasticity is important for functioning of the lungs and cardiovascular system. In bats and birds, this maintenance has another important role. To be aerodynamically effective, a flying animal clearly requires a tight skin. Wrinkles in the web of a bat or floppy feathers on a flying bird would not be a characteristic of survival. Thus it is reasonable to assume that flying species have evolved improved systems for maintenance of elasticity. A secondary effect would be a contribution to species longevity, because of improved maintenance of lung and cardiovascular systems. Land-based species are subjected to less severe selection for maintenance of, skin elasticity and would not thus have evolved the improved maintenance and accompanying contribution to longevity.

This may partially account for the high ratio of longevity versus body weight in bats and birds as compared to other animals. If correct, it might be useful to compare elastic fibre maintenance in bats and birds with that of humans. Extending the speculation to the molecular realm, it might be found that improved maintenance included systems for elastin and collagen replacement and/or in situ repair. A detailed understanding of the systems might lead to strategies for better elasticity maintenance in humans, manifesting in cardiovascular, lung and skin tone improvements.

330

ROUND TABLE DISCUSSION: REMARKS OF THE MODERATOR

Bentley Glass

Division of Biological Sciences
State University of New York at Stony Brook
Stony Brook, NY 11794

Being myself a prime example of the aging process, I think it might be useful to recall some previous symposia on aging in which I have participated. The first of these was in Gatlinburg, Tennessee, in 1956. There followed a symposium organized by the AAAS in 1960, one by the Gerontological Society in Puerto Rico, and the previous Brookhaven Symposium in 1984. In comparison with my recollections of these summations of the current state of the art, the Brookhaven Symposium of 1986 presents us with enormous advances in methodology and the advent of research on a new variety of organisms, especially Caenorhabditis elegans. Nevertheless, a few reminiscent comments may be helpful as we attempt to summarize our findings. On this occasion we miss a good number of the oldtimers in the study of aging: George Sacher, of course, to whom this symposium is dedicated: Alex Comfort, Nathan Shock, Howard Curtis, Leo Szilard, Bernard Strehler, and many others, to say nothing of such great oldtimers as H. S. Jennings, Raymond Pearl, and C. M. McCay. New insights must always be interpreted in the light of older demonstrated knowledge. Even abandoned theories of aging have their value in keeping us on the right road.

I welcome to studies on aging of new organisms, such as Caenorhabditis elegans, that remarkable little transparent nematode. Yet I take considerable pleasure in noting that the older paragon of laboratory work, the fruitfly Drosophila melanogaster, is well represented here by a variety of interesting new approaches to old problems. My own modest contributions to the study of aging were conducted with Drosophila, hence the pleasure.

I note, in particular, a paucity of interchange of ideas between clinical gerontologists and biological scientists. A two-way flow of information and ideas here would be very helpful. The present Symposium, so void of clinical gerontologists, makes me wonder whether we biologists have the influence our findings ought to provoke in health care and medical treatment.

Furthermore, there is a tendency to forget, or ignore, the findings of earlier times. It is fitting that this Symposium should be dedicated to George Sacher, a participant in a number of the symposia I have mentioned in beginning my remarks. His emphasis on the importance of homeostatic systems in aging was of prime importance, as was also his abiding interest in the influence of exposure to high-energy radiation on the aging process. As respects the former concern, we may note that McClearn's concept of "vitality" in the present symposium must surely be related to these homeostatic mechanisms. I would, however, caution that it would be well to avoid using the term "vitality" in this connection, for fear of a grave misunderstanding. It is surely not to be implied that anyone here endorses the outworn concept of "vitalism," in the sense of some non-physical, non-chemical life-force. No, the meaning intended is that a complex of physicochemical mechanisms of a homeostatic nature operate in some way as a unit important in the aging process. I am reminded of the genetic homeostasis postulated by I. M. Lerner as being a buffering of the genotype by means of dominance modifiers and suppressor genes, that act to protect the normal phenotype from alteration within the ambience of the usual environment.

Sacher was also deeply interested in the life-shortening produced by exposures to high-energy radiation. Although that aspect of our subject has been intentionally excluded from the present agenda, as having been one of the subjects of the preceding Brookhaven Symposium on Aging, there are interactions and relationships between the effect of high-energy radiation on aging and other causes of life-shortening, or lengthening, that make it perilous to ignore such matters altogether. Thus Kirkwood's theory of an "accumulation of somatic defects and a disposable soma" takes us back to the earlier theories, in order to consider their similarities as well as possible differences.

In particular I call to mind, in contemplating McClearn's concept of a kind of unitary "vitality" that is diminished or increased by a variety of causes, an experiment that has been unjustifiably neglected by modern workers, an experiment that to my mind is unsurpassed for the elegance of its design and the thoroughness of its execution. Yet I cannot find it discussed to in any of the works of recent times on the nature of aging. I refer to a experiment on the life-shortening of mice exposed to X-rays, performed by Patricia Lindop and Joseph Rotblat in 1961. Strehler, in his exhaustive treatment of the subject of aging in the second edition of his book, Time, Cells, and Aging (1977), has cited only the first, incomplete report of their study and not the second, far more significant paper published by them in Nature 189: 645-648 (1961). Allow me therefore to quote from my summary of this experiment in a volume recently written:

> Using mice all of a particular age and belonging to a homogeneous genetic strain, they compared groups unirradiated with others irradiated with doses of X-rays ranging from 50 to 780 roentgens (rads). The mice were followed through life until all had died, and each one was then autopsied to determine the cause of its death. The shortening of life produced by the irradiation was found to be directly and linearly proportional to the size of the administered dose. There was not the slightest indication that the smallest dose administered produced less than the expected amount of effect. In other words, there was no indication of any threshold below which the radiation fails to shorten life, even though the 50 rad dose is well below the level that produces any visible symptoms. Moreover--a point to be emphasized--the deaths which occurred were from the usual causes characteristic of this strain of mice, and not from any unusual causes attributable to the radiation. It is as if the radiation had merely advanced the time of death from the usual causes, quite as if it had removed a segment of the life span at the time when the irradiation was administered and left the irradiated animals biologically older than their chronological age would indicate!

(Bentley Glass, Progress or Catastrophe, pp. 220-221. Praeger, New York. 1985).

There is more, but this excerpt should be sufficient to indicate that there is past evidence to support the idea advanced in this symposium that there is some sort of "vital" unit that is subject to life-shortening (or possibly life-lengthening) agents as a single entity. We may be well-advised to search for a variety of causes of life-shortening that act upon this entity in an exactly similar fashion, in the hope of identifying it.

On the other hand, the conflicting evidence that has been presented in this symposium (by Donald Ingram) with respect to the relation of the effect on life span of the size/body weight parameters when examined intraspecifically (inverse proportionality) and interspecifically (inverse proportionality) suggests that the genetic mechanisms involved must be quite different, and that intraspecific and interspecific variation in life span are quite distinct.

With these rather random and informal reflections on our new evidence and our older conceptions, let me turn to our rapporteurs for a more orderly critique.

THE FUTURE OF AGING RESEARCH

Rajindar S. Sohal

Department of Biology
Southern Methodist University
Dallas, TX 75275

Usually the task of a Rapporteur is to summarize the ideas presented by various speakers and to provide, predict or speculate about the future directions of research. However numerous ideas about the nature of the aging process were presented at this Symposium and they do not fit within neat categories. Nor could I catalogue or even recall all of them. Furthermore, it would be very presumptious on my part, and perhaps inherently unfair to some people, to say that these particular ideas are worthy of notice while others can be ignored. I will let you be the judge of the relative appeal of the various points of view that have been expressed.

Now, as a Rapporteur, should I prophesize about the future? Frankly, I do not wish to create such a trap for myself because, first, I am not a guru and, secondly, I really do not know what the future of aging research will be, or even should be. Permit me to ask: did I know fifteen years ago what I shall be doing in my own laboratory in 1986? In fact, the general or specific notions I had about the future at that time did not turn out to be the case. In my view, history clearly instructs us about the hazards of predictions, specially in science. Could anyone have predicted in 1950 or 1960 what the status of biological knowledge would be in 1986 or what projects would yield the most rewarding results? I hope you will agree that in science, the future direction is always determined by the information at hand, and not by some grand planning. The term "discovery" itself implies the unknown nature of the potential find.

Such pitfalls, however, have not deterred some, especially governmental agencies, from engaging in clairvoyance or in overly exaggerating the future impact of a scientific finding. I can recall an official report written by the staff of the National Institute on Aging in the early seventies which stated that the most significant finding, that would be invaluable in solving the riddle of aging, was the Hayflick phenomenon of limited cell division potential in vitro. It was believed that a universal in vitro model of aging had become available and was waiting to be exploited. After 15 years, it is realized that their statement was an overly optimistic and perhaps misplaced enthusiasm. The results are not as rosy as the predictions were. Another example which comes to mind is the Progeria model, which was very confidently touted as a model of accelerated aging in humans. It was felt that aging is under the control of a few genes. Again, the reality turned out to be quite sobering. The point I wish to make is that it is futile and perhaps arrogant to make predictions concerning the most fruitful directions or future discoveries in science.

I think it will be safer and perhaps more profitable if I provide you with my personal view of the current situation in gerontology and then express what I would like to know in the immediate future, while being prepared and eager to be excited by unknown fruits of research that presently are beyond my imagination.

I think some of you will agree with me that these are highly muddled times for gerontologists. We neither know nor agree on the underlying causes of the aging process. Nor do we know how to measure the rate of aging in biochemical terms. What is known in considerable detail, however, are the manifestations of aging. For example, age-related changes in parameters such as cell structure, enzyme activities, amounts of proteins, cellular and organ functions, DNA damage and repair, to name a few, have been amply studied. Without deriding the significance of any of these studies in any way, one can ask whether the manifestations of aging are ever going to tell us what the nature of the underlying mechanism of aging is? In my opinion, the reason why organisms undergo functional loss with age cannot be determined on the basis of cataloging the changes accompanying aging; the most important goal of gerontological research is to understand the underlying mechanism(s) of aging. Not what happens with age, but why, and how does the mechanism of aging operate? To achieve this ultimate goal, I would like to pursue the following lines of investigations.

1. First, I would like to know how to measure the rate of aging. If specific biochemical markers of aging are identified, then it may be possible to conduct studies on the genesis of such markers, which can help elucidate the mechanism of aging. Whether or not such biomarkers will ever be found or if they even exist is a matter of speculation. It is very possible that aging has no distinct or unique biomarkers, and may simply be an attrition of function rather than a qualitative change.

As some of you may know, I have been searching for biomarkers of aging long before it became a fashionable pursuit. In my opinion, the relative usefulness of different biomarkers varies. A useful biomarker should provide a clue about the possible mechanism of aging. For example, in the housefly, the stamina or duration of a single non-stop flight declines after 4 days of age and I can reasonably tell the age of the fly from its flight duration (Sohal and Runnels, 1986). However, this functional loss is a generalized expression of aging and is not instructive about the nature of the underlying aging mechanism. In contrast, I also detected that the rate of n-Pentane exhalation by flies in vivo increases linearly with age (Sohal et al., 1985). n-Pentane is a product of free radical-induced lipid peroxidation, suggesting that aging is associated with increased oxidative stress. This biomarker thus may be useful in understanding the potential mechanism of aging.

2. Another intellectual wish of mine is to develop proper controls for aging studies. If experimental regimes could be found that truly alter the rate of aging, then the trivial, time-related changes occurring in cells and tissues could be separated from those that are specific to physiological age, or are reflective of the life expectancy of the animals. Although low caloric intake has been claimed to retard the rate of aging in mammals, it is also possible that what these studies indicate is that overeating brings about the early onset of disease and death. We have identified variation of metabolic rate as an experimental regime to vary the life span of poikilotherms, but I shall not exploit this opportunity to familiarize you with my own work. In general terms, at present, we do not know

how to alter the rate of aging, partly because we really do not know how to measure aging rates.

3. I would also like to know, what is the relationship between development and aging? Are these two separate processes, or is aging a continuation of development? Do the same inducers bring about cellular differentiation and cellular senescence? Recently we postulated that changes in redox state and ionic distribution induced by oxygen free radicals play a causal role in cellular differentiation and senescence (Sohal and Allen, 1986). According to this hypothesis, differentiation and senescence occur in response to a continuum of oxidative stress. If development and aging share a similar mechanism or are controlled by the same constellation of genes, an understanding of the mechanism of aging would become a more achievable goal.

4. Another desire I have is to know the relationship between the genetic and the stochastic factors in aging. Specifically, what is the relative contribution of the genetic and stochastic factors in aging? A tired old controversy in gerontology, that has always sounded to me as naive or silly, is whether aging is programmed or is a product of stochastic events. Rhetorically one can ask, is there any biological characteristic which is not genetically controlled? The real question is whether or not there are a series of genes whose de-repression or repression at specific periods during life controls the events governing aging, or whether longevity is dependent on the overall efficiency of protective and reparative mechanisms. A resolution of this matter would help identify the longevity determinants, whether they be antioxidant enzymes or DNA repair enzymes or something else. In other words, it is important to know what kind of damage, if any, is most crucial to the aging process and how this damage affects the switching or modulation of genes.

It is my hope that this Symposium has stimulated new thoughts in the mind of its attendees.

REFERENCES

Sohal, R. S., Muller, A., Koletzko, B., and Sies, H., 1985, Effect of age and ambient temperature on n-pentane production in adult housefly, Musca domestica, Mech. Ageing Dev., 29:317-326.

Sohal, R. S., and Allen, R. G., 1986, Relationship between oxygen metabolism, aging and development, Adv. Free Radical Biol. and Med., 2:117-160.

Sohal, R. S., and Runnels, J. H., 1986, Effect of experimentally prolonged life span on flight performance of houseflies, Exp. Geront., 21:509-514.

SURVIVAL ANALYSIS:

LESSONS FROM QUANTITATIVE GENETICS

Lindon J. Eaves

Department of Genetics
Medical College of Virginia
Richmond, VA 23298

INTRODUCTION

Symposia such as this provide a unique opportunity to evolve interdisciplinary strategies for solving scientific problems. Quantitative and behavioral genetics illustrate the wealth of natural experimental material to be obtained from the study of individual differences and the correlations between relatives. The study of natural variation and familial resemblances can help us understand the genetic and environmental regulation of any process and there are areas of theory and knowledge which suggest models, methods and paradigms which would be valuable in analysing the processes underlying aging. It has become increasingly clear that the timing of onset of disease is correlated in families (Farrer and Conneally, 1985), but that there are important individual differences in age-dependent processes, the elucidation of which may help us understand more about the genetic and environmental control of aging. In my brief discussion I want to summarize the basic issues of genetic analysis of individual differences and then suggest how some of the mathematical models geneticists have devised might be used to study aging.

WHAT CAUSES VARIATION?

Studies of variation in micro-organisms, higher plants, mammals and primates, including humans, have revealed the complexity of genetic and environmental effects which create variation within a population: some of the main sources are summarized in Table 1. A detailed discussion of the significance of each of these aspects is given by Mather and Jinks (1983) and Morton (1982).

Kinship Data- The Raw Material Of Quantitative Genetic Analysis

Whatever the trait being studied, whether it is continuous like stature or blood pressure, or discontinuous like hypertension, there is no genetic analysis without some kind of kinship data. Exactly what kinds of families are studied will depend on the specific questions being asked, but may include ordinary nuclear families, half-sibships, extended pedigrees, twins and the relatives of twins, adoptees and their biological and foster relatives. The task of genetic analysis is to determine in terms of genetic and environmental effects, the single best explanation which

Table 1. Basic Components of Variation Within Populations

---

1. Genetic

    a) due to identifiable genetic markers and linked genes
    b) due to latent genetic effects still to be identified
        - single genes of large effect;
        - many genes of small cumulative effects:
            - additive, dominant and epistatic genetic effects.

2. Environmental
    a) independent environmental covariates
    b) correlated between relatives: e.g., social interaction and
        cultural inheritance
    c) uncorrelated between relatives: random, accidental and residual
        effects.

3. Genotype-environmental
    a) Genotype x environment interaction: genetic control of sensitivity
        to environmental change.
    b) Genotype-environment correlation: genetic effects on the quality of
        environment.
    c) Developmental changes in genetic and environmental effects
    d) Assortative mating

---

accounts for the observations on the pedigrees. Typically, for this purpose geneticists use the method of maximum likelihood. We seek the parameter values under a given model for gene frequencies, gene effects, polygenic and environmental components of variance which maximize the likelihood of the observations. If the data on the ith kinship with k members
comprise the vector of observations $x_i = (x_{i,1}, x_{i,2} \ldots x_{i,k})$ and the
likelihood of the ith kinship is $l(x_i)$ then the likelihood of the whole set
of n kinships is:

$$l(x) = \prod_i l(x_i) .$$

The precise form of the likelihood of a kinship will depend on the
biological and social relationships between members of the kinship and upon
the model of inheritance assumed. When kinships are not randomly sampled,
but are secured through systematic selection of affected individuals the
likelihood must be modified to reflect the method of ascertainment
(Cavalli-Sforza and Bodmer 1971, Appendix II; Elston and Yelverton, 1975;
Morton, 1982). There is a substantial genetic literature on the kinds of
genetic models used and the implications of their likelihood functions
(Elston and Stewart, 1971; Lange et al., 1976; Eaves et al., 1978; Eaves,
1982; Ott, 1985).

Frequently, the data include one or more covariates, Y, measured on
the family members, which might encompass measures of exposure to salient
environmental factors or to relevant demographic covariates, such as age
and sex. The likelihood then may be formulated conditional on the values
of the covariates and the model extended to include parameters describing
the impact of the covariates and their interaction with other genetic and
environmental effects (Eaves, 1982, 1984, 1987; Eaves et al., 1987; Kendler
and Eaves, 1986).

For my purposes here the details of genetic and environmental models do not matter. The important points for the "survival analysts" to appreciate are: 1) every trait that geneticists have studied show substantial variation within populations; 2) only a small fraction of that variation can usually be attributed to measureable covariates; 3) much of the variation remaining after covariates have been excluded is substantially correlated between family members; 4) an enormous literature exists on how these correlations between relatives can be analyzed and interpreted in terms of genetic and environmental effects; and 5) any mathematical model or statistical method for aging or survival which fails to allow for these effects is headed for disaster in the court of empiricism.

MODELLING SURVIVAL IN KINSHIPS

Assume that we have failure times on a typical kinship of k members. We allow some of these measures to be follow-up times for those family members who were studied or withdrew prior to failure. Let the vector of failure/follow-up times be $t=(t_1, t_2 ... t_k)$, $0 \leq t_i < \infty$. Let the ith element of the vector z be 1 if t_i denotes failure time, and 0 if it represents follow-up time without failure. We may also allow for a series of covariates measured for each family member. Let y_i denote the vector of covariates for the ith family member. The task of analyzing the genetics of survival boils down to computing the likelihood of the failure/follow-up times under an appropriate model for individual differences and family resemblance in risk, conditional on the values of any salient covariates.

We let the hazard rate for the ith individual be $0 < \lambda_i < 1$. That is, for the period of study, we assume that the hazard rate is constant for a given individual. From data already presented at this symposium, we know that this assumption is false at the level of population statistics. Here, we only assume that it is constant within an individual and that such apparent temporal changes in λ as are found in average population statistics can be accounted for by individual differences which can be specified in an appropriate genetic model. The hazard rate for the ith individual is a function of covariates, y_i, and a residual, latent variable x_i which reflects unmeasured, but nevertheless substantial genetic and environmental effects that can be detected and analyzed.

Given a uniform hazard rate, the probability that the ith individual will survive to time t_i is simply:

$$s(t_i, \lambda_i) = e^{-\lambda_i t_i}.$$

The likelihood of the observed failure/follow-up time for the ith individual, given individual hazard rate λ_i, is thus:

$$l(t_i, \lambda_i) = \lambda_i^{z_i} s(t_i, \lambda_i),$$

and the likelihood of the k members of the family, is the product:

$$l(t, \lambda) = \prod_i l(t_i, \lambda_i)$$

Unfortunately, the individual hazard rates, λ, of the family members are unknown. However, we can assume a functional relationship between the unknown individual hazard rates on the one hand, and covariates, Y, and latent variables x, on the other. Although the individual values cannot be known, their distribution within and between kinships can be specified in terms of the parameters of a set of alternative genetic models. Let $\Phi(x)$ be the probability distribution function (PDF) of the latent variables in kinships identical in structure to that for which the likelihood is required. Typically, this is assumed to be multivariate normal if there are no individual genetic or environmental effects which stand out against the background of polygenic and random environmental effects (Lange et al., 1976). Otherwise, it might be assumed that Φx denotes a mixture of multivariate normal distributions with mean vectors characterized by the average values of individual genes of major effect on the trait (Lalouel et al., 1983).

The likelihood of the vector of failure/follow-up times, when the individual hazard rates are unknown but are assumed to be functions of latent variables with multivariate distribution $\phi(x)$ is the multiple integral:

$$\int_{-\infty}^{\infty} \cdots \int_{-\infty}^{\infty} \Phi(\underline{x}) \prod_i l\,(t_i,\, \lambda_i)\, dx_k \cdots dx_l$$

where λ_i, $l(\,t_i,\, \lambda_i)$ and $s(t_i,\, \lambda_i)$ are defined earlier in terms of the latent variable x_i and the covariates y_i. The likelihood of an entire set of independent randomly chosen kinships is then the product of the likelihoods of the individual kinships.

Model-Fitting: Is It Practicable?

Given a particular set of kinship data, in theory, the likelihood over all kinships can be evaluated and maximized numerically with the parameters of the genetic model for Φx, and the parameters representing the additive and non-additive effects of covariates. In principle, there is no problem with kinships of variable structure, since genetic theory enables us to specify a separate PDF for each as a function of the specific relationships in the kinship (Lange et al., 1976). Ideally, we would like to compare a number of alternative models for kinship resemblance in survival by likelihood-ratio methods. For example, three major hypotheses of progressive complexity which may be compared by likelihood-ratio tests are: 1) constant hazard rate for all individuals after allowance is made for covariates; 2) variable hazard rate caused by random effects which are not transmitted in families; and 3) variable hazard rates which are correlated between family members with a pattern characteristic of polygenic inheritance. More subtle models can also be specified which, in principle, are testable with the right choice of kinships. Although for simplicity we have assumed that the hazard rate is constant for each individual, different functional relatiohships between age and hazard rate could be specified without seriously changing the structure of the problem. If more than one parameter is required to specify the relationship between age and hazard-rate within an individual, then we have to recognize that some or all of these parameters might display individual differences and family resemblance. In principle, such models can also be explored by likelihood methods, but it is too early to say whether they will be practically informative.

The simplicity of the theory should not blind us to practical problems which may restrict our implementation of this simple idea. The accurate numerical evaluation of multidimensional integrals for more than two or three dimensions generally requires a great deal of time on the computer. Experience has shown that the most general model, involving major genes and family resemblance of residual effects, is virtually intractable for cases similar to ours with any but the smallest kinships. However, existing algorithms might deal with those cases where the multiple integral can be expressed as a weighted sum or product of unidimensional integrals. Examples where such simplification is possible are hypothesis number 2 above, and cases in which family resemblance is attributable to one or, at most, two genes of large effect (Ott, 1985). Further, we can make substantial progress by studying genetically informative families of size 2 for which numerical analysis is still possible, although it is time-consuming (Eaves et al., 1987). For example, a large body of data on failure in identical and non-identical twins could be used for testing basic hypotheses about the causes of heterogeneity in individual hazard rates. With a large sample of twins, the well-known model-fitting approaches to quantitative twin data might be extended to analyse variation in survival and failure (Eaves, 1982). Among the hypotheses which can be tested within twin data are: 1) is "survival" familial?; 2) is the familial component of survival environmental or genetic?; 3) do the same genes (or environments) affect survival in both sexes?; and 4) are some genotypes especially sensitive to the effects of measured environmental risk factors? The basic theory I outlined might encourage those interested in the analysis of human survival to address these issues in the next generation of empirical studies.

ACKNOWLEDGEMENT

This research is supported by grants AG04954, GM30250 and GM32732 from the National Institutes of Health.

REFERENCES

Cavalli-Sforza, L. L., and Bodmer, W. F., 1971, "The Genetics of Human Populations," Freeman, San Francisco.
Eaves, L. J., 1982, The utility of twins, in: "The Genetic Basis for the Epilepsies," V. E. Anderson, W. A. Hauser, J. K. Penry, and C. F. Sing, eds., Raven Press, New York.
Eaves, L. J., 1984, The resolution of genotype x environment interaction in the segregation analysis of nuclear families, Genet. Epidem., 1:215.
Eaves, L. J., 1987, Including the environment in models for genetic segregation, Psychiat. Rev., in press.
Eaves, L. J., Last, K. A., Young, P. A., and Martin, N. G., 1978, Model-fitting approaches to the analysis of human behavior, Heredity, 41:249.
Elston, R. C., and Stewart, J., 1971, A general model for the analysis of pedigree data, Hum. Heredity, 21:523.
Elston, R. C., and Yelverton, K. C., 1975, General models for segregation analysis, Am. J. Hum. Genet., 27:31.
Farrer, L. A., and Connealley, P. M., 1985, A genetic model for age of onset in Huntington disease, Am. J. Hum. Genet., 37:350
Kendler, K. S., and Eaves, L. J., 1986, A etiologic model for psychiatric illness incorporating genetic and environmental risk factors, Archs. Gen. Psychiat., 18:64ff.
Lalouel, J. M., Rao, D. C., Morton, N. E., and Elston, R. C., 1983, A unified model for complex segregation analysis, Am. J. Hum. Genet., 35:816.
Lange, K. L., Westlake, J., and Spence, M. A., 1976, Extensions to pedigree analysis III. Variance components by the scoring method, Ann. Human Genet., 39:485.
Mather, K., and Jinks, J. L., 1983, "Biometrical Genetics: The Study of Continuous Variation" (3rd ed.), Chapman Hall, London.
Morton, N. E., 1982, "Outline of Genetic Epidemiology," Karger, New York.
Ott, J., 1985, "Analysis of Human Genetic Linkage," Johns Hopkins University Press, Baltimore, London.

PARTICIPANTS

ARKING, Robert
 Dept. of Biological
  Sciences
 Wayne State U.
 Detroit, MI 48202

BAKER III, George T.
 American Association
  for Advances in Health
  Care Research
 14628 Carona Drive
 Silver Spring, MD 20904
BERGAMINI, Ettore
 Institute of General
  Pathology
 Via Roma 55
 I-56100 Pisa
 Italy
BERKOVICH, Simon
 Dept. of Electrical
  Engineering and Computer
  Science
 George Washington U.
 Washington, DC 20052
BEVERTON, Raymond J. H.
 Dept. of Applied Biology
 U. of Wales Institute
  of Science and Technology
 P.O. Box 13
 Cardiff CF1 3XF
 United Kingdom
BRICELJ, Monica
 Marine Sciences
  Research Center
 State U. of New York
 Stony Brook, NY 11794

CALVO, Lou
 Germaine Monteil
  Cosmetiques Corp.
 450 Comac Road
 Deer Park, NY 11729
CASTANEDA, Mario
 Inst. of Biomedical Res.
 U. of Mexico
 P.O. Box 70228
 04510 Mexico, D. F., Mexico
CHEAL, MaryLou
 Dept. of Psychology
 Arizona State U.
 Tempe, AZ 85287
CHRISTIAN, Robert R.
 Biology Dept.
 East Carolina U.
 Greenville, NC 27834-4353

DUNMORE, Cheryl
 Biology Dept.
 Brookhaven National Lab.
 Upton, NY 11973

EAVES, Lindon J.
 Dept. of Genetics
 Medical College of Virginia
 Richmond, VA 23298-0001

GLASS, Bentley H.
 Div. of Biological Sciences
 State U. of New York
 Stony Brook, NY 11794

GRIGLIATTI, Thomas A.
Dept. of Zoology
U. of British Columbia
2075 Wesbrook Mall, Vancouver
British Columbia V6T 2A9
Canada

HART, Ronald W.
Dept. of Health Education
  and Welfare
National Center for
  Toxicological Research
(HFT-1)
Jefferson, AR 72079

HIRSCH, Henry R.
Dept. of Physiology and
  Biophysics
U. of Kentucky
College of Medicine, M.S. 507
Lexington, KY 40536-0084

HOLTZMAN, Seymour
Physiology Dept.
New York College of
  Osteopathic Medicine
Old Westbury, NY 11568

HUGHES, Donald H.
Regulatory Services Division
Corporate Research and
  Development
The Procter and Gamble Co.
Ivorydale Technical Center
Cincinnati, OH 45217

INGRAM, Donald K.
Room 4-E-13
Gerontology Research Center
Natl. Institute on Aging
Frances Scott Key
  Medical Center
Baltimore, MD 21224

JODLOS, Susan
Estee Lauder Inc.
Research Park
125 Pinelawn Road
Melville, NY 11747

JOHNSON, Thomas E.
Dept. of Molecular
  Biology and Biochemistry
U. of California
Irvine, CA 92717

KALLMAN, Klaus D.
Osborn Laboratories of
  Marine Sciences
New York Aquarium
Boardwalk W. 8th St.
Brooklyn, NY 11224

KIRKWOOD, Thomas B. L.
Natl. Institute for
  Medical Research
The Ridgeway, Mill Hill
London, NW 7 1AA
England

KONDO, Sohei
Atomic Energy
  Research Institute
Kinki University, Kowakae
Higashi-Osaka
Osaka 577, Japan

LINTS, Frederick A.
Dept. of Genetics
Catholic U. of Louvain
B-1348 Louvain-la-Neuve
Belgium

LUCKINBILL, Leo S.
Dept. of Biological Sciences
Wayne State U.
Detroit, MI 48202

MAMONE, Tom
Estee Lauder Inc.
Research Park
125 Pinelawn Road
Melville, NY 11747

MANGEL, Walter F.
Biology Dept.
Brookhaven National Lab.
Upton, NY 11973

McCLEARN, Gerald
Institute for the Study
  of Human Development
The Pennsylvania State U.
University Park, PA 16802

McDOWELL, Bruce W.
Accelerator Development Dept.
Brookhaven National Lab.
Upton, NY 11973

MERKER, Philip C.
Pharmacology and Toxicology
Vicks Research Center
Richardson-Vicks, Inc.
Shelton, CT 06484

MILLER, Arnold R.
Dept. of Biological
  Sciences
U. of Denver
Denver, CO 80208

MORSTIN, Krzysztof
Safety and Environmental
  Protection Div.
Brookhaven National Lab.
Upton, NY 11973

ORMISTON, Brian
Medical Dept.
Brookhaven National Lab.
Upton, NY 11973

PENNA, Fred
Estee Lauder
Research Park
125 Pinelawn Road
Melville, NY 11747
PROSSER, C. Ladd
Dept. of Physiology
and Biophysics
U. of Illinois
Urbana, IL 61801
PROTHERO, John W.
Dept. of Biological
Structure, HSB SM-20
U. of Washington
School of Medicine
Seattle, WA 98195

REICH, Edward
Dept. of Pharmacology
State U. of New York
Stony Brook, NY 11794-8651
RUDENKO, Larisa
Biology Dept.
Brookhaven National Lab.
Upton, NY 11973
RUSSELL, Richard L.
Dept. of Biological Sciences
U. of Pittsburgh
Pittsburgh, PA 15260
RYBICKA, Krystyna
Dept. of Applied Science
Brooklyn National Lab.
Upton, NY 11973

SETLOW, Richard B.
Biology Dept.
Brookhaven National Lab.
Upton, NY 11973
SMITH, James R.
Dept. of Virology
and Epidemiology
Baylor College of Medicine
1 Baylor Place
Houston, TX 77030

SMITH, Walter
Estee Lauder
Research Park
125 Pinelawn Road
Melville, NY 11747

SMITH-SONNEBORN, Joan
Dept. of Zoology
and Physiology
Box 3166
University Station
U. of Wyoming
Laramie, WY 82071
SOHAL, Rajindar S.
Dept. of Biology
Southern Methodist U.
Dallas, TX 75275
SPROTT, Richard L.
Natl. Institute on Aging
Building 31, Rm 5C11
Natl. Institutes of Health
9000 Rockville Pike
Bethesda, MD 20205
STODOLSKY, Marvin
Div. of Health Effects
Research
Office of Health and
Environmental Res., ER 72
GTN Rm F-207
U.S. Department of Energy
Washington, DC 20545
STONE, John P.
Pilgrim Psychiatric Center
P.O. Box A
Brentwood, NY 11717
SUTHERLAND, Betsy
Biology Dept.
Brookhaven National Lab.
Upton, NY 11973

TEMPLETON, Alan R.
Dept. of Biology
Washington U.
St. Louis, MO 63301
THOMPSON, Keith H.
Biology Dept.
Brookhaven National Lab.
Upton, NY 11973
TOTTER, John R.
Institute for Energy Analysis
Oak Ridge Associated U.
P.O. Box 117
Oak Ridge, TN 37831-0117

WILLIAMS, Darrell D.
Regional Primate Research
Center Field Station
U. of Washington
Medical Lake, WA 99022

WILLIAMS, George C.
Dept. of Ecology
and Evolution
State U. of New York
Stony Brook, NY 11794

WITTEN, Matthew
 Dept. of Community Health
 U. of Louisville
 Louisville, KY 40292
WOODHEAD, Avril D.
 Biology Dept.
 Brookhaven National Lab.
 Upton, NY 11973
WRIGHT, Barbara E.
 Dept. of Microbiology
 U. of Montana
 Missoula, MT 59812

Flour beetle
  lifespan, 270
Flux map, 119
Free radicals, and aging, 336
Fusion studies, 285
  inhibition of DNA synthesis,
    285-286

Gene expression
  temporal pattern, 194,202
Gene regulation, 138
Generation time, 80,89
Genetic abnormalities
  and age, 214
Genetic approach, 91
Genetic correlations
  with lifespan, 94,98
Genetic switches
  and aging, 5,13
Genetic program
  for aging, 193
Geotaxis, 205
Gerbils, 145-146
Germ line, 103
  immortality of, 209,214
  selective mechanisms, 215-216
Gompertz plots, 5,170,300
Group-housed rodents
  and survival, 267
Growth
  cessation of, 149
  duration of, 276-277
  and food supply, 176
  and temperature, 178
Growth rate, 112-113

H2 locus, 106
Haplotypes, 101,107
  and cholesterol, 132
Hayflick limit, 24,27
Hazard rate, 341
Heterosis
  and lifespan, 92
Hibernation
  and longevity, 68
Homeoboxes, 18
Homeostasis, 322,328
Humans
  mortality, 124,236
Humidity ecotone, 127
Hybrid mice
  longevity, 265
Hybrid vigor, 94

Immortality
  of protozoa, 101,105-107
  of cells, 213
Immune System
  and aging, 106

Inbred mice
  longevity, 265
Inbreeding, 104
  depression by, 94
Inclusive fitness, 13
Infinite versus finite
  lifespan, 107
Inflection time, 311
Inhibitor mRNA, 287
Inhibitor protein
  from quiescent cells, 287-288
Interactive information, 321
Integral equations, 189
Integrative systems analysis, 122
Interventions
  in aging, 17
Intrinsic information, 321
Intrinsic rate
  of increase, 211-212

Juvenile hormone, 15,126

Kidney weight
  and lifespan, 54,70
Killer genes, 202
Kinetic models, 115-116
Kinship data, 339

Large gap repair, 106
Larval density
  and developmental
    homeostasis, 5
Lethal mutations
  on X chromosome, 195
Lethal phase, 197
Life extension mutants, 2
Life-history traits
  evolution of, 92,94
Life-time Cohort Egg Production
  168-170,182
Lifespan
  heritability of, 94
  and growth duration, 276-277
  and protein intake, 267
  unicellular organisms, 104
Lifespan data
  systematic bias, 49
Likelihood ratio test, 342
Lipofuscin
  and aging, 40,46
  in posterior intestine, 46
Liver weight
  and lifespan, 70
Long-lived stocks,
  of nematodes, 91
Longevity, 105
  and behavior loss, 203,205-206
  and body weight, 247
  of _Drosophila_ larvae, 195